Clinical Gynecologic
Oncology

Per Kolstad

Clinical Gynecologic Oncology
The Norwegian Experience

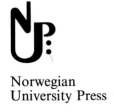

Norwegian
University Press

Norwegian University Press (Universitetsforlaget AS), 0608 Oslo 6
Distributed world-wide excluding Scandinavia by
Oxford University Press, Walton Street, Oxford OX2 6DP

London   New York   Toronto
Delhi   Bombay   Calcutta   Madras   Karachi
Kuala Lumpur   Singapore   Hong Kong   Tokyo
Nairobi   Dar es Salaam   Cape Town
Melbourne   Auckland

and associated companies in
Beirut   Berlin   Ibadan   Mexico City   Nicosia

© Universitetsforlaget AS 1986
Cover design: Tor Berglie

British Library Cataloguing in Publication Data

Kolstad, Per
    Clinical gynecologic oncology: the Norwegian experience
    1. Generative organs, Female—Cancer—Norway
    I. Title
    616.99'465'009481   RC280.G5

    ISBN 82-00-07672-5

Printed in Denmark
by P. J. Schmidt A/S, Vojens

Contents

Foreword

by Hans Ludwig

In this book Per Kolstad summarizes the broad experience of his entire professional life. He does so in a very precise and factual style covering the whole field of gynecologic oncology. The Norwegian Radium Hospital, opened in 1932, was until recently the one and only institution in Norway devoted to the treatment of gynecological cancer in a population of around 2 million women, and it still remains one of the leading institutions in gynecologic oncology in the world. Its reputation for excellence is not only due to the fact that the long-term treatment results achieved there are outstanding, but also to the brilliant organization of the referral system, to the cooperation with the Norwegian Cancer Registry, to the follow-up of patients once treated, to the scientific design of treatment protocols, and to its publication policy. Professor Kolstad directed the Department of Gynecologic Oncology during that institution's most expansive period, he himself being one of the rare clinicians with personal competence in surgery, external and intracavitary radiotherapy, and chemotherapy.

He beautifully describes his own procedure of radical surgery in stage Ib/IIa cervical cancer, the Oslo method of radiotherapy, and what kind of philosophy the strict treatment protocols of the Oslo institution should follow in the light of present world-wide insight. Even in the more rare cases like melanoma of the vulva, adenocarcinoma of the cervix uteri, sarcoma of the uterus, endodermal sinus tumor of the ovary, dysgerminoma, or malignant tumors of the female urethra, specific figures derived from his own institution are given, and they include the information gathered during sometimes decades of follow-up. Who else could write a book on the firm basis of 93 collected publications – 43 of them with the leading participation of the author – about specialized oncologic problems experienced in one's own in-

stitution? Nevertheless, the text is full of references to current world-wide practice and to the relevant literature, bringing each chapter into the appropriate historical frame and revising dogmatic options here and there because they are found not to be based on true grounds.

The collection of large numbers of treatments and follow-ups in cases of the most widespread gynecologic tumors leads to sound statements and very useful clinical recommendations. The book is also a plea for a continuation of the 'Annual Report On The Results Of Treatment In Gynecological Cancer', a publication once started in 1937 under the auspices of the League of Nations and continued since 1958 under the responsibility of the International Federation of Gynecology and Obstetrics. There are parallel trends in Oslo and in the analyses of the Annual Report about other areas in the world, and there are a few other cases in which the trends are to a certain extent contradictory, giving rise to questions, e.g. in the prognosis of adenocarcinoma of the cervix, in the long-term results of borderline tumors of the ovary, or in the 'radioisotope versus whole abdominal irradiation' issue in early ovarian cancer. Some kind of reporting about world-wide experience in the treatment of gynecological cancer, like 'the Norwegian experience' put down so brilliantly in this book, might have been a worthy goal for the promoters of the Annual Report. Their message was that, without proper staging, any secure comparability of therapeutic statistics will not be possible.

The problem of individualization of cancer treatment versus standardization according to a protocol is under discussion at present. Per Kolstad is in favor of a data-based standardization of treatment, wherever such data are available. He regrets when he is unable to provide the reader with sufficient facts and when even his large collection of data fails to give appropriate standards, so that one must have recourse to individualization. On the other hand, he advocates a periodical revision of standardized treatment recommendations, and his book is a rich source of arguments against some traditional beliefs in gynecologic oncology.

This book should come into the hands of all gynecologic oncologists and be passed on to those in training. It is unique in its composition of facts from thoughtful observation of female cancer patients, from evaluation of diagnostic procedures like colposcopy, colpophotography, cytology and tumor markers, from a scientific basis in epidemiology, histology and experimentation and, most valuable, from clear-cut results attained by proceeding according to strict treatment protocols and controlled clinical trials.

The Norwegian experience with the treatment of gynecologic tumors does not conceal the fact that there is still no breakthrough in our understanding of what cancer is, nor is there any spectacular improvement of the overall survival figures, except when very early stages of gynecologic cancer are treated. But considerable steps towards a better outcome for all cancer patients have been made in the last decade. The progress is gradual. How to proceed most effectively without putting aside the individual needs of the suffering patient can be learned from reading Per Kolstad's excellent book.

Basel July 1986
Professor Dr. Hans Ludwig
Head of the Department of Gynecology and Obstetrics, University of Basel

Author's Preface

Gynecologic oncology today is a well recognized subspeciality within the field of gynecology and obstetrics. In 1976 George Morley giving the Presidential Address at the yearly meeting of the Society of Gynecologic Oncologists said, "On their shoulders we stand", and certainly we are all indebted to a number of great men who, during the last five decades, have clearly shown that gynecologic cancer patients need special attention and care with regard to work-up, treatment and follow-up.

A large number of excellent monographs and textbooks on gynecologic oncology have appeared during the last two decades. It may therefore be questioned what is the purpose of the present publication. The answer is first and foremost that the development of gynecologic oncology in Norway has been unique. Centralization of the treatment of gynecologic cancer started as far back as the early 1930s when the Norwegian Radium Hospital was opened. Throughout the years this relatively small, private hospital has grown into a comprehensive Cancer Center. A Gynecologic Oncology Department was founded in the late 1930s. It has become one of the largest units in the world within this field, covering today 2/3 of a population of about four million people. Since the opening of the hospital, follow-up has been almost one hundred per cent.

The chiefs of the Gynecologic Oncology Department have always had responsibility for the work-up and for all types of treatment: surgery, intracavitary radium, external irradiation, radiocolloid therapy, and also in the later decades,

chemotherapy and hormone therapy. The large material of different types of gynecologic cancer made it possible, relatively early, to start randomized clinical trials which have given us most valuable information. And, since from the very beginning the medical record system was designed for a complete follow-up, our statistics on e.g. treatment results should deserve international interest. The compulsory cancer registration system which was introduced in Norway in 1952 has made our statistical studies still more reliable.

In this work, the author passes on to his colleagues throughout the world information about the Norwegian experience with a system of centralized treatment, and also a system where the gynecologic oncologist has responsibility for all types of treatment. Therefore I have written this book which reflects the treatment results in more than 30,000 patients seen over a period of 50 years.

Another reason for presenting data from a Scandinavian country is the influence Forsell, Heyman and Kottmeier at the Radiumhemmet have had on the developments within the field of gynecologic oncology throughout this century.

Last, but not least, this publication is a tribute to one single person, Dr. Reidar Eker, who throughout his lifetime devoted all his efforts to building a comprehensive Cancer Center around the Norwegian Radium Hospital. This Center today consists of the Hospital, with a unique clinical material, a Cancer Research Institute, and a Cancer Registry which covers the total population of Norway.

Oslo September 86
Per Kolstad

Acknowledgements

It is impossible to adequately acknowledge all those people who in some way focused attention on the work of the Gynecologic Oncology Department of the Norwegian Radium Hospital.

I have to begin, however, by thanking Professor Oddmund Koller for providing a first class insight into what may be described as clinical scientific curiosity. Without his natural inquisitiveness, this book would never have been written. Koller's method of colpophotography was developed in the mid-1950s and today, 30 years later, it has still not been surpassed by any other method of photography of benign, preinvasive and invasive lesions of the lower genital tract of women. This method forms much of the basis of my own understanding of the evolution of malignant disease.

My sincere thanks are extended to Dr. Reidar Eker, former Managing Director of the Cancer Center. Dr. Eker was for many years Head of the Laboratory for Pathology and also President of the Norwegian Cancer Society.

Much of the histopathologic and cytologic material presented in this work is due to an intimate collaboration with two persons working in the Laboratory for Pathology, Dr. Kari Høeg, Head of the cytopathologic section, and Dr. Vera Abeler. For many years Dr. Abeler has been responsible for reviewing our large materials of gynecologic cancer, and for placing the different cases in strictly defined histopathologic categories. Her help has been invaluable.

During my years as Head of the Department of Gynecologic Oncology, I started a number of clinical and experimental studies. But having also administration duties, the education of doctors, students and nurses, terms of office on several different hospital, university, medical society and cancer society committees, I had to call on the staff of the Department to help review our series for publication in international journals. All those who helped me in this respect are gratefully acknowledged.

I am grateful also in this connection to all those persons working in our service departments, especially Dr. Liverud, the former Head of the Radiodiagnostic Department.

We are fortunate at our hospital to have the Cancer Registry of Norway on the premises. Many of the valuable data found in this book have been collected from publications from this Registry. Throughout the years I have had many stimulating discussions with the former Chief of the Cancer Registry, Dr. Einar Pedersen, his Assistant Chief, Dr. Phil. Knut Magnus, and the Data Processing Chief, Aage Andersen.

Throughout the years I have travelled to numerous countries around the world, visiting famous hospitals and institutes. It is impossible for me to acknowledge all the people I have met and who have increased my understanding of gynecologic oncology, but one person I cannot forget is the late Professor Hans-Ludvig Kottmeier of Radiumhemmet, Stockholm. He brought me into the international medical world in a way that today is almost unbelievable.

My respects go to Emeritus Professor Howard Ulfelder, Chairman of the Cancer Committee of the International Federation of Gynecology and Obstetrics for so many years. Thanks also to the members of this committee.

Mrs. Gunnel Stormorken typed the manuscript. The diagrams, curves and photographs were expertly reproduced by Helge Vereide and his staff at the Laboratory for Photography at the Norwegian Radium Hospital.

My sincere thanks go to the Norwegian Cancer Society for generous financial support during the last 25 years.

Last, but not least, I thank my wife, Otti, for her patience with me during the many years of researching and writing which occupied most of my time.

Heads of the Gynecologic Oncology
Department 1932–1984

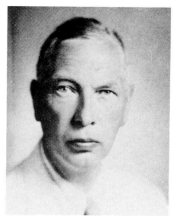

Dr. med. K. Skajaa, 1932–38.

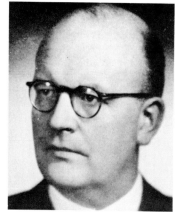

Dr. med. E. Schjøtt-Rivers, 1938–52.

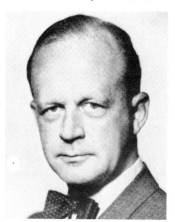

Dr. med. T. Dahle, 1953–57.

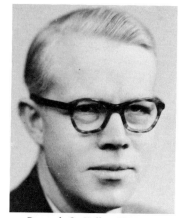

Dr. med. O. Koller, 1957–67.

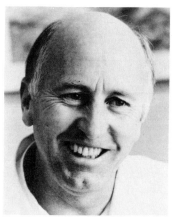

Dr. med. P. Kolstad, 1967–84.

1

Historical survey

In 1898 Dr. Heyerdahl of the city of Oslo, at that time called Kristiania, purchased a radiodiagnostic machine. He was without doubt one of the first physicians in Scandinavia who clearly appreciated the great potentialities that roentgenrays might have within the field of medicine. In 1913 along with Dr. Huitfeldt, he opened the Kristiania Radium Institute, and together they began treating different types of carcinomas, including carcinoma of the cervix, with radium. This Institute may be regarded as the forerunner of the Norwegian Radium Hospital. In 1916 Heyerdahl and Huitfeldt initiated a country-wide fund-raising campaign with the aim of building a hospital designed for the treatment of cancer with radium and roentgen-rays. The campaign was a great success, but because of the First World War, the depression following the war, and also discussions about the localization of the institute, the building of the hospital was delayed until 1929. In 1932 the Norwegian Radium Hospital could open its doors for cancer patients who were referred from all over the country. A second fund-raising effort in 1931 made it possible to buy 2 grams of radium from Radium Belgé. Eight certificates for some of the radium still in use are signed by Madame Curie (Fig. 1.1).

The accepted treatment for carcinoma of the cervix in Scandinavia in the 1930s was radiotherapy, and from the very beginning, this tumor type represented a relatively large percentage of the patients being admitted. A consultant in gynecology, Dr. Skajaa, was therefore attached to the hospital. He was responsible for the radium applications in cervix cancer, and also for the surgical and surgical-radiological treatment of other types of gynecologic malignancies. In 1936 he was appointed head of a separate Department of Gynecology, and it may be correct to state that from this year the speciality of gynecologic oncology

started its development in Norway. The second chief of the department, Dr. Schjött-Rivers, followed Dr. Skajaa in 1938, and worked in the hospital for 15 years. Later he became a member of the Board of the hospital and had a great influence on the further development of the Department of Gynecologic Oncology.

When it opened, the hospital had a total of 71 beds, but this soon proved to be insufficient. A first expansion was finished in 1941, and at that time it was decided that the Department of Gynecology should occupy about 30 out of a total of 110 beds. After the Second World War a new fund-raising made a second expansion of the hospital possible, and the number of gynecologic beds was increased to 90. However, only ten years later the waiting-lists for cancer patients being referred was once more found to be too long. After a thorough analysis of the cancer situation in the country (1), the Government and Parliament raised the money for a third expansion; this was completed in 1980. At present the Norwegian Radium Hospital has 440 beds, 110–120 of which are allotted to the Department of Gynecologic Oncology. Within the confines of the hospital are the Cancer Registry of Norway, which began its work in 1951, and a research institute which was opened in 1954. Altogether these three institutions represent a modern, comprehensive Cancer Center. In the hospital there are Departments of Clinical Oncology and Radiotherapy, Hematology, Lymphology, Surgery, Urology, Gynecology, Radiodiagnostics, Anesthesiology, Histopathology, Cytopathology, Clinical Biochemistry, Nuclear Medicine and Medical Physics. In the Research Institute there are sections for Biochemistry, Immunology, Biophysics, Ultrastructural Pathology, Genetics, Tissue Culture, Carcinogenesis and an animal stable designed especially for the breeding of athymic nude mice.

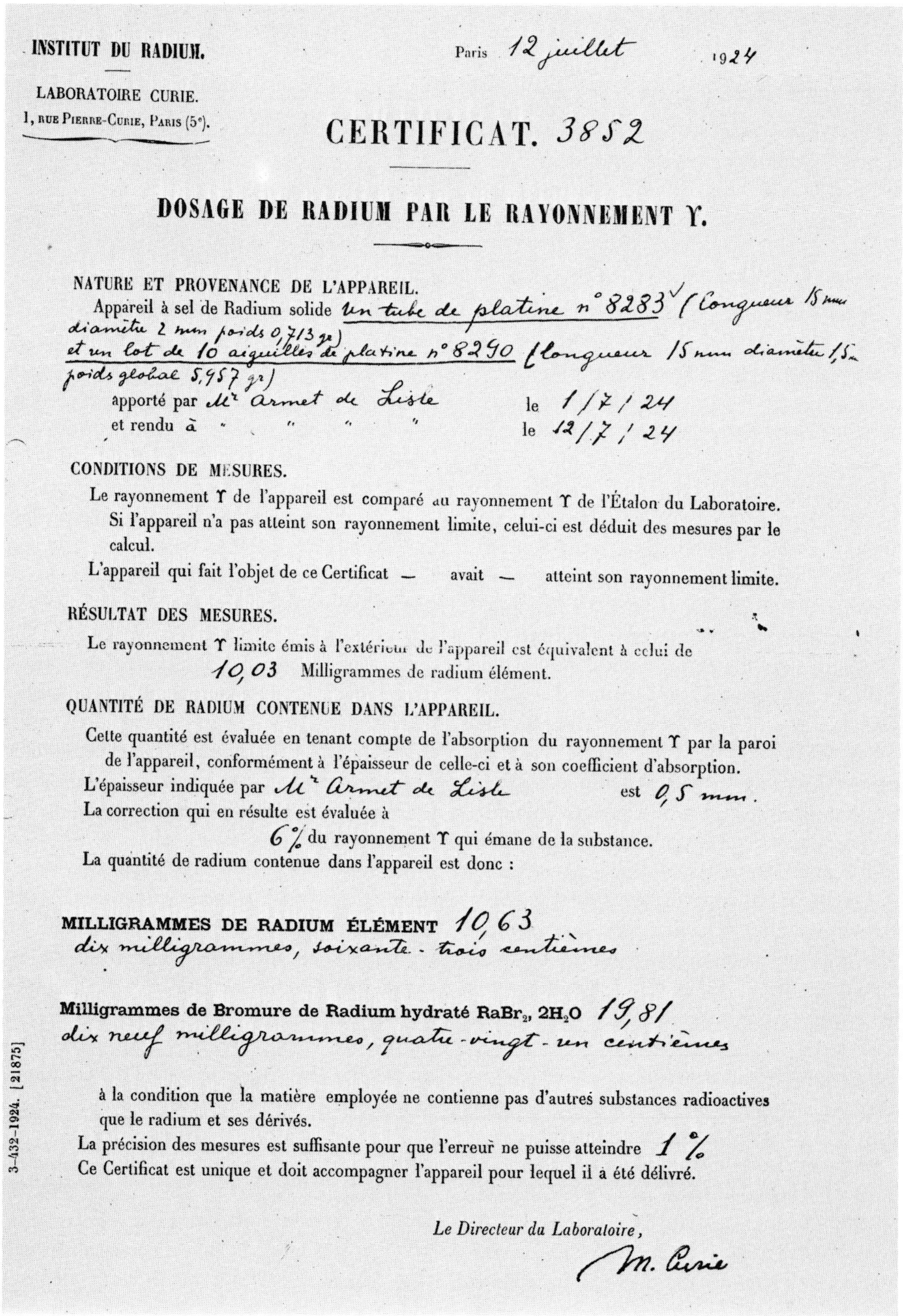

INSTITUT DU RADIUM.

LABORATOIRE CURIE.
1, RUE PIERRE-CURIE, PARIS (5ᵉ).

Paris *12 juillet* 1924

CERTIFICAT. 3852

DOSAGE DE RADIUM PAR LE RAYONNEMENT ɣ.

NATURE ET PROVENANCE DE L'APPAREIL.
Appareil à sel de Radium solide *un tube de platine n° 8283 (longueur 15 mm diamètre 2 mm poids 0,713 gr) et un lot de 10 aiguilles de platine n° 8290 (longueur 15 mm diamètre 1,5 poids global 5,957 gr)*
apporté par *Mᵉ Armet de Lisle*   le *1 / 7 / 24*
et rendu à   "   "   "   le *12 / 7 / 24*

CONDITIONS DE MESURES.
Le rayonnement ɣ de l'appareil est comparé au rayonnement ɣ de l'Étalon du Laboratoire.
Si l'appareil n'a pas atteint son rayonnement limite, celui-ci est déduit des mesures par le calcul.
L'appareil qui fait l'objet de ce Certificat — avait — atteint son rayonnement limite.

RÉSULTAT DES MESURES.
Le rayonnement ɣ limite émis à l'extérieur de l'appareil est équivalent à celui de
10,03 Milligrammes de radium élément.

QUANTITÉ DE RADIUM CONTENUE DANS L'APPAREIL.
Cette quantité est évaluée en tenant compte de l'absorption du rayonnement ɣ par la paroi de l'appareil, conformément à l'épaisseur de celle-ci et à son coefficient d'absorption.
L'épaisseur indiquée par *Mᵉ Armet de Lisle*   est *0,5 mm.*
La correction qui en résulte est évaluée à
6 % du rayonnement ɣ qui émane de la substance.
La quantité de radium contenue dans l'appareil est donc :

MILLIGRAMMES DE RADIUM ÉLÉMENT *10,63*
dix milligrammes, soixante-trois centièmes

Milligrammes de Bromure de Radium hydraté RaBr₂, 2H₂O *19,81*
dix neuf milligrammes, quatre-vingt-un centièmes

à la condition que la matière employée ne contienne pas d'autres substances radioactives que le radium et ses dérivés.
La précision des mesures est suffisante pour que l'erreur ne puisse atteindre *1 %*
Ce Certificat est unique et doit accompagner l'appareil pour lequel il a été délivré.

Le Directeur du Laboratoire,

M. Curie

3-432-1924. [21875]

Fig. 1.1. Radium certificate for 10 mg radium still in use at the Gynecologic Oncology Department and signed by Madame Curie on July 12, 1924.

The staff of the Department of Gynecologic Oncology has always consisted of gynecologic oncologists. Today there are five senior staff members (one chief and four assistant chiefs) and eight residents. The residents have usually passed the Board of Obstetrics and Gynecology before they are accepted for training in the more specialized part of gynecologic oncology which is being carried out in the hospital.

The staff of the department is responsible for brachy- and external radiotherapy, surgery, chemotherapy and hormone treatment of all patients being admitted. There has, however, always been a close cooperation between the gynecologists and the specialists working in the Departments of Radiotherapy and Medical Physics when planning the radiotherapy of gynecologic patients. Furthermore, the Department of Gynecologic Oncology also works in close contact with all other departments and sections in the hospital and the Research Institute.

From the very beginning, surgery has been an integrated part of the treatment of gynecologic malignancies. As early as the 1940s, surgery was performed not only for endometrial and ovarian carcinomas, but also in cases of early cervix cancer. The tradition of combined radium irradiation and surgical treatment of carcinoma of the cervix Stage I has continued for more than 40 years. Today afterloading brachyradiotherapy with cobolt sources is in focus.

Chemotherapy and hormone therapy were introduced in the early 1960s, at first for palliation, but also with the aim of achieving a permanent cure of an otherwise incurable disease.

When the hospital opened in 1932, strict follow-up routines were introduced. Norway is a small country with a stable population, a fact which has influenced the completeness of the follow-up (see later). At present the Department of Gynecologic Oncology has information about more than 30,000 gynecologic cancer patients who were being treated during the 50 years 1932–82. For the great majority of these patients histopathologic slides and paraffin blocks of the biopsy specimens are also available, from which new sections can be cut and stained. The medical records, the histopathological material, and also since 1951 a vast number of cytopathologic slides, have throughout

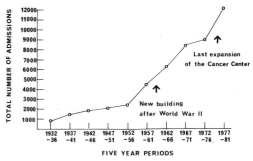

Fig. 1.2. Total number of admissions to the Gynecologic Dept. in 5-year periods (1932–81).

the years formed a firm basis for clinical research. In 1968 controlled clinical trials on a randomized basis were introduced for the major tumor types. Both the retrospective and especially the prospective clinical studies serve as "production control" for the work being carried out.

There has been a steady increase in the work load during the 50 years which have passed since the hospital opened (Fig. 1.2). During the first 25 years, 7,520 new patients with gynecologic malignancies were admitted. In the 25 years from 1957 to 1982 the number amounted to 25,569 patients, so that the total number of patients on file up to 1982 is 33,089. Today, the average yearly number of new patients is approximately 1,200. A large percentage of the cases are re-admitted for follow-up or for further treatment, either as part of the primary treatment plan, or for therapy of recurrent disease. The total yearly number of admissions amounts to about 2,500–2,600 cases.

Up to about 1965–70 the main cancer type was carcinoma of the cervix, followed by endometrial carcinoma. During the past 20 years, however, there has been a remarkable increase in patients with ovarian cancer being referred. This tumor type must certainly be regarded as our major treatment problem today. Fig. 1.3 shows the distribution of these three major gynecologic tumors during the years from 1950 to 1982.

The Norwegian Radium Hospital is still the main cancer center in Norway. However, during the last two decades the concept of regionalized health care has been put into action. One new center has been developed at the University of Bergen covering western Norway, and a second

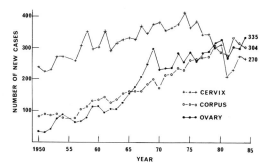

Fig. 1.3. Numbers of new cases of carcinoma of the cervix, corpus and ovary in the period 1950–84.

is under construction at the University of Trondheim, covering the central part of the country. A third cancer center is being planned for northern Norway at the University of Tromsö (Fig. 1.4). In future the Norwegian Radium Hospital will serve as the Regional Cancer Center for eastern and southern Norway where about 60% of the population are concentrated. In addition, the hospital will be responsible for the evaluation and treatment of rare and special cases from the whole country. The regionalization of health care will reduce our clinical material somewhat, but it seems that a Department of Gynecologic Oncology of at least 110–120 beds will be necessary for the number of patients expected to be referred.

In addition to clinical research, which has been carried out to an increasing degree since the hospital opened, in the last 20 years, combined experimental and clinical research projects have also been made possible by grants from the Norwegian Cancer Society. Foreign fellows from Europe, America, Asia and Australia have been involved in this work. Through these combined projects, an intimate cooperation has developed between the Department of Gynecologic Oncology and the Research Institute.

Of importance for the diagnostic and therapeutic policy of the department is, of course, not only the experience accumulated through own investigations, but also the most valuable information acquired through international connections and conferences. Every year the staff of the department travel to other countries in Europe, to the United States; even countries in the Far East and Australia have been visited. Communication and exchange of experience and knowledge within all fields of medicine certainly are and will continue to be of the greatest importance for our achievements.

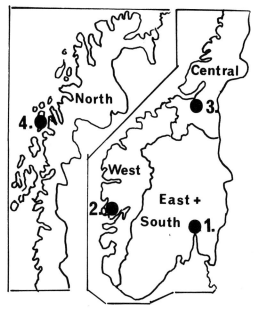

Fig. 1.4. Locations of the four regional centers for cancer treatment in Norway: 1. Oslo, 2. Bergen, 3. Trondheim and 4. Tromsø.

2
Classification and staging

In 1928 the Cancer Commission of the Health Organization of the League of Nations was called upon to consider a proposal that an international study be made of the value of radiotherapy of cancer. Carcinoma of the cervix was found to be the most suitable tumor for the study as this disease, even then, was being treated successfully both by surgery and radiotherapy. The Cancer Commission recognized that reliable information regarding the results obtained by different treatment methods could be achieved only if the results were recorded in a uniform way. The task of formulating rules designed to facilitate the presentation of exact and comparable statistics was entrusted to Dr. J. Heyman, Dr. A. Lacassagne and Dr. F. Voltz. Their pioneer work within this field was adopted and published in 1929 (1). They reported their methods of treatment and the five-year results obtained in radiotherapy of carcinoma of the cervix at the Radiumhemmet, Stockholm, the Curie Foundation, Paris, and the University Gynecological Clinic, Munich.

The matters which they considered to be of particular importance were:

1. The classification of the different varieties of uterovaginal carcinoma.
2. The grouping of cervix carcinoma into different stages according to the extent of the growth.
3. The data which are essential in a statistical report together with the methods which should be employed in calculating results.
4. A scheme for setting out the details of the techniques employed.

It is amazing, so many years later, to read the report by Heyman, Lacassagne and Voltz (1). It is both clear and complete and, without doubt, can be considered the foundation upon which later rules for classification and stage grouping of gynecologic cancer have been built.

In 1934 at a conference in Zürich the World Health Organization decided that analyses of the results of treatment by radiotherapy in cervix cancer should be issued annually. The first *Annual Report on the Results of Radiotherapy in Cancer of the Uterine Cervix* was published in 1937. Six clinics submitted their data, and Heyman was the editor (2). Three volumes of the *Report* were issued before the Second World War and the League of Nations bore the financial responsibility. In 1938 Heyman published an atlas illustrating the division of cancer of the cervix into four stages (3). This atlas might well be used today with only small modifications.

The work on the *Annual Report* came to a standstill during the war, but it was resumed in 1945 thanks to financial support from the British Cancer Campaign, the Donner Foundation in Philadelphia and the Cancer Society in Stockholm. In 1958 the International Federation of Gynecology and Obstetrics (FIGO) assumed patronage of the *Annual Report,* and the Federation's Cancer Committee is today responsible for it being published every third year. It is sponsored by a series of gynecologic and cancer societies from all over the world. Professor James Heyman, Stockholm, was the first editor till his death in 1956, when he was succeeded by Professor Hans-Ludvig Kottmeier who continued Heyman's work until he died in 1982. There is no doubt that without these two great men and their never-failing interest in an international cooperation concerning classification and staging of gynecologic cancer, we would have been far from the universal agreement which exists today.

The first seven volumes of the *Annual Report* described results achieved by radiotherapy only. In 1951 Meigs initiated the inclusion of cervix cancer treated by surgery, and in 1953 the scope of the *Report* was widened to include cases of endometrial carcinoma. Carcinoma of the ovary was first presented in 1973, carcinoma of the vulva in 1979, and in 1985 malignant trophoblastic disease was also included. Since all the major types of gynecologic cancer are now reported, the name has been changed to the *Annual Report on the Results of Treatment in Gynecological Cancer.* At the present time about 130 major institutions from all over the world submit their data every third year. The Norwegian Radium Hospital has taken part in this international work since the hospital opened in 1932.

The continuous efforts of the Editorial Board of the *Annual Report* have been rewarded by universal acceptance of the principles they have set forth, but also by an established concordance pledged by the TNM Committee of the International Union against Cancer (UICC), the American Joint Committee on Cancer Staging and End Results Reporting (AJC), the World Health Organization and the Cancer Committee of FIGO. The agreements achieved are mainly due to the work by Professor Howard Ulfelder. Accordingly, all the above-mentioned committees have adopted the same classification in the two dialects (FIGO staging and TNM). The TNM system (T = Tumor, N = Nodes, M = Metastases) was developed by Pierre Denoix between the years 1943 and 1952 (4). In 1950 the UICC appointed a Committee on Tumor Nomenclature and Statistics, followed in 1954 by a special Committee on Clinical Stage Classification and Applied Statistics. In 1958 the first recommendations for the clinical stage classification of breast and larynx cancer were published. Since then TNM classifications for more than 30 sites have been approved by a series of national committees and international organizations, among which is the American Joint Committee (AJC). The AJC was organized in 1959, and in 1977 a detailed *Manual for Staging of Cancer* was published (5). This manual is based on the TNM system. Instructions for the reporting of cancer survival and end results are given in detail. It is also recommended that one should use a so-called "Host Performance Scale after Treatment", and special "Oncology Data Forms".

Most gynecologic oncologists prefer the FIGO clinical staging system. It has been found to be as useful and also simpler than the TNM system for the different types of gynecologic cancer and it is easier to get comparable statistics. The FIGO system will be used throughout this book. In the following, the general rules for classification and staging of malignant tumors in the female pelvis as described in the eighteenth volume of the *Annual Report* (6) are presented (with some modifications). Detailed definitions will be found in the respective chapters.

CLASSIFICATION OF MALIGNANT TUMORS IN THE FEMALE PELVIS

Carcinoma of the cervix

Cases should be classified as carcinoma of the cervix if the primary growth is in the cervix. All histological types must be included, except for the rare sarcomas.

Carcinoma of the corpus

A case should be classified as carcinoma of the corpus uteri when the primary growth is in the corpus. Cases of uterine sarcoma, pure or mixed, and choriocarcinoma, should be reported separately.

Every gynecologist and pathologist knows that there are cases in which it is clinically as well as histologically difficult to decide whether the cancer is primarily a cancer of the corpus uteri or a cancer of the ovary. As a rule, it is possible to decide from the history of the patient and from the clinical examination which tumor is likely to be the primary one. In rare cases this may be impossible, however. Such cases might be included in the statistics on carcinoma of the corpus as well as in the statistics on ovarian cancer.

Occasionally it may be difficult to decide whether the origin of the growth is in the corpus or in the cervix. If a clear decision cannot be made at e.g. fractional curettage, hysteroscopy or hysterography, an adenocarcinoma should be allotted to carcinoma of the corpus and an epidermoid carcinoma to carcinoma of the cervix.

Carcinoma of the vagina

Cases should be classified as carcinoma of the vagina when the primary site of the growth is in the vagina. Tumors present in the vagina as secondary growths from either genital or extragenital sites should be excluded from registration.

A growth that is limited to the urethra should be classified as carcinoma of the urethra.

Carcinoma of the ovary

Cases should be classified as carcinoma of the ovary when the primary growth is a malignant epithelial tumor, and its primary site is in the ovary (see also under carcinoma of the corpus).

Carcinoma of the vulva

Cases should be classified as carcinoma of the vulva when the primary site of the growth is in the vulva. Tumors present in the vulva as secondary growths either from a genital or extragenital site should be excluded from registration. Malignant melanoma should be reported separately.

A carcinoma of the vulva which has extended to the vagina should be considered as carcinoma of the vulva.

Carcinoma of the urethra

Cases should be classified as carcinoma of the urethra when it is evident that the primary site of the growth is in the urethra.

It is important to separate cases of carcinoma of the external urethral os from cases originating deeper in the urethra. At present the Cancer Committee of FIGO has not proposed a stage-grouping for carcinoma of the urethra. The TNM system has to be used.

CLINICAL STAGING OF GYNECOLOGICAL CARCINOMA

The staging should be based on careful *clinical examination* and should be performed before any definitive therapy. It is desirable that the examination be performed by an experienced examiner and *under anesthesia.*

Where *ovarian cancer* is concerned, staging should be based on *clinical findings and surgical exploration.* The histology is to be considered in the staging as is cytology as far as effusions are concerned. It is desirable that a biopsy is taken from suspicious areas above the pelvis, from the omentum, the intestines, from the colonic gutters, or from the peritoneum of the diaphragm.

The clinical staging must not be changed later and should never be postponed. It is not permitted to change the *clinical staging* on the basis of subsequent findings, even if there has been an obvious "mistake" in the staging.

When it is doubtful to which stage a particular case should be allotted, the earlier stage should be chosen.

Opinions differ as to which findings should serve as the basis for clinical classification and staging of carcinoma of the uterus and carcinoma of the vagina. In order to obtain a correct and uniform classification and staging, the Cancer Committee of FIGO considers it important that only such examinations be used as can be carried out at any hospital by the physicians and surgeons. The following examinations fulfill these requirements: Inspection, palpation, colposcopy, biopsy, endocervical curettage, conization, cystoscopy, proctoscopy, intravenous urography, and X-ray examinations of lungs and skeleton.

Findings by examinations such as lymphography, arteriography, venography, laparoscopy, receptor studies, etc., are of value for planning treatment, but they should have no influence on the staging. Positive laparoscopic biopsies may influence the staging of ovarian carcinoma. These examinations are not carried out as a routine and the interpretation of the results is not uniform.

The clinical staging of carcinoma of the cervix should be based on the examinations mentioned above. A conization or amputation of the cervix should also be regarded as a clinical examination, and an invasive carcinoma of the cervix diagnosed in this way should be registered as invasive carcinoma Stage Ib.

Patients with carcinoma of the cervix who have been operated upon under the wrong diagnosis and where more than Stage Ib is found in the removed uterus cannot be given a clinical stage.

It is important to follow the above principles in order to secure comparability of therapeutic statistics. The Editorial Committee is well aware of the fact that the clinical observations do not always agree with the anatomical findings and that many patients classified as for instance, Stage I or Stage II carcinoma of the cervix or the corpus, at operation might be found to have metastases to the lymph nodes or spread of tumor beyond the pelvis. It may also be found in rare cases that clinical Stage III carcinoma of the cervix proves to be operable. In order to secure reliable uniformity, such incidents should have no influence on the *clinical staging*. However, in the presentation of Stage III carcinoma of the corpus, we indicate that a differentiation between surgical-pathological and clinical Stage III might be advisable.

3
Registration

Official *mortality* statistics for many years comprised the best material for studies of trends in the occurrence of cancer. Important changes in the incidence of various forms of cancer are reflected in the mortality rates. An example is the increase in mortality from lung cancer which was noted in the 1930s and which has continued to date. Mortality statistics have also been used as a basis for studies of group variations in cancer mortality within countries, and in investigations of the cancer risk within certain populations and occupations. It is obvious that the official mortality statistics have been, and still are, of the greatest value in the description of, and research into, cancer as a health problem.

A more complete picture of the cancer situation in a defined population can, however, only be achieved by exact *morbidity* statistics. For this purpose regional or national cancer registries have been established in a large number of countries throughout the world. The first national cancer registration in Norway was started as early as in 1907 and continued for almost twenty years. The purpose of this registration was clearly spelled out in a report which appeared in 1916 covering the first five-year material (1):

> Fundamentally, investigations of the incidence and geographical distribution of a disease, its time trends, and its distribution by age, sex and social class, always aim at throwing light on the cause of the disease in order to make possible its prevention and cure. Such investigations are of great importance as they may throw light upon environmental factors that have influence on the occurrence of the disease. Knowledge of the environmental conditions under which the disease occurs may lead to discovery of real causal factors in a gradually narrowing field. However, statistical investigations of this kind

alone cannot be expected to provide the final solution to a biological problem such as that of the causation of cancer. The final solution must come from more direct (experimental) observations.

The view expressed in this statement reflects the fact that an understanding of the principles of epidemiology was more disseminated among the medical profession in Scandinavia, and certainly also in other countries, at the beginning of this century than is generally realized today. Some of the reports from this first attempt at cancer registration in Norway are remarkable for the number and kind of details described. However, on the whole, the material was incomplete and heterogeneous, and it was realized that it was impossible under the existing conditions to obtain really satisfactory registration of the recognized cases in the population. The project was well beyond the resources of that time, and it had to be abandoned.

After the Second World War, in 1948, the newly created Norwegian Cancer Society appointed a committee with the aim of considering the establishment of a permanent Cancer Registry of Norway. The report from the committee was submitted to the Director-General of the Health Services in Norway in 1950, and in October 1951 it was decided that compulsory cancer registration should be introduced into the country, becoming effective as of 1 January 1952. The Cancer Registry of Norway was launched as a joint project by the Ministry of Social Affairs, the Central Bureau of Statistics, the Norwegian Radium Hospital and the Norwegian Cancer Society. Finance was for many years the responsibility of the Norwegian Cancer Society, the Ministry of Social Affairs covering only approximately 10% of the budget. During the last decades the situation has changed, and the Ministry has taken over the main responsibility for the yearly budget of the Registry, the Norwegian Cancer Society supporting specific research projects only.

The registration covers the total population of Norway, at present approximately 4.2 million people, and is based on compulsory reporting of all new cases of cancer diagnosed after 1 January 1952. In addition, all tumors (benign or malignant) of the central nervous system, all papillomas of the urinary tract, and all cases of carcinoma in situ of the cervix are included. According to the rules laid down, reports are required from: (1) all hospitals, (2) all institutes of pathology, and (3) all departments of radiology. New cases seen in hospital outpatient departments which are not admitted to the wards should also be reported. In this way a case will usually be reported from two or even three sources, making the registration more complete and accurate. A new report is to be submitted every time a cancer patient is admitted to hospital for his/her malignant disease. The reports are usually completed when the patient leaves the hospital. Some hospitals prefer to send in the original medical records of cancer patients at regular intervals for abstracting in the Cancer Registry.

The Registry is located within the premises of the Norwegian Radium Hospital, and there has always been close cooperation between these two institutions. The Registry enjoys unlimited access to the very detailed patient records of the hospital, and the hospital enjoys access to the expertise and the data of the Registry.

Computerization of cancer registration started in 1966. The entire material accumulated since 1953 is now stored in a computer. Files are updated every three months, and at the same time two sets of microfilms are produced, one set arranged according to the names of the patients in alphabetical order, and one set by the personal identification number which since 1960 has been assigned to every citizen of Norway. Opportunities for record linkage are therefore now exceptionally good. The Cancer Registry also has access to computerized data on all deaths, from all causes, in the Norwegian population since 1951, and to microfilms covering the entire current population of the country.

During the first years after the Cancer Registry was established, priority was given to epidemiological studies of the incidence rates of different types of cancer, and of variations which they exhibit in different segments of the population. Incidence data have since been reported at regular intervals (2), and thus studies of variations of the incidence of specific tumors have been made possible (3). Also, extensive studies of the survival of cancer patients over a longer period of time have been published (4).

Although such studies based on data from regional or national cancer registries are often claimed to be inaccurate because details about staging, treatment and follow-up may be lacking, they may give a valuable overall picture of the cancer situation in the population. Last, but not least, today the role of environmental factors in the causation of cancer is in focus in the ongoing studies of the Cancer Registry of Norway.

It is obvious, however, that statistical studies carried out in specialized hospital departments such as the Department of Gynecologic Oncology of the Norwegian Radium Hospital, may bring out details that can never be reached by routine reporting to a regional cancer registry. The most perfect cancer registration cannot replace the accurate investigation of different treatment methods by carefully designed clinical trials. A prerequisite for such trials is an adequate medical record system. This was fortunately realized when the hospital opened in 1932. The medical records were typewritten, important details marked out in red letters, and the aim was for a complete follow-up. The patients have been examined at regular intervals in the Outpatient Department of the Radium Hospital, in local hospitals, by private specialists in gynecology or surgery, or by the patient's own family physician. Reports on almost all patients have been received at regular intervals from all over the country, and in the case of death, special investigations as to the cause of death have been carried out. Today it can be claimed that a complete follow-up of almost all patients admitted as far back as 1932 is available.

The hospital has always required the histopathologic biopsy material from patients first seen in other hospitals. Therefore it has also been possible to keep both histopathologic slides and paraffin blocks from the majority of the patients being admitted, whether their admittance was for example, for additional treatment after primary surgery in a local hospital, or for primary and definitive treatment in the Norwegian Radium Hospital.

The different registration systems and follow-up routines described above form the basis of the clinical observations which are described in this book.

4
Dystrophia vulvae

In 1976 the International Society for the Study of Vulvar Disease (ISSVD) published a new nomenclature for some common vulvar lesions (1). Up to that time a confusing number of different terms had been used especially for white lesions, but also for red and mixed white-red lesions. Well known are such terms as leukoplakia, diffuse or localized, leukoplakic vulvitis, kraurosis, lichenification, atrophic dermatitis, erythroplasia, dysplasia, carcinoma in situ and Bowen's disease.

In earlier days white lesions were usually regarded as definitely premalignant, mostly because white (leukoplakic) areas are often found adjacent to squamous cell carcinoma of the vulva. However, white lesions are common, and vulvar carcinoma is rare. It may be claimed that neither retrospective nor prospective studies have solved the question of the real malignant potential of white vulvar lesions. The ISSVD has tried to introduce a new terminology which can neutralize the bias associated with the different terms mentioned above. This classification is shown in Table 4.1.

Dystrophy denotes a disturbance of nutrition. Jeffcoate (2) first applied this term to vulvar white lesions. The ISSVD has recommended (1) that the term dystrophy should be used for all white lesions and some white-red lesions encountered in the vulvar region, and that a distinction should be made between atrophic (hypoplastic) dystrophy,

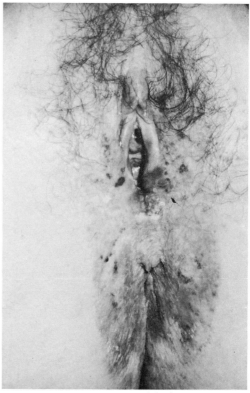

Fig. 4.1. Typical appearance of lichen sclerosus and atrophicus. Atrophy of the clitoris and the labia with constriction of the introitus. The skin around the vulva and anus is parchment-like with subepithelial bleedings due to itching and scratching.

Table 4.1. New nomenclature for vulvar dystrophies

I.   Hyperplastic dystrophy
     A. Without atypia
     B. With atypia
II. Lichen sclerosus
III. Mixed dystrophy (lichen sclerosus with foci of epithelial hyperplasia)
     A. Without atypia
     B. With atypia

hypertrophic (hyperplastic) dystrophy and mixed dystrophy.

CLINICAL FEATURES AND HISTOLOGY

Clinically, atrophic dystrophy is characterized by pruritus of long standing, an atrophic, parchment-like skin and increasing stenosis of the introitus and to a greater or lesser extent a disappearance of the clitoris. The lesion may only surround the introitus, but frequently has a figure-of-eight or hour-glass appearance involving the skin of both the vulvar and the perianal region (Fig. 4.1). The histologic characteristics are those of lichen sclerosus and atrophicus, with a thin epithelium with loss of the epithelial folds. The dermis beneath the squamous epithelium has a characteristic homogeneous, acellular hyalinized appearance, and chronic inflammatory cells are found deep in the homogeneous zone. Hyperkeratosis or parakeratosis may be present, but often the keratin layer is normal.

Hypertrophic dystrophy is clinically also characterized by pruritus of long standing, but instead of atrophy, inspection reveals thickened gray or white plaques located in the vulvar skin and/or the mucosa (Fig. 4.2). Biopsies from hypertrophic dystrophy show acanthosis with elongation and blunting of the epithelial folds (rete pigs). Marked hyperkeratosis is usually present, and there is a mild to severe inflammation within the dermis. In contrast to pure atrophic dystrophy, mild, moderate or severe atypia may sometimes accompany hypertrophic dystrophy (see Chapter 7), and these lesions therefore must be considered potentially premalignant.

In mixed dystrophy one finds areas with both the above-mentioned forms of dystrophy, and therefore in the part of the lesion dominated by hypertrophy, atypia may be present in some cases.

The atypical features in hypertrophic and mixed dystrophy include keratinized cells, abnormal nuclei, mitosis throughout the epithelium and not only in the basal layer, and a shift in the nuclear-cytoplasmatic ratio. An increased density of the cells is sometimes noted, as are alterations in the overall architecture of the epithelium. Atypia of some degree is found in approximately 5% of the hypertrophic and mixed dystrophies (3).

It is not within the scope of this book to give a detailed description of the clinical, histologic and therapeutic problems encountered in cases of lichen sclerosus. We have not made any thorough studies of this disease, but we agree with the description given by Friedrich (3). In our experience it is a disease of postmenopausal women. Lichen sclerosus is seldom found in those who are pre-

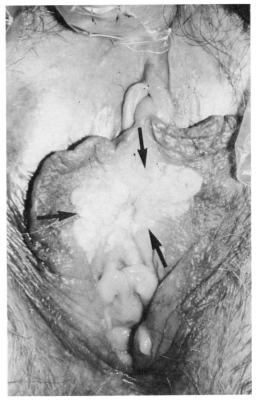

Fig. 4.2. Hypertrophic dystrophy with hyperkeratosis (arrows).

menopausal and extremely seldom in young women. What is important from an oncologic point of view is the unfinished discussion of the possibility that atrophic dystrophy is a premalignant disease.

There is no doubt that lichen sclerosus is found in a large percentage adjacent to invasive vulvar carcinoma. In a long-term follow-up of 160 cases of lichen sclerosus, Stening (4) found that 9.4% developed vulvar carcinoma in the course of an average of eight years. Furthermore, lichen sclerosus was the major cause of diffuse leukoplakia which was present in 72% of 204 cases of invasive squamous cell carcinoma of the vulva. Way (5) is also of the opinion that white lesions are premalignant. In contrast to this stands the statement by Friedrich (3) that "without the admixture of atypical foci of hyperplasia, lichen sclerosus has essentially no premalignant potential". We have no spesific follow-up studies that can prove or dis-

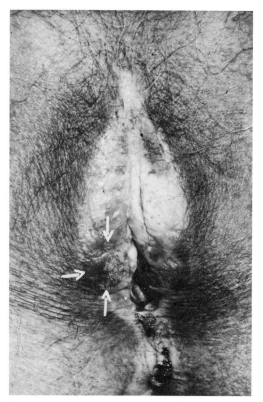

Fig. 4.3. Atrophic dystrophy with white, atrophic skin and a small invasive carcinoma (arrows).

prove the above-mentioned statements. However, we agree that if there is an admixture of hypertrophic dystrophy, and especially if biopsies show foci of atypia, the lesion certainly may be prema-lignant, as are all similar lesions of pure hypertrophic dystrophy with atypia. Areas of atypia may be revealed by Collin's Toluidine-blue test (1% Toluidine-blue followed by cleansing with 1–3% acid). However, this is not a reliable test.

TREATMENT

The type of treatment applied may be of some importance for lichen sclerosus to develop into mixed dystrophy and eventually to invasive carcinoma. If lichen sclerosus is left untreated and pruritus not combated, the result may be mixed dystrophy with atypia. In the author's experience, topical application of 3–5% testosterone ointment seems to be the most effective treatment today. In the initial phase, hydrocortisone ointment may give immediate relief of intense itching, but such treatment should not be carried out for a prolonged period. On the other hand it has been claimed that testosterone treatment can give permanent control of lichen sclerosus (3). The ointment should be applied twice or three times a week and can be continued for several years. Even with this treatment, however, it is my experience that pruritus may recur. In such cases, as well as before treatment starts, one should always search for fungus infection. Also vaginitis should be combated, and even if estrogen ointment applied to the vulva is of no use, atrophic colpitis will disappear, as will secretions which are keeping the vulva wet. Furthermore, the vaginal bacterial flora will change towards normal.

5

Condylomata acuminata

The most common form of virus-induced tumors in the vulva is condyloma acuminatum. The lesion is readily recognized under macroscopic inspection, presenting as multiple, finger-like, sharply pointed ("acuminate") warts located in the labia majora. Without treatment the warts may spread to the labia minora, the perianal region, the vagina and the cervix. The warts are benign in the vast majority of cases. Under certain circumstances, and especially in long-standing disease, a premalignant condition may develop, and even invasive epidermoid carcinoma of the vulva originating in condylomata acuminata have been reported (1, 2).

EPIDEMIOLOGY

In Norway, as in other countries in the Western world, the frequency of condylomas has increased during the last few decades. The disease is caused by a sexually transmitted, DNA-containing virus (HPV 6 or 10), and a proper name is therefore venereal warts. The common wart, verruca vulgaris, is caused by a closely related virus, and may affect the same areas as condylomata acuminata. It is sometimes difficult to differentiate between the two lesions, but it should be remembered that verruca vulgaris has the same appearance as when occurring in other sites of the body, that is smaller and flatter compared to the typical venereal warts.

Typically, condylomata acuminata are located in the anogenital region, often in connection with poor perineal hygiene, moisture and vaginal discharge. In most countries neither condylomas nor Herpes virus II lesions are reportable diseases, so it is impossible to present any exact incidence figures for these, today, very common venereal infections. This situation may be changed in the course of a few years. Both gynecologists and dermatologists recommend that the same rules for the reporting of gonorrhea and syphilis should be applied for venereal warts and Herpes virus II infections. In Norway, Herpes genitalis became a reportable disease in 1983.

Condylomata acuminata are usually found in sexually active women during their fertile years frequently during pregnancy. However, cases occur in children and in postmenopausal women with no history of sexual contact. The explanation may simply be that the virus has an extremely variable incubation period ranging from some weeks up to several months or even years. It may also be that an asymptomatic carrier state exists. Spread from toilet seats or from mother to child is also a possibility. The growth and spread of the warts are enhanced by pregnancy and the use of oral contraceptives. Estrogen usage alone does not seem to promote growth.

PATHOLOGY

Condylomata are usually multiple and exhibit a wide variety of macroscopic appearances. Young lesions are typically finger-like, sharply pointed, and have a gray or white color due to a superficial coating of keratin. They are unevenly distributed, first on the labia majora, later in the perianal region and on the labia minora. With time they become confluent and pigmented, either red, because of the abundancy of capillaries within the papillomatous projections, or often almost dark brown because of the accumulation of pigment in the thick layer of squamous cells covering the vessel-containing stromal papillae (Fig. 5.1). Long-standing condylomata may take on large, sometimes enormous proportions as shown in Fig. 5.2. Most venereal warts are so typical that the diagnosis is obvious. But biopsy is always indi-

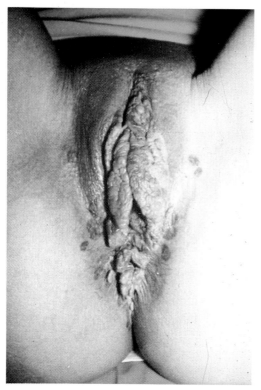

Fig. 5.1. Long-standing condylomata acuminata with confluency and development of pigmented areas.

ta acuminata, it is necessary, especially in large, confluent lesions to examine a substantial number of microscopic sections. Stening, in his series of 204 cases of epidermoid carcinoma of the vulva, found that six cases had developed from condylomata (3). We have also found cases of intraepithelial carcinoma in surgical specimens of confluent condylomata. After having become alert to the possibility, two cases of epidermoid vulvar carcinoma most probably developing from verrucous lesions have been observed. It must be emphasized, however, that condylomatous venereal warts have a low potentiality for developing into invasive carcinoma.

cated, especially in somewhat atypical lesions, and in all lesions which are not treated by surgery, but by destructive methods like electrocoagulation or laser evaporization.

The histologic features depict a papillomatous lesion covered by a thick, acanthotic squamous epithelium thrown into numerous folds, and supported by abundant stromal papillae (Fig. 5.3). The stratum corneum is only slightly thickened with parakeratotic cells, while the stratum spinosum shows hyperplasia, papillomatosis and acanthosis. Many mitotic figures may be found. The picture may resemble carcinoma in situ, but the polarity of the cells is preserved throughout the whole thickness of the epithelium. In the upper half of the epidermis, a marked vacuolization of the cells can be seen. The basement membrane is intact, although it can be distorted.

Because both intraepithelial neoplasia and invasive carcinoma can develop from condyloma-

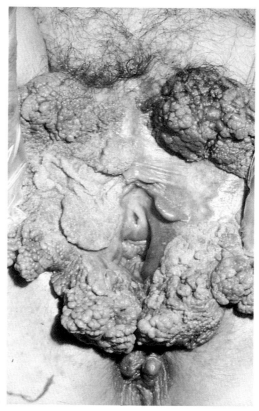

Fig. 5.2. Enormous condylomatous lesion in a 60-year-old woman. She had had her disease for at least 12 years before consulting a doctor. Microscopic examination showed no sign of malignancy.

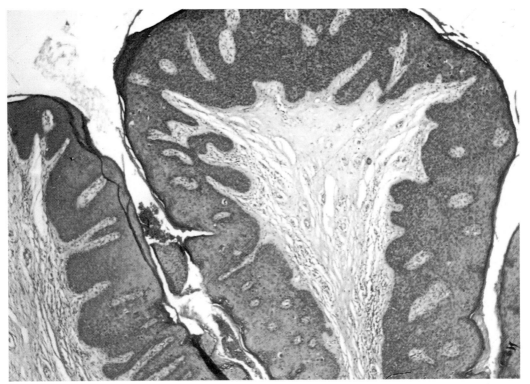

Fig. 5.3. Microscopic picture of condyloma. The papillomatous projections are covered by a thick, acanthotic epithelium supported by numerous stromal papillae.

DIAGNOSIS

The patients usually complain of pruritus and wetness in the vulvar region. Secondary infection may bring about a foul odour. The itching is not as intense as in atrophic vulvar dystrophy. Therefore it may take many years before a doctor is consulted. The lesions shown in Fig. 5.2 had been recognized by the patient for at least twelve years.

The diagnosis can usually be made by macroscopic inspection, and if only a few small warts are present, they can be treated without histological confirmation. But in larger, confluent lesions, multiple biopsies or multiple sections of a surgical specimen are mandatory. And in all cases a thorough examination of the vagina and the cervix for other venereal diseases or cancer should be performed.

TREATMENT

Small warts may effectively be treated by podophyllin 20–25%, but not if they are located in the vagina or on the cervix. Podophyllin sets up an intense chemical inflammatory reaction when used intravaginally. Concomitant vaginitis should be adequately treated. Frequently the vaginal or cervical warts then disappear. Larger vulvar warts can be treated by electrocoagulation during local anesthesia. After such treatment, however, there may be a dramatic soreness which makes it necessary to use anesthetic creams or strong pain-relieving tablets for a few weeks. After having purchased laser equipment, we have found that evaporation by the laser beam gives much better cosmetic results than electrocoagulation, and the soreness is definitely less pronounced. Laser evaporation can be used not only in the vulva, but also in the perianal region, the vagina and the cervix. We have abandoned surgery of extensive lesions because of the scarring and impaired sexual function which usually follow such treatment. Condylomata located in the perianal region treated by surgery may result in stricture of the anus. It is of course also necessary when laser treatment is decided upon to eradicate concomitant vaginitis and vulvitis. Anesthetic cream should also be prescribed.

FOLLOW-UP

It is often difficult to eradicate all warts in one session. Two or three sessions, 3–4 weeks apart, may be necessary, when podophyllin, electrocoagulation or laser are used. When recurrences occur, it may be necessary to examine the sexual partner and treat him. Even if no lesion is found on the penis, it is advisable that he use a condom during intercourse for a period of time.

6
Paget's disease of the vulva

In 1874 Sir James Paget described the cutaneous excematoid lesion which bears his name (1). His original description was of the disease affecting the nipple and the areola of the breast, with an associated subjacent ductal carcinoma of the mammary gland. Later he found the same lesion affecting the penis, and others have reported cases affecting the anus, the axilla, the umbilicus and the external ear canal. The most common sites for extramammary Paget's disease are areas where apocrine sweat glands are concentrated, the axilla, the anus, but particularly the vulva. It should be noticed that the mammary gland may be regarded as a modified apocrine gland.

EPIDEMIOLOGY

Paget's disease of the vulva is exceedingly rare, and this necessarily limits extensive personal experience. The first case was reported by Dubreuilh in 1901 (2). Since that time a number of case reports have appeared in the literature. In the last decades more extensive studies of the clinical behavior, histologic features and pathogenesis of Paget's disease of the vulva have been published (3).

Meaningful incidence figures cannot be produced. In our own series of 18 cases we found that between 1939 and 1972 there was approximately one case of Paget's disease for every 53 patients with vulvar carcinoma, or a frequency of approximately 20/1000 invasive carcinomas of the vulva (4).

One patient was 38 years of age when the diagnosis was made, the other 17 were all postmenopausal, 72% being more than 60 years of age. The mean age was 64.7 years. Friedrich states from an extensive review of the literature that the median age is 65 years (5).

In collected series a high incidence of associated or prior malignancy especially of the breast and genital organs has been reported. In the series of 18 cases from the Norwegian Radium Hospital, three patients had at some time diagnosed cancer elsewhere. One was radically treated several years previously for adenocarcinoma of the breast. Another was treated by surgery and irradiation for a Stage Ia serous carcinoma of the ovary three years before the onset of vulvar disease, and the third had an epidermoid carcinoma of the cervix uteri concomitant with the onset of vulvar disease.

DIAGNOSIS

Itching, often accompanied by soreness, and sometimes by a burning sensation, are the most common symptoms. In spite of this it is typical that there is a definite patient delay of up to several years. In our series there was a mean delay of 22 months before professional help was sought.

The lesions are often described as erythematous and eczematous with a flecking, white hyperkeratosis. Others may be crusted or papillary, sometimes with superficial ulceration. The margins are generally well defined macroscopically, but it must be emphasized that the underlying microscopic lesion usually extends many centimeters outside these margins. The physical appearance of Paget's disease of the vulva is often confused with benign cutaneous lesions. Because of this, proper treatment, based on histologic diagnosis, was in our series delayed on average 20.6 months, frequently for several years.

The size of the lesion can vary from small foci on one labium major to extensive areas involving mons, clitoris, urethra, labia majora, anus, and inner aspects of both thighs. Labia minora may also be involved, but no lesion will be found limited to hairless areas, The vagina is not affected. Some examples of the macroscopic appearance

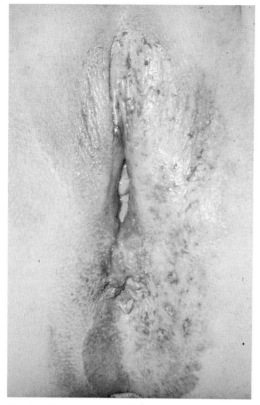

Fig. 6.1. Excematous type of Paget's disease with partly pigmented or red areas; the skin appears partly atrophic and white.

are shown in Figs. 6.1 and 6.2. There is no doubt that after having studied a few cases of Paget's disease of the vulva, it is possible to suspect the diagnosis, a fact which leads to an early biopsy. Since the series of 18 cases was published, we have seen six more patients with this lesion, and in all of these there was a suspicion of Paget's disease before biopsies were taken.

HISTOLOGY AND HISTOGENESIS

There is always a variable degree of epidermal acanthosis and hyperkeratosis, sometimes also small areas of parakeratosis. The characteristic Paget cells are easy to recognize and pathognomonic. They have a pale, vacuolated, clear to slightly basophilic cytoplasm and vesicular nuclei with a prominent nucleolus. The nuclear/cytoplasmic ratio is approximately 1:3. The Paget cells

are found either singly or in groups or bands, and are most often located in the basal part of the epidermis (Fig. 6.3). The Paget cells may also form intraepidermal gland-like hair follicles (Fig. 6.4.).

Mucinous material may be found in some Paget cells, but not in all. In our series the number of cells giving a positive histochemical reaction varied considerably between cases. In addition, the intensity of the staining reaction varied from cell to cell and among groups of cells.

The histogenesis of Paget's disease has caused much controversy. When the lesion affects the breast, it is claimed that there is always a subjacent malignancy. The original view was that the cutaneous lesion represents an intraepithelial invasion of cancer cells from an underlying intraductal carcinoma. This explanation cannot be valid in Paget's disease of the vulva. In agreement with earlier studies, we found that 11 out of 18

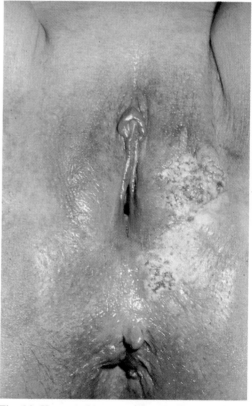

Fig. 6.2. Hypertrophic type of Paget's disease with hyperkeratosis and small areas with superficial ulceration.

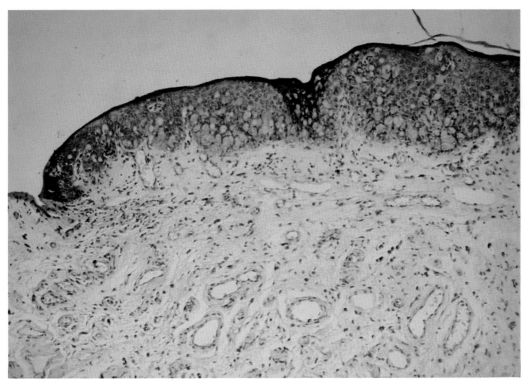

Fig. 6.3. Microscopic picture of typical Paget cells. These are pale, vacuolated with a slightly basophilic cytoplasm and grow in bands mostly in the basal part of the epidermis.

cases showed no signs of an underlying adnexal gland atypia or carcinoma.

Today there seems to be a growing consensus of opinion that Paget's disease is a type of intra-epithelial cancer (5). It is important to keep in mind, however, that in approximately one third of the cases of vulvar Paget's disease, a concomitant adnexal gland carcinoma will be found. Electron microscopic studies have contributed significantly to the present concept of the histogenesis of Paget's disease. All cells of the epidermis and its adnexal structures are derived from the embryonic stratum germinativum of the ectoderm. Cells from this layer may develop along a variety of pathways and become epidermal squamous cells, sweat gland or sebaceous gland cells, hair follicles, etc. The Paget cells appear to represent an unusual abnormal differentiation of the stem cell. This explains the usual location of Paget cells which are first noted adjacent to the more or less undifferentiated basal cells, both in the epidermis and in the adnexal structures.

TREATMENT

Before any decision upon therapy is made, a thorough search for an associated carcinoma of the genital tract and the breast should be performed. A malignant tumor at any of these or other sites, for example the gastro-intestinal tract, will have preference over Paget's disease of the vulva.

It is our experience that radiotherapy has no place in the primary treatment of Paget's disease, neither have chemotherapy, cryosurgery or laser vaporization. A wide surgical excision is to be preferred. The depth of the excision should take into account the possibility of a concomitant carcinoma of apocrine or eccrine glands. In the majority of cases surgery will consist of vulvectomy with removal of the epidermis, the corium and the underlying fat tissue. The incision must be well outside the visible lesion, at least 3 cm from the margin, because Paget cells at the periphery of the lesion can be found adjacent to the basal cells without any changes in the overlying skin. Mul-

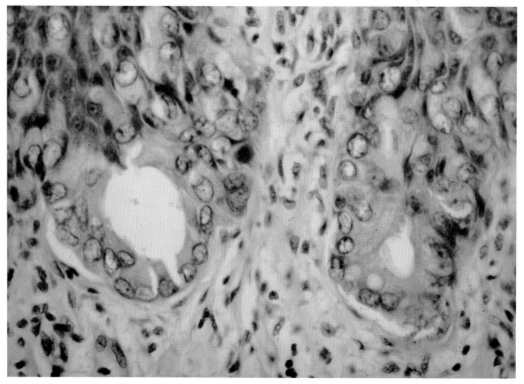

Fig. 6.4. Paget cells forming glandular structures. Note the prominent nucleoli.

tiple sections of the surgical specimen should be examined microscopically to confirm that the margins are free, and also to rule out an underlying carcinoma. If the lesion is not removed with ample free margins recurrence is bound to occur, although frequently many years after primary therapy. If adnexal gland carcinoma is revealed, additional ipsilateral or bilateral inguinal lymphadenectomy should be carried out according to the site of the lesion. In tumors located strictly to one labium majus, ipsilateral lymphadenectomy may be sufficient.

In our own series, 15 patients underwent surgical excision in an attempt at definitive therapy. Nine of these had margins involved by Paget cells, even though the surgeon in eight of these nine cases claimed to have performed a wide, "radical" excision. No patient with involved margins has failed to have a recurrence, while none of the six patients with free margins has had a local recurrence.

Seven of the 18 patients had either adnexal gland carcinoma (two cases), adnexal gland atypia (two cases) or vulvar adenocarcinoma with metastases (two cases). In one case only limited histologic material was available, and no associated carcinoma could be found in the vulvar specimen, but she had lymph node metastases. Six of these seven patients died of carcinoma. The interval from the first attempt at definitive treatment to death varied from 4 to 156 months.

Because of patient delay and doctor's delay, Paget's disease of the vulva is often very extensive and a wide amount of skin has to be removed. Large surgical defects may thus be produced. We have found that in the plastic management of such defects, full-thickness rotational flap grafts as recommended by Julian, Callison and Woodruff (6) may be useful (Fig. 6.5 and 6.6).

Paget's disease of the vulva is notoriously chronic and subject to repeated local recurrences. If there are no signs of adnexal gland carcinoma

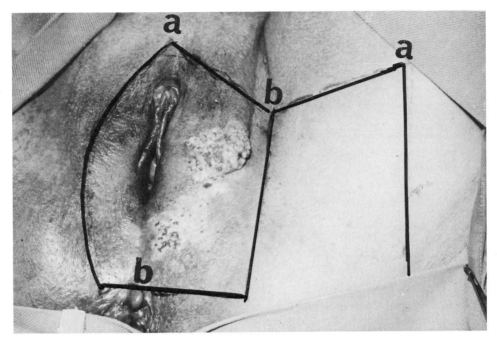

Fig. 6.5. Incision lines for surgical treatment of the lesion shown in Fig. 6.4.

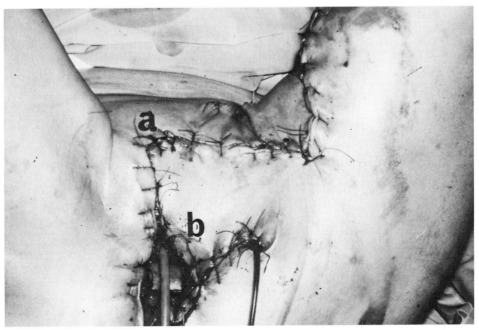

Fig. 6.6. Rotational flap covering the area of skin removed.

in the primary vulvectomy specimen, recurrent sites constitute only a local threat. As emphasized by Friedrich, they are symptomatic and may enlarge to encompass wider areas. Surgical management by repeated excision has traditionally been used, but extensive scarring may result. Friedrich therefore recommended that for such recurrent cases, the experimental methods of laser vaporization or topical chemotherapy with 5-fluorouracil may be considered (5). We have no personal experience with these methods.

FOLLOW-UP

Because of the high frequency of recurrences, routine follow-up is of extreme importance. It should be remembered that recurrences are on average detected about two years after primary therapy. Regular visits should therefore be scheduled at three-month intervals, for two years. Preferably the patient should have a follow-up of yearly visits for the rest of her life. In our series the longest interval between primary therapy and the first recurrence was 14 years.

7
Vulvar intraepithelial neoplasia

In 1967 Richart (1) introduced the term "Cervical Intraepithelial Neoplasia" (CIN) into gynecologic oncologic terminology. In the opinion of the present author it is about time that similar terminology were used for premalignant lesions of the vulva. The term "Vulvar Intraepithelial Neoplasia" (VuIN) would comprise lesions which up to now have been listed as hypertrophic or mixed dystrophy with atypia, atypical epithelial hyperplasia, erythroplasia of Queyrat, Bowen's disease, dysplasia, and carcinoma in situ. All these lesions have a potential of becoming invasive, although of different degree, but diagnostic measures, treatment and follow-up will be identical. The ISSVD has proposed that all these lesions should be included in the term "carcinoma in situ". A better alternative in the author's opinion is "vulvar intraepithelial neoplasia" (VuIN).

EPIDEMIOLOGY

It is impossible to produce any prevalence or incidence figures for VuIN. There are no screening methods to detect the disease, and cases being reported to cancer registries depend totally upon the alertness of the physician performing gynecologic examination of a substantial number of females, and on his willingness and ability to take biopsies from appropriate areas of the vulva.

There are several studies which seem to indicate that the frequency of VuIN is increasing, and that the disease is found more frequently in the younger age groups than 20–30 years ago (2, 3).

During the years 1956–74, 29 cases of verified carcinoma in situ (4) and 424 cases of invasive squamous cell carcinoma of the vulva were admitted to our hospital, which gives only 6.8 cases of VuIN to 100 invasive carcinomas. Throughout the last three decades invasive vulvar carcinomas have shown an incidence rate of 2.5/100,000 females in Norway. This indicates an incidence rate of VuIN of approximately 0.2/100,000 women. This is certainly not a true incidence figure. There are too many indications that a large percentage of VuIN lesions are not detected because the physician does not have any knowledge of this disease. In the United States an incidence rate of carcinoma in situ of the vulva of 0.53/100,000 has been reported (5). The percentage of VuIN developing into invasive carcinoma is much less than for example the CIN lesions.

Today there is an increasing awareness of this entity and more biopsies are being taken from small vulvar lesions. However, this is possibly not the only explanation of the reported slight increase in vulvar intraepithelial neoplasia. Another explanation may be the increase in viral lesions of the lower genital tract in women which seems to have occurred in many countries throughout the world. The most common of these are the Herpes virus type II and the papilloma viruses, which are all sexually transmitted. There is no doubt that genital flat papillomas and condylomas are premalignant. This is recognized by gynecologists, dermatologists and histopathologists.

PATHOLOGY

The macroscopic or clinical picture of vulvar intraepithelial neoplasia is highly variable. White, gray, pink, red and brown lesions may hide an underlying VuIN microscopic picture. The lesions may be single, multiple or confluent. They may be located to any part of the vulva, labium major or minus, the clitorial region or the perineum. However, there are certain hallmarks stressed by Friedrich (6). With few exceptions the lesions are papular or raised above the surrounding skin and they have a roughened surface. This can best be studied by using a magnifying glass of 2-4 ×, or a colposcope preferably at one of the lower magnifications of 4-6 ×.

Usually VuIN shows parakeratosis or hyperkeratosis when examined microscopically. Keratosis can also be diagnosed clinically, and should always raise suspicion of a preinvasive lesion.

Friedrich has introduced three so-called "P-factors", namely: Parakeratosis, Papule formation and Pigment incontinence. One or more of these factors is always found in hypertrophic or mixed dystrophy, atypical epithelial hyperplasia, erythroplasia, Bowen's disease, dysplasia or carcinoma in situ—or as proposed here—in all examples of VuIN. Papule formation is possibly most important, while parakeratosis and keratosis can often be found in benign lesions. Pigment incontinence is probably most often found in premalignant lesions developing as a result of a papilloma virus infection.

The microscopic features of VuIN are similar to those of premalignant lesions at other sites of squamous cell origin. The normally layered architecture of the epithelium is destroyed. There is an architectural disorientation which involves either part of the surface epithelium (VuIN grade I or II), or virtually the whole thickness of the epidermis (VuIN grade III) (Fig. 7.1). If the surface layers show parakeratosis or keratosis, this should not interfere with the grading of the lesion. In cases of parakeratosis the most superficial cells are flat and show retention of nuclear chromatin in the otherwise acellular keratin layer of the epithelium. The atypical cells are often enlarged with abnormal nuclei, multiple nuclei, and there is pleomorphism and hyperchromasia. There can be formation of so-called "corps rond", round bodies, which are formed by large, hyperchromatic nuclei with a light halo around. Mitotic figures are found high up in the epithelium and some abnormal mitosis may be encountered. There is a shift in the cytoplasmic/nuclear ratio. On rare occasions precocious maturation and formation of squamous pearls are seen near the tip of the rete pigs. The significance of this last observation in cervical lesions is that it frequently occurs just prior to early invasion. Whether the same is true in vulvar lesions remains to be proved.

DIAGNOSIS

The most important factor for an early diagnosis of vulvar intraepithelial neoplasia is the alertness

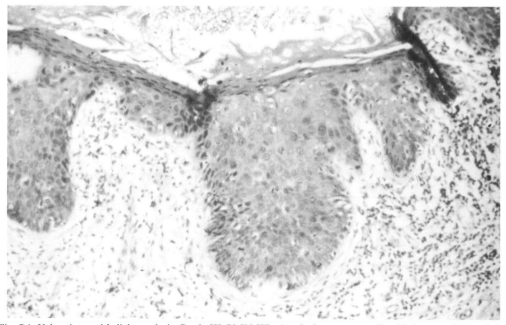

Fig. 7.1. Vulvar intraepithelial neoplasia Grade III (VuIN III). Atypical squamous cells with large nuclei involving the whole thickness of the epithelium. Note parakeratosis and hyperkeratosis at the surface.

of the clinician. His awareness that even a seemingly innocuous lesion should be biopsied, and that frequently multiple biopsies are necessary, is the best assurance of success. Collin's toluidine blue test may help in finding the biopsy sites, but it is an unspecific method.

Fortunately, most preinvasive lesions of the vulva give symptoms. Itching, usually combined with soreness, or the recognition of a raised plaque or papule are the most common complaints. Such symptoms should always lead to a gynecologic examination. It is sad to state that some physicians still prescribe antipruritic ointment without having inspected and palpated the vulva. Such an attitude cannot be excused even in a large and busy private practice.

Cytology and/or colposcopy may give additional information. However, these methods are not of the same importance in vulvar as in vaginal and cervical lesions. VuIN is frequently covered by keratotic epithelium which prevents exfoliation of malignant cells. At the same time keratosis is non-translucent and the underlying colposcopic pattern cannot be seen. A certain percentage of the VuIN lesions are wet, especially red lesions located to the inner side of the labia minora or to the urethral area. Such wet lesions exfoliate cells which can easily be studied in cytologic smears. At the same time characteristic colposcopic pictures can be seen. The same criteria for making a correct colposcopic diagnosis as used in cervical intraepithelial neoplasia are applicable in VuIN (see p. 72). Colposcopy may pin-point the most atypical part of the lesion where the biopsy should

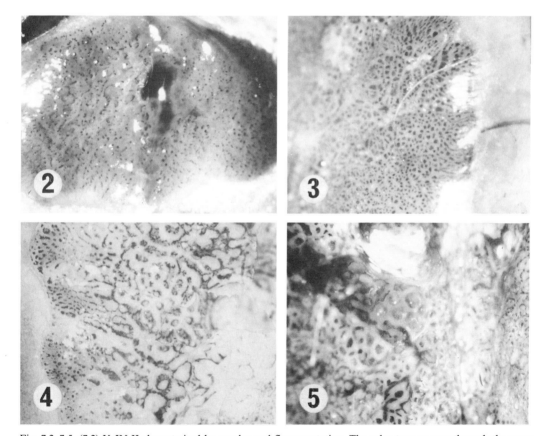

Fig. 7.2–7.5. (7.2) VuIN II characterized by regular and fine punctation. The color tone as seen through the green filter is dark. (7.3) VuIN II–III. Both fine and coarse punctation vessels, dark color tone, but smooth surface. (7.4) VuIN III with both fine and coarse punctation vessels and irregular mosaic. (7.5) VuIN III with suspicion of early stromal invasion. The punctation vessels are coarse and irregular, and the surface of the lesion slightly nodular.

preferably be taken. Better translucency of the surface epithelium resulting in a clearer colposcopic picture can be obtained by application of physiological saline, or in some dry lesions, some sort of skin oil. Acetic acid 3% may reveal acetowhite epithelium which should always be biopsied.

It should be pointed out that the vascular atypia is much less conspicuous in many vulvar lesions compared with similar cervical or vaginal lesions. Therefore, there is a chance of underdiagnosing early invasive carcinomas. In Figs. 7.2, 7.3, 7.4 and 7.5, examples of the colposcopic patterns of wet vulvar lesions are shown.

TREATMENT

Vulvar intraepithelial neoplasia is not infrequently found concomitant with vaginal or cervical premalignant or malignant lesions. It is therefore mandatory that a thorough gynecologic, cytologic and colposcopic examination of the total lower genital tract be performed before a decision on therapy is made.

Confusion has existed as to the malignant potential of VuIN. After a meticulous review of the medical literature, Friedrich (6) concluded that there are few proven cases reported of invasive squamous cell carcinoma developing from carcinoma in situ of the vulva. Most authors today agree that it is not necessary to treat these lesions with radical surgery or radiotherapy. Much more conservative measures can be used. Simple vulvectomy has been recommended for many years because of the possibility of multiple foci. This was also the case in our own series of 29 patients, 20 of whom were subjected to vulvectomy (Table 7.1). Six cases from the later

years were treated with local excision and two with hemivulvectomy. The patients have been followed-up for a period of 3–20 years. The only recurrence was detected after 62 months in a patient initially treated with hemivulvectomy. Histologic examination of the initial specimen showed carcinoma in situ in the resection border at the site where the recurrence developed. Re-excision was performed, but histologic examination once more revealed atypical epithelium at the resection border. The patient this time received topical application of 5-fluorouracil cream. Four years later, however, early invasive squamous cell carcinoma was detected in the same region. A complete local excision of the lesion was performed. The patient is without signs of disease five years after the last resection.

The experience from this series, and from other studies reported in the literature, shows that vulvar intraepithelial neoplasia has an excellent prognosis. Regarding treatment, some authors recommend simple vulvectomy, others "skinning" vulvectomy, and some prefer local excision (6). In young patients topical 5-fluorouracil 5% has been tried. Our experience with this latter type of therapy is limited, and we are not able to state its value, although we have observed complete disappearance of in situ carcinoma of the vulva in a few cases. The follow-up of these patients is, however, too short for us to reach any definite conclusion about the value and safety of topical 5-fluorouracil. Judging from the literature, the success rate is relatively low and the recurrence rate high. In recent years, laser evaporization has been recommended. We have little experience with this sort of therapy. It should always be kept in mind that an excisional biopsy is much safer, as the ultimate histological diagnosis of the lesion will then be revealed.

In conclusion, vulvar intraepithelial neoplasia is an innocent condition that should not be overtreated by mutilating surgery. In our opinion, the standard treatment should include a wide local excision in order to obtain an accurate histologic evaluation of the entire lesion. Unnecessary removal of the clitoris or the whole vulva should be avoided. Topical 5-fluorouracil or laser treatment should be restricted to young women for whom surgery is found not feasible, which will in practice

Table 7.1. Treatment methods and recurrence

Treatment group	Total No.	Recurrence	Death
Excision	6		
Hemivulvectomy	2	1	
Vulvectomy	20		
Radical vulvectomy with lymphadenectomy	1		
Total	29	1	0

be very few patients. If multiple lesions are present, simple vulvectomy with preservation of the clitoris may be the treatment of choice.

FOLLOW-UP

Multiple foci are not uncommon in vulvar intraepithelial neoplasia. Three out of 29 cases (10%) in our own series had multiple lesions. Since treatment today is usually conservative with preservation of as much as possible of the labia and clitoris, regular visits should be scheduled for the patients so that recurrence or new lesions can be detected as early as possible. We recommend follow-up visits every six months the first and second year, and thereafter once yearly, preferably for the rest of the patient's life. In patients who have had VuIN, the vulva may be regarded as a potential neoplastic field. New lesions may develop many years after the first focus was detected, not infrequently because of new outbursts of virus infection.

8
Epidermoid carcinoma of the vulva

STAGING

Stage 0. – Carcinoma in situ, vulvar intraepithelial
neoplasia (VuIN).

Stage I. – Tumor confined to the vulva–2 cm or
less in diameter. Nodes are not palpable, or are
palpable in either groin, not enlarged, mobile
(not clinically suspicious of neoplasm).

Stage II. – Tumor confined to the vulva–more
than 2 cm in diameter. Nodes are not palpable,
or are palpable in either groin, not enlarged,
mobile (not clinically suspicious of neoplasm).

Stage III. – Tumors of any size with: (1) adjacent
spread to the lower urethra and/or the vagina,
the perineum, the anus, and/or (2) nodes palpable in either or both groins, enlarged, firm
and mobile, not fixed, but clinically suspicious
of neoplasm.

Stage IV. – Tumors of any size: (1) infiltrating the
bladder mucosa, and/or the upper part of the
urethral mucosa, and/or the rectal mucosa,
and/or (2) fixed to the bone, or other distant
metastases. Fixed or ulcerated nodes in either
or both groins.

EPIDEMIOLOGY

The age-adjusted incidence rate of vulvar carcinoma in Norway was 2.5/100,000 in the years
1972–76. The incidence in the different age groups
is shown in Fig. 8.1. The highest rates are found
in the age groups over 70 years, and extremely
few cases are reported under the age of 40 years.
In a series of 445 cases of epidermoid carcinoma
treated in our hospital, 54.6% were above 70
years, and only 7% under 50 years.

Carcinoma of the vulva comprises 0.9% of all
female malignancies in the country, and 4.0% of
all gynecologic malignancies. There has been a
slight, but not significant increase in the incidence

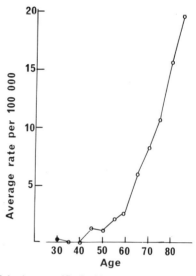

Fig. 8.1. Age specific incidence rate in patients with
carcinoma of the vulva in Norway in the period 1972–76.

rate since the Cancer Registry of Norway started
collecting data in 1952. This is probably a reflec-
tion of the increased longevity of the population.
The average life expectancy for Norwegian females today is 79.3 years.

The Norwegian Radium Hospital today receives approximately 80% of all cases detected in
the country. During the first 25 years, from 1932
to 1956, 409 patients were referred for treatment,
while in the next 25 years, the number increased
to 702, probably because of a higher referral rate,
but also due to an increase in the population of
older age groups.

Survival studies performed by the Cancer
Registry of Norway have shown a significant improvement in prognosis from the years prior to
1962 to the years after 1968 (Fig. 8.2). Since the
majority of the patients in this period were treated
in our hospital, this improved prognosis most
probably reflects the fact that from the early

1960s, radical vulvectomy with bilateral lymph-adenectomy was introduced as standard treatment. Before this time treatment was less radical and varied much from case to case, and many patients were treated by radiotherapy only.

There has not been any significant change in stage distribution during the last 30 years. In the eighteenth volume of the *Annual Report* (1) the hospital reported 255 patients being treated in the 10-year period 1966–75, 31.4% of whom belonged to Stage I, 31.4% to Stage II, 31.7% to Stage III and 5.5% to Stage IV.

PATHOLOGY

The macroscopic appearance of epidermoid carcinoma of the vulva may be described as either ulcerating (endophytic) or hypertrophic (exophytic). A third type, the so-called non-ulcerating, nodular tumor is often not an epidermoid carcinoma, but a tumor of the Bartholin's gland, an adenocarcinoma of adnexal apocrine or eccrine glands, or a cylindroma. These tumors usually have an intact epithelial lining, but can be palpated as firm or hard nodules.

Ulcerating epidermoid growths are by far the commonest. They can be described as endophytic or inverting with varying degrees of ulceration forming an excavation or crater. The ulcer may often have markedly everted edges (Fig. 8.3). Adjacent to the tumor, lichen sclerosus will be found by macroscopic inspection or by microscopy of the edges of the growth in about 50–70% of the cases.

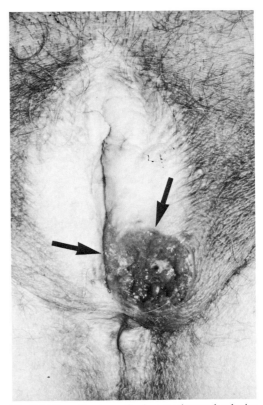

Fig. 8.3. Ulcerating type of vulvar carcinoma developing in a large area of lichen sclerosus.

Hypertrophic tumors usually have a distinct macroscopic appearance. In these cases there seems to be no or minor relationship to previous lichen sclerosus. The growth is typically papillomatous, and may in rare cases develop from condylomata acuminata. Hypertrophic epidermoid carcinoma shows its proliferative activity externally, and may reach massive proportions (Fig. 8.4).

The term "kissing ulcers" (Fig. 8.5) is used to describe two separate tumors, one on each labium exactly opposite each other. In older literature it is implied that one was due to implantation of cancer cells from the other. Another theory is that both sides of the vulva are subjected to the same etiological factors at the same time, and thus the rare "kissing ulcers" are examples of two primary tumors arising at the same time. The fact that separate multiple tumors are relatively common, in Stening's series 23% (2), while kissing ulcers are rare, points in favor of the latter theory.

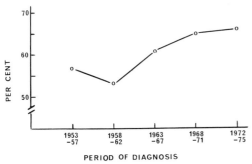

Fig. 8.2. Five-year survival rate for patients with carcinoma of the vulva in Norway in the period 1953–75 (see text).

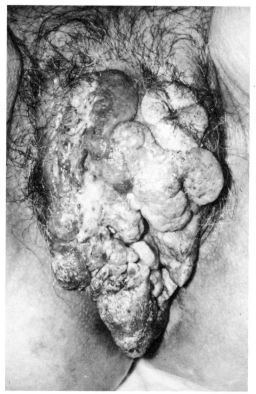

Fig. 8.4. Proliferating, cauliflower-like vulvar carcinoma of massive proportions.

Tumors arising in the dense tissue of the clitoris tend to be smaller than those developing in the loose tissue of the labia (Fig. 8.6). They are frequently of a nodular type before spread to the adjacent preputium occurs.

The vast majority of vulvar malignancies are classified as epidermoid carcinomas. When cases of intraepithelial neoplasia, basal cell carcinoma, Bowen's disease and Paget's disease are included in the statistics, the distribution by histologic type in a series of 613 cases is as shown in Table 8.1.

Different classification and grading systems have been proposed for epidermoid carcinoma of the vulva. Highly and moderately differentiated lesions are commonly regarded as having a better prognosis than the poorly differentiated tumors. Way (3) classified the lesions into differentiating, anaplastic and giant cell tumors, the latter having an extremely poor prognosis. The tumors may also be described as large cell keratinizing, large cell non-keratinizing and small cell non-keratin-

izing, the majority belonging to the first group. Keratin production and pearl formation is a distinct feature of most vulvar carcinomas (Fig. 8.7). In the smaller tumors, Stage I lesions, it is important to make a thorough search for vessel invasion (Fig. 8.8). If no vessel invasion is found, a more conservative approach to surgical therapy may be chosen.

LYMPH DRAINAGE FROM VULVA

A precise knowledge of the lymphatic system of the vulva is of utmost importance to the surgeon who is treating cancer of this organ. About 40–50% of the patients have metastases to the regional lymph nodes when they are first seen, all stages being taken into account.

The tissues of the vulva have an abundancy of lymph vessels which *primarily* drain to the groin lymph nodes. They all represent a common group of lymph nodes which are divided into two main groups, the superficial and the deep inguinal

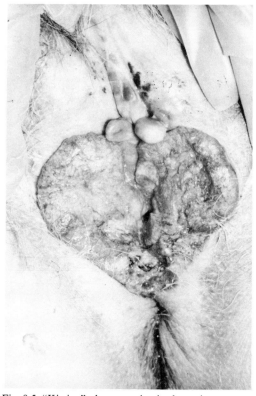

Fig. 8.5. "Kissing" ulcers meeting in the perineum.

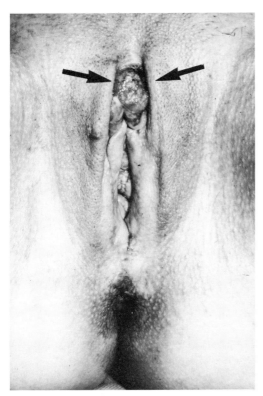

Fig. 8.6. Small carcinoma of the clitoris.

Table 8.1. Distribution by histologic type in 613 cases of malignant tumors of the vulva

Histologic diagnosis	Total No.	Per cent
Squamous cell carcinoma	445	70.6
Carcinoma in situ	56	9.1
Malignant melanoma	49	8.0
Basal cell carcinoma	28	4.6
Paget's disease	13	2.1
Bowen's disease	6	1.0
Adenocarcinoma	6	1.0
Cylindroma	5	0.8
Others	5	0.8
Total	613	100.0

nodes. The superficial nodes are located alongside the inguinal ligament and around the upper part of the great saphenous vein and its branches. The deep nodes are located subfascially between and along the femoral vessels. The uppermost of these deep nodes are located high up in the femoral canal posteromedial to the femoral vein, the deep femoral node or the node of Cloquet or Rosenmüller.

From the lymph nodes in the groin, vessels pass to the *secondary* regional nodes of the vulva, the pelvic nodes. These can be divided into the external, the internal and the common iliac chain (Fig. 8.9). The external iliac chain comprises a lateral, an intermediate and a medial chain. The lateral chain consists of nodes located lateral to the external iliac artery with the most distal node called the lateral lacunar node. The intermediate chain is found in front of and between the external iliac artery and vein, and is usually removed together with the lateral chain during operation. The lymph nodes on the medial and posterior side of

the iliac vein, between the vessels and the obturator nerve, are called the medial external iliac chain or the obturator nodes. The most distal node of this chain is found partly within the femoral canal and is often called the medial lacunar node, which is identical with the upper deep femoral node (node of Cloquet or Rosenmüller).

From the lateral and intermediate external chains lymph vessels pass on mainly to the common iliac nodes located lateral, anterior and posterior to the common iliac vessels. In addition, the lymph from the medial external chain drains to the parietal group of the internal iliac lymph nodes. This group consists of the presacral nodes located medial to the common iliac vessels, and

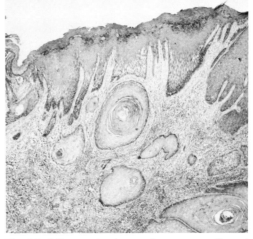

Fig. 8.7. Microscopic picture of squamous cell carcinoma of the vulva with typical keratin production and pearl formation.

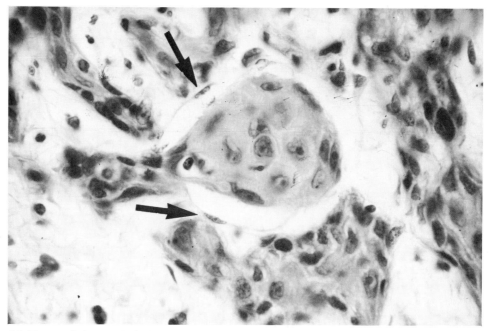

Fig. 8.8. Tumor cells in an endothelial lined space. The nuclei of the endothelium can clearly be seen (arrows).

the gluteal nodes located deep in the pelvic alongside the internal iliac vessels. However, many anastomoses exist between the above-mentioned lymph vessel chains.

It has been claimed that tumors located anteriorly in the midline of the vulva, especially the clitoreal tumors, have a direct lymphatic pathway to the medial external iliac and the internal iliac lymph nodes. More recent clinical and experimental studies do not support this theory. In our own series of 100 cases where routine pelvic lymphadenectomy was performed (4), seven cases were found to have spread to the pelvic nodes. In only one of these seven cases were concomitant metastases to the lymph nodes in the groin not found. The groin nodes were not subjected to serial sectioning. Way, in 1960 (5), described three cases with pelvic node involvement which appeared to occur in the absence of inguinal node involvement. However, further and more extensive studies involving serial sectioning of the inguinal node material, revealed metastases that had been overlooked at the first examination (3). Way's total series comprised 250 cases.

In our own Department an experimental investigation of the lymph drainage from the vulva has been performed. In a series of 54 patients with cervical cancer Stage Ib with normal vulva, the radioactive colloid ^{99m}technesium was injected in labium majus, labium minus, glans clitoris and the perineum (Fig. 8.10) (6). All patients underwent radical surgery with bilateral pelvic lymphadenectomy. The uptake of radioactive colloid in the lymph nodes was recorded both in vivo by a scintillation method and in the removed lymph nodes with a well counter. The different node groups were kept separate from each other, as were the medial and lateral lacunar nodes, the first pelvic node stations after the inguinal nodes. No direct pathway was found from the clitoris to the pelvic lymph nodes. Both the clitoris and the perineum were found to have a bilateral lymph flow. No other differences were found in relation to other injection sites.

It is well documented that tumors located exclusively on one side may metastasize to both the ipsilateral and contralateral groin. Spread to the same side is by far the most frequent. However, in cases with unilateral tumor and inguinal metastases, Way (3) found that 20% had contralateral metastases. Our own figure is 15% (7). Contralateral metastases alone were found in 5% and

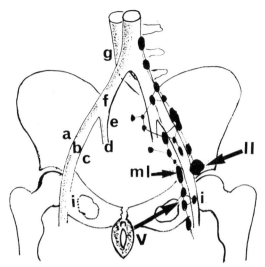

Fig. 8.9. Lymphatic drainage of vulva. v: vulva, i: inguinal nodes, a, b, c: lateral, intermediate and medial external nodes, d: internal iliac nodes, e: presacral nodes, f: common iliac nodes, g: periaortic nodes, ml: medial, and ll: lateral lacunar node.

2% in the two studies, respectively. We agree with Way that the spread of vulvar cancer is quite simple:

1. Most tumors situated on the left side of the vulva spread to lymphatics in the left groin.
2. Most tumors situated on the right side spread to lymphatics in the right groin.
3. Vulvar tumors involving the midline or both sides of the vulva can spread to both groins.
4. In a few cases of strictly unilateral tumors, contralateral spread may occur, especially when the ipsilateral nodes are already affected and there is a blockage of the lymph stream.
5. There is no evidence of spread to the pelvic nodes without first involving the inguinal nodes, and the often quoted statement that the clitoris drains directly to the pelvis is inaccurate.

The chance of bilateral spread is the background for the general recommendation that bilateral lymphadenectomy should always be performed even when the tumor is strictly unilateral.

SYMPTOMS

The question of an early diagnosis of vulvar carcinoma has never been thoroughly discussed. There are no specific or conspicuous symptoms which may alert the patient to seek medical advice at an early stage. It is characteristic that in a period when 424 cases of invasive vulvar carcinoma were treated in our hospital, only 29 cases of VuIN were seen. Of the invasive lesions, less than 30% were in the clinical Stage I.

The most prominent symptom is pruritus, which frequently may be due to a preceding lichen sclerosus et atrophicus. Pruritus therefore may be of long standing and is often neglected both by the patient and the doctor. Itching may also be due to vaginal discharge, either because of monilial infection or senile vaginitis. In rare cases it may be due to diabetes. Nevertheless, pruritus is a symptom that should alert the doctor to search for a preinvasive or invasive tumor. In our own series, itching and soreness was the main complaint in about 40% of the cases.

The second most common symptom is simply that the patient has recognized a small lump or an ulcer. About 10% of patients do not seek advice for their pruritus until they are aware of the presence of a tumor or ulcer. By the time the patient is referred for treatment, between 40 and 50% of them describe a lump in the vulva.

Bleeding is usually a late symptom and is most often found in clinical Stages II–IV. When bleeding occurs, it is slight and usually due to necrosis

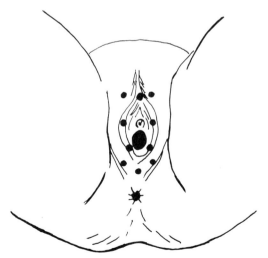

Fig. 8.10. Injection sites for ⁹⁹ᵐtechnesium colloid in the vulva (see text). (Redrawn after T. Iversen (6)).

of the superficial parts of the tumor with erosion of the vessels developing in the tumor itself.

Pain is relatively uncommon and is mostly a complaint of patients with advanced disease involving the bony pelvis or nerve roots. It is strange that even extremely large, fungating lesions may be almost without pain. Sometimes an acute or subacute cellulitis is set up, and then the pain of inflammation may be present.

Disturbance of urination may occur in lesions affecting the urethra, and disturbance of defecation in tumors involving the anal sphincter.

Ulcerating growths are always secondarily infected not only with aerobic, but also often with anaerobic bacteria. Foul odour may in such cases sometimes be the only presenting symptom. It happens that the patient's husband or other close relatives insist upon a consultation with her doctor, because of the excessively foul odour.

DIAGNOSIS

More than ⅔ of the patients have an advanced Stage II–IV tumor when they are first seen. This is often due to a definite patient delay (Fig. 8.11). Many patients are reluctant to allow medical inspection of a vulvar tumor, partly because of ignorance due to the rarity of the disease, partly because of shyness or embarrassment. Some women even admit that they waited a long time before consulting a doctor due to the fact that they were afraid of cancer. In our own series 55%

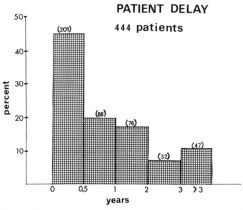

Fig. 8.11. Patient delay in 444 women with vulvar carcinoma.

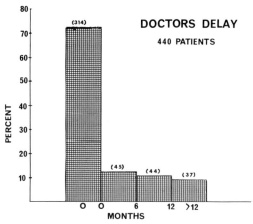

Fig. 8.12. Doctor's delay in 440 women with vulvar carcinoma.

of the patients presented for advice more than six months after the onset of symptoms and 35% waited for more than one year. This experience is in agreement with that of many other authors.

Regrettably, there is also a definite doctor's delay in making a correct diagnosis, almost always because of failure to examine the patient at the first consultation (Fig. 8.12). In a series of 440 patients, gynecological examination with biopsy was performed immediately in 72% of the cases. In 12% biopsy was delayed for a few months. It is sad it must be admitted that in as many as 16% of the cases, the doctor's delay was more than six months.

We agree with Way (3) that it is doubtful whether patients with vulvar carcinoma will in the future be educated to the point where their reluctance to seek medical advice can be overcome. However, the message for the doctor is clear: Always examine thoroughly every patient complaining of vulvar disorder, such as soreness and itching. Furthermore, biopsies should be used much more freely to reveal both VuIN and frank invasive carcinoma. Every lump or ulcer in this region should be examined microscopically.

GROIN PALPATION

The value of clinical palpation of the groin is challenged by most authors. It is well known that when examined microscopically, obviously enlarged nodes may be found not to contain cancer and, conversely, that even in very thin patients non-palpable nodes may contain cancer. Therefore it has been suggested that it is better to use a postoperative staging system in which the spread to the lymph nodes is verified by histologic examination (8, 9). In our own institution the value of groin palpation in epidermoid carcinoma of the vulva has been studied in a series of 258 patients with Stage I–III disease which were treated with radical vulvectomy and bilateral groin lymphadenectomy (10). In 99 of these cases pelvic lymphadenectomy was also performed. Metastases to the groin lymph nodes were found in 100 patients (38.8%). In 36 of these, the lymph nodes were not clinically suspicious. This gives a false negative rate of 36%. In 40 out of the 258 cases the groin lymph nodes were suspected to be involved, but this could not be verified by microscopic examination. This gives a false positive rate of 15.5%. It is tempting to conclude that groin palpation is of no value in the preoperative evaluation of patients with epidermoid carcinoma of the vulva. However, a comparison of the group of patients with microscopic metastases ("micrometastases") with the group of patients with palpable suspicious nodes which showed containing cancer ("macrometastases") reflected a significant difference in prognosis between the two groups (Fig. 8.13).

Table 8.2. Correlation between histologic and lymphographic findings in a total of 102 inguinal and pelvic lymph node regions

| Lymphographic findings | Histologic findings | | | |
| | Inguinal region | | Pelvic region | |
	Negative	Positive	Negative	Positive
Negative	35	6	32	1
Uncertain	7	0	9	0
Positive	6	1	5	0
Total	48	7	46	1

The message is that enlarged suspicious lymph nodes may give valuable information about the best treatment method and prognosis. This information is lost if one relies upon a postoperative staging system only. An important prognostic indicator is also the occurrence of fixed and/or ulcerated groin nodes (Stage IV). In such cases it may be of value to give preoperative irradiation with or without chemotherapy (11).

LYMPHOGRAPHY

There are differences of opinion about the value of lymphography in the treatment of vulvar carcinoma. Some authors claim that the accuracy of lymphography is high, while others are less enthusiastic. Fuchs in 1969 (12) surveyed the literature and described his own series. He concluded that the method is of little value where the inguinal nodes are concerned.

Our own experience comprises a series of 27 cases of epidermoid carcinoma and two cases of malignant melanoma in which lymphography was performed preoperatively (13). A modification of the technique described by Kinmoth et al. (14) was used with etiodol as contrast medium. In eight patients etiodol combined with chlorophyll was injected on one side, while etiodol only was used on the other. This was done in order to see if the green staining of the nodes could be of some help to the surgeon during the lymph node dissection. It was also of interest to study the effect of chlorophyll on the quality of the lymphograms.

The correlation between histologic and lymphographic findings in a total of 102 inguinal and pelvic lymph node regions is shown in Table 8.2.

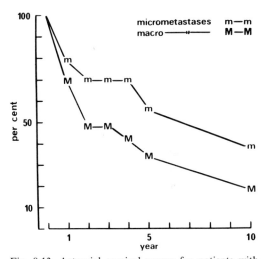

Fig. 8.13. Actuarial survival curves for patients with non-palpable (m) and palpable (M) groin metastases. From (11) and reproduced by courtesy of Academic Press Inc.

It was disappointing to find that lymphography revealed only one of the seven cases with metastases in the inguinal node group. The false positive rate was 6 out of 48 inguinal regions and 5 out of 46 pelvic regions. This false positive rate was due to fibrolipomatous degeneration. In addition, the number of lymphograms labelled "uncertain" in the two regions were 7 and 9 respectively.

Chlorophyll dissolved in contrast medium consistently disclosed considerable retention in the lymphatic vessels. This often lasted for more than one week and made the interpretation of the lymphograms difficult. Extravasation of the contrast medium also occurred. In addition, the surgeon failed to be impressed by the green staining of the nodes. This was particularly true for the groin nodes, both superficial and deep, because dissection in this region is performed en bloc.

It may be concluded that lymphography is of little or no value in revealing lymph node metastases from vulvar carcinoma. The number of false positive and false negative findings are too high. Neither is staining of the lymph nodes with chlorophyll of value.

INDIVIDUALIZED TREATMENT OF STAGE I CARCINOMA

Since Stanley Way in 1948 (15) described the anatomy of lymphatic drainage of the vulva and his radical operation for carcinoma, the majority of surgeons and gynecologists dealing with this relatively rare disease have preferred radical vulvectomy, groin and pelvic lymphadenectomy. There is no doubt that this is a mutilating procedure, es-

pecially in the younger age groups. In later years, therefore, less radical procedures have been suggested by several authors, especially when dealing with small, unilateral tumors. The term "microinvasive carcinoma" of the vulva has been suggested for lesions with stromal infiltration less than 5 mm (16). Our own experience with such small tumors was published in 1981 (17). The aim of this clinical and histopathological study was to determine whether it was safe to treat patients with small vulvar carcinomas on a more individualized basis.

During the years 1956–74, 117 patients with epidermoid carcinoma of the vulva Stage I were referred to the Norwegian Radium Hospital. The histopathological material was reviewed and reclassified into large cell keratinizing, large cell non-keratinizing, and small cell non-keratinizing types. The depth of stromal infiltration was measured from the tumor surface. In cases with infiltration less than 1 mm and with an intact epithelial-stromal border, the infiltration was measured from this. Careful search was made for blood and/or lymph vessel invasion. The edges of the specimens were scrutinized for tumor involvement.

There were 33.5% large cell keratinizing, 19.7% large cell non-keratinizing, and 6.8% small cell non-keratinizing carcinomas. No relationship was found between cell type and recurrence.

The depth of infiltration varied over a large scale from below 1 mm up to 15 mm (Table 8.3). As many as 80 showed an invasion into the underlying stroma of less than 5 mm, and could thus be called microcarcinomas according to Wharton, Gallager and Rutledge (16). No clear-cut relation-

Table 8.3. Carcinoma of the vulva Stage I: Correlation of tumor depth with clinical outcome

Depth of infiltration (mm)	Total No.	Vessel invasion	Recurrence			Deaths of cancer
			Vulva/ vagina	Inguinal	Distant	
0 –0.9	23	–	2	–	–	–
1.0–1.9	12	4	–	2	–	2
2.0–2.9	13	1	–	–	–	–
3.0–4.9	32	7	5	2	1	6
5.0–8.9	28	3	2	3	–	2
9.0–15.0	9	4	3	–	–	–
Total (%)	117 (100)	19 (16.2)	12 (10.3)	7 (6.0)	1 (0.9)	10 (8.5)

ship between depth of infiltration, recurrences and death from cancer was found, except for the fact that lesions with less than 1 mm of invasion showed no vessel invasion and no inguinal metastases.

The significance of vessel invasion in the primary lesion in relation to lymph node metastases is illustrated by the series of 76 patients who underwent radical vulvectomy and lymphadenectomy (Table 8.4). Of 15 women with vessel invasion in the primary lesion 6 had lymph node metastases, while only 2 of the 61 women without demonstrable vessel invasion had such metastases. It is also important that of 8 histologically verified groin metastases, 7 were located on the same side as the primary tumor. Bilateral metastases were only found in one case which showed invasion of tumor cells in lymphatic vessels. Six out of 19 cases with invasion of lymph vessels died from cancer as compared to only 4 out of 98 cases with no invasion.

Pelvic lymphadenectomy was performed in 22 cases, none of which had metastases to the pelvic nodes. In these women the frequency of recurrence was the same as in the women treated with only groin lymphadenectomy. The 5-year crude survival rate was 79% for the total number of patients, 85% for those without vessel invasion, and 52% for those with vessel invasion.

It seems reasonable to recommend that one should always have an excisional biopsy in Stage I carcinoma of the vulva, and the depth of infiltration and evidence of vessel invasion should be checked before deciding upon final therapy. Hemivulvectomy or, in younger patients, even a wide excision may be sufficient treatment when the tumor infiltrates less than 1 mm and if there is no vessel invasion. If the infiltration is deeper than 1 mm, and the tumor is unilateral, hemivul-

vectomy without removal of the clitoris should be combined with ipsilateral inguinal lymphadenectomy. If the tumor is located in the midline and/ or if vessel invasion is found, it is necessary to perform vulvectomy with bilateral inguinal lymphadenectomy. As to the question of the possible entity called microcarcinoma of the vulva, the only subgroup that might be so defined would be tumor with an infiltration depth of less than 1 mm.

TREATMENT OF STAGES II, III AND IV CARCINOMA OF THE VULVA

The use of radical surgical resection of the vulva and its regional lymphatics was proposed as early as 1912 by Basset (18). Taussig in 1940 (19) published an analysis of 155 cases treated by radical vulvectomy and groin dissection. Way in 1948 (16) described the anatomy of the lymphatic drainage of the vulva and its influence on the radical operation for vulvar carcinoma. His vast experience with the treatment of this disease was compiled in a monograph in 1982 (3). Stening, in 1949, visited Way and adopted his method of treatment. Stening's life-long work with vulvar disease is described in his book *Cancer and Related Lesions of the Vulva* (2). For the last twenty years the concept that epidermoid carcinoma of the vulva should be treated by radical vulvectomy and bilateral lymphadenectomy has been accepted by most authorities throughout the world. However, in the last decade there has been growing concern about the necessity for this radical procedure, especially in the early Stage I lesions. Our own attitude to this problem has already been discussed.

Although we agree that surgery should be the main treatment of vulvar carcinoma, radiotherapy may also have its place in selected cases.

In the years 1956–74, 126 Stage II, 155 Stage III and 26 Stage IV lesions were treated (4). In the earlier years of the study period, treatment varied from simple vulvectomy to radical vulvectomy with inguinal and pelvic lymphadenectomy. Some patients were only given external irradiation. Altogether 121 patients did not receive standard treatment. The results were definitely poor, with a total of 62.8% deaths from cancer.

The results of radical surgery with lymph-

Table 8.4. Vessel invasion and lymph node metastases

Status of vessels	Total No.	Lymph node No.	metastases %
Invasion	15	6	40.0
No invasion	61	2	3.3
Total	76	8	10.5

Table 8.5.

Treatment	Total No.	Recurrence Local	Recurrence Inguinal	Recurrence Distant
Radical vulvectomy and bilateral inguinal lymphadenectomy	82	15	4	4
Radical vulvectomy, bilateral inguinal lymphadenectomy and irradiation	26	6	5	3
Radical vulvectomy, inguinal and pelvic lymphadenectomy	72	15	1	8
Radical vulvectomy, inguinal and pelvic lymphadenectomy and irradiation	6	4	1	
Total	186	40	11	15
Per cent	100	21.5	5.9	8.1

adenectomy are illustrated in Table 8.5. Of a total of 186 cases, 108 were treated with radical vulvectomy and bilateral groin dissection; 26 of these also received external irradiation because of metastases. In 78 cases the surgical procedure included pelvic lymphadenectomy, 6 of which also received radiotherapy.

Our greatest problem has been the large number of local recurrences. Altogether 40 patients (21.5%) had a recurrence in the vulvar region. Six out of these 40 patients had tumor infiltration in the resection borders. Of another six patients with involved margins, five died from intercurrent disease during the follow-up period. It is remarkable, however, that as many as 34 patients developed a local recurrence in spite of free margins on the primary operation specimen. This observation is in agreement with the experience of many other authors (19, 20, 21).

Of the 11 patients with inguinal recurrences, only one did not have inguinal lymph node metastases at the time of operation. Fifteen patients (8.1%) developed distant metastases. In Fig. 8.14 the great influence of metastases on the outcome of treatment is illustrated. Here we have included the Stage I lesions treated with radical surgery, but excluded the Stage IV lesions. Altogether 258 patients in Stages I, II and III underwent radical vulvectomy with bilateral lymphadenectomy. In

158 patients no metastases were found, and they had a 5-year survival rate, close to the expected survival rate. In the group with metastases the survival rate was only about 50% of the expected rate.

In seven patients metastases were found in the pelvic lymph nodes, and only one of these survived for more than 5 years.

A total of 72 patients were treated with both groin and pelvic lymphadenectomy, while 82 patients in Stages II, III and IV were operated with radical vulvectomy and bilateral groin lymphadenectomy only. The 5-year corrected survival rates for these two groups were 53% and 59% respectively. It seems justifiable to conclude that we cannot support the theory that additional pelvic lymphnodectomy will increase the survival rate in Stages II, III and IV. Many authors still recommend that pelvic lymphadenectomy should be done in all patients with epidermoid carcinoma of the vulva. Even in cases with pelvic metastases, approximately 20% 5-year survival has been achieved (2, 3).

In our total series of Stages I, II, III and IV lesions treated with radical surgery including bilateral lymphadenectomy, 53 out of 100 patients with metastases had a unilateral tumor. The localization of metastases in these cases was: (1) Only ipsilateral lymph node metastases in 83%, (2) bi-

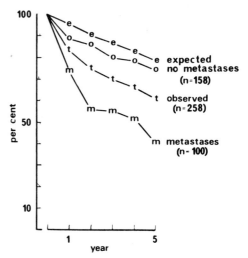

Fig. 8.14. Actuarial survival curves for 258 patients with vulvar carcinoma Stages I–III, respectively, with or without groin metastases. From (7) and reproduced by courtesy of T. Iversen.

lateral lymph node metastases in 15%, (3) only contralateral metastases in 2% (1 patient).

In unilateral tumors, Stages II, III and IV, the risk of bilateral metastases increases with increasing stage. In selected cases of Stage II, the procedure recommended by Morris (23) might possibly be followed. In his opinion, in unilateral vulvar cancer, if the ipsilateral inguinal nodes are negative then the risks from routine contralateral node dissection appear to exceed the benefit.

IRRADIATION AND CHEMOTHERAPY

Our results with radiotherapy of epidermoid carcinoma of the vulva have been poor. Eight out of 15 cases treated with vulvectomy only and irradiation of the groin died from cancer. Out of 38 patients who received irradiation treatment only, 31 died from cancer. It must be admitted, however, that this last group represented a negative selection of patients with large tumors, and not all of these were suitable for radical surgery. Furthermore, it must be emphasized that most of our cases were treated with conventional X-ray therapy, and it is a common observation that the vulvar skin tolerates this type of irradiation poorly. With modern high voltage technique it is easier to give an adequate dose both to the primary tumor and to the regional lymph nodes. The primary tumor can also be treated with high-energy electrons. This type of treatment has become popular especially in some centers in Germany (22). In Sweden, a combination of electrocoagulation and irradiation was the treatment of choice for many years (23). Combined therapy and therapy on a more individualized basis seem to give results equal to that of radical surgery only.

Some promising reports concerning the combination of bleomycin with irradiation in the treatment of head and neck and laryngeal epidermoid carcinomas, prompted us to try this method in patients with inoperable vulvar carcinoma (11). Our treatment schedule in such cases was introduced in 1975 and is shown in Table 8.6. In the 4-year period 1975–78, nine patients with inoperable disease received primary treatment with bleomycin and radiotherapy. Two were treated with vulvectomy and bilateral lymphadenectomy two weeks after combined chemoradiotherapy. It was

Table 8.6. Carcinoma of the vulva. Combined radiotherapy-chemotherapy

1. week:
   1. day – 30 mg bleomycin i.v. + 300 rad
   2. day – 30 mg bleomycin i.v. + 300 rad
   3. day – 30 mg bleomycin i.v. + 300 rad
   4. day – 30 mg bleomycin i.v. + 300 rad
   5. day – 30 mg bleomycin i.v. + 300 rad

2. week: No treatment

3. week: As the first week
   Total dose: $30 \times 6 = 180$ mg bleomycin
   $300 \times 10 = 3000$ rad
   Surgery 4–6 weeks later
   If surgery is not planned:
   Total dose: 220–270 mg bleomycin
   3900–4500 rad

considered that the other patients would not benefit from secondary surgery, and in these cases treatment was mainly given for palliation. In the same period, six patients with recurrences which were not operable were treated similarly.

The overall results in this very poor prognostic group of patients were not spectacular. Seven of the 15 patients, however, demonstrated more than 50% regression of the tumor. In two cases the effect was modest, and in six patients the effect was minimal. Recurrences developed a few months after treatment had been completed in 11 out of the 15 patients. Only one of the two patients who underwent surgery, survived for more than five years.

At present, combined treatment with chemotherapy and radiation can be used for palliation, but radiotherapy alone may give the same results.

COMMENTS

The majority of surgeons and gynecologists dealing with epidermoid carcinoma of the vulva today prefer radical surgery. Radical surgery in this connection means:

1. Removal of the primary tumor with ample free margins, the labia minora and majora and the clitoral region.
2. Removal of a skin flap containing the lymphatic vessels draining the vulva to the groin lymph nodes.
3. Removal of part of the skin covering the groin and the fossa ovalis, the underlying subcutane-

ous tissue with the superficial and deep groin lymph nodes. The operation is made *en bloc*.
4. In addition some surgeons also prefer to remove the pelvic lymph nodes.

There is no doubt that this operation is mutilating, especially in the younger age groups. The immediate postoperative course is frequently complicated with sloughing of the skin, necrosis and infection. The reported percentage of wound breakdown is from 30 to 60%. Debilitating and marked lymphedema has been reported in from 5 to 10%. All patients experience some degree of swelling of the legs. Fortunately, lymphedema is classified as trivial in more than ⅔ of the cases. It is important to remember that lymphedematous limbs may be subject to attacks of streptococcal skin infection. If this infection is not immediately combated with sulfonamide or penicillin, elephantiasis may be the result. It is necessary to start treatment as soon as possible and continue with antibiotics for a long period of time, preferably 2–3 months.

Sexual activity may also be a problem after radical vulvectomy, especially in the younger age groups. The operation leads to the extirpation of the Bartholin's gland and the clitoris. Furthermore, the patients may suffer from contracture of the introital orifice. Nevertheless, Way (3) reports five women who became pregnant after radical surgery. Dahle in 1959 (24) published a similar case from the Norwegian Radium Hospital. Since only about 10% of patients with vulvar carcinoma are premenopausal, the problem of pregnancy following vulvectomy is a very small one. The problem of sexual activity, however, is larger. It must also be remembered that radical surgery in old and often debilitated patients carries with it a certain postoperative mortality rate. During the last decade, therefore, several authors have challenged the view that radical vulvectomy with bilateral lymphadenectomy is the only appropriate way of treating vulvar carcinoma. A more conservative, or at least individualized, therapeutic approach has been recommended. Today there is considerable evidence that before deciding upon the type of therapy, the following factors should be taken into account:

1. The stage of the disease. Lesions classified as Stage I may be much more conservatively treated than Stages II, III or IV disease.
2. The size of the tumor. Especially in Stage II the size of the primary lesion may influence the extent of the surgical intervention.
3. The location of the primary tumor. Epidermoid carcinoma of the vulva follows a predictable pattern of spread directly to the groin nodes, and secondly to the pelvic lymph nodes. Strictly unilateral tumors spread to the ipsilateral regional nodes. Tumors involving or located to the midline, clitoral region or posterior commissure may spread to both groins. There are no direct pathways from either of these regions to the pelvic lymph nodes.
4. Fixed or ulcerated nodes in the groin are a grave prognostic sign. Radiotherapy with or without chemotherapy may be the treatment of choice, either as a preoperative measure or with the aim of giving palliation.
5. Involvement of the urethra/bladder or the anus/rectum must be treated according to the extent of tumor involvement, either by resection of the lower urethra or the rectum, or by exenterative procedure. The place of radiotherapy in such cases must also be discussed.
6. Groin recurrences are only found in patients with clinically suspicious and histologically proven positive groin nodes.

   Postoperative radiotherapy should be considered in such cases. Patients with occult metastases, that is, metastases in non-palpable or unsuspicious nodes, seldom experience groin recurrence.
7. The survival rate after positive pelvic lymphadenectomy has been reported to vary from approximately 10 to 25%. In our own series one out of seven patients with positive pelvic nodes survived five years. Metastases to the pelvic nodes are found only in cases with positive groin nodes. If the medial and/or lateral lacunar nodes do not contain metastases, the deeper pelvic node will usually be unaffected.

When facing the individual case of epidermoid carcinoma of the vulva, these seven factors should be remembered.

9
Malignant melanoma of the vulva

Malignant melanoma of the vulva is a rare disease. Most published series present limited numbers of patients collected over a considerable period of time. Even in large oncologic units it is difficult to obtain adequate experience in handling this disease. Staging and treatment principles are still under discussion. Particularly controversial is the value of groin lymphadenectomy.

In the 19 year period 1956–74, 49 patients were admitted to the Norwegian Radium Hospital with primary malignant melanoma of the vulva. In all but one patient the histological diagnosis was based on excision biopsies. In 1984 a histopathological and clinical study of this series was performed (1).

The tumors were reclassified according to Clark's histological classification of malignant melanoma (2). Furthermore, the maximum tumor thickness was measured with an ocular micrometer according to the method described by Breslow (3). The maximum diameter of the tumor in the histological slides was also recorded. Search was made for blood and lymph vessel invasion.

After the histological revision 11 patients were rejected from the study. Five of these had naevus cell tumor without clear evidence of malignancy. In three cases the malignant melanoma in the vulva represented metastases. In one case a diagnosis of undifferentiated carcinoma was made, and in two cases there was insufficient material for revision. This left 38 patients for further evaluation.

The mean age of the series was 67 years with a range from 42 to 83 years. Only two patients were younger than 50 years. It should be mentioned that the five patients who were revised as compound naevus cell tumors without clear evidence of malignancy, had a significantly lower mean age (30 years). *We are of the opinion that one should be reluctant to accept a diagnosis of malignant*

melanoma of the vulva in a patient younger than 40 years.

From the clinical examination at the time of primary treatment, 31 patients were considered to have localized disease and seven to have inguinal lymph node metastases. In five cases the assumed lymph node metastases were histologically verified.

Of the 38 patients, 8 were treated with local excision, 12 with vulvectomy and 18 with combined vulvectomy and groin lymphadenectomy. In two cases additional radiotherapy was given after surgery, and in one patient radiotherapy was given as the only treatment. The actuarial survival among the total series is shown in Fig. 9.1. Most deaths occurred during the first two years of follow-up. The 5-year survival was close to 40%. Although death from malignant melanoma occurred even after ten years, the risk of fatal outcome after two years is about the same as for the

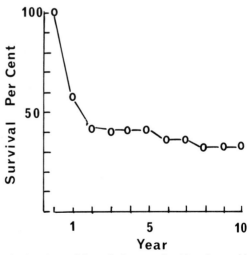

Fig. 9.1. Actuarial survival curves for 38 patients with malignant melanoma of the vulva. Reproduced by courtesy of V. Abeler and T. Iversen.

Table 9.1. Correlation between tumor thickness, vessel invasion and clinical outcome

Tumor thickness in mm	Total no.	Vessel invasion	Recurrence (local and distant)	Death from MM
0–0.9	3	–	1	1
1–2.9	7	1	4	4
3–4.9	5	1	4	3
5–9.9	9	5	5	5
10–14.9	4	3	3	3
15–20.0	8	5	6	6
Total	36*	15	23	22

* The exact tumor thickness and diameter could not be established in two patients, which are therefore here excluded.

Table 9.2. Relation of type of treatment to clinical outcome

Treatment	Total No.	Vulva/vagina	Recurrence Inguinal	Distant	Unknown	Deaths from MM
Local excision	8	2	1	3	2	8
Vulvectomy	12	2	1	3	–	5
Vulvectomy with groin lymphadenectomy	18	2	1	5	3	11
Total	38	6	3	11	5	24

general female population. A total of 27 patients was considered to have melanoma of the so-called superficially spreading type (SSM) and five of nodular type (NM), whereas six remained unclassified (UM). The last two groups had a poorer prognosis than those patients with superficially spreading melanoma. Altogether 15 out of 27 patients with SSM died from their disease as compared to four out of five with NM and five out of six with UM.

Table 9.1 presents the relationship between tumor thickness, vessel invasion and recurrence or death. Of the patients with depth of infiltration less than 5 mm 8/15 died from melanoma compared to 14/21 of those with deeper infiltration. This difference is not statistically significant. It should be pointed out that we also observed one death out of three patients with infiltration less than 1 mm.

Frequency of vessel invasion correlated positively with tumor thickness. A higher rate of death from malignant melanoma was found among patients with vessel invasion than in those without.

No significant correlation was found between tumor size and recurrence or death. Of patients with a largest tumor diameter less than 1 cm, 8/13 died from malignant melanoma compared to 10/15 and 4/8 of those with a tumor diameter of 1–1.9 cm and larger than 2 cm, respectively.

Among 18 patients treated with groin lymphadenectomy, lymph node metastases were found in four, all of whom died from malignant melanoma.

Table 9.2 shows the relation of the type of treatment to the outcome. All eight patients where local excision only was performed, died from malignant melanoma. If vulvectomy was performed, there was a better prognosis. Five out of 12 died from their disease. Additional groin lymphadenectomy did not seem to improve the prognosis as 11 out of 18 died from malignant melanoma. Morrow and DiSaia (4) collected a series of 322 cases from the literature between 1927 and 1974. These authors conclude that the minimum acceptable treatment for vulvar melanoma, irrespective of the lesion size or depth of invasion, is total vulvectomy and bilateral groin lymphadenectomy. Our results do not agree with this. We therefore do not recommend routine prophylactic groin lymphadenectomy. This is in agreement with a WHO study of 553 patients with Stage I melanoma of the limbs. The patients were randomized prospectively to receive elective regional node dissection versus nodal observation (5). No difference in survival between the two groups was noted.

If during the follow-up period there are clinical signs of metastases to the groin, we perform groin lymphadenectomy. A local recurrence is usually treated with re-excision. In inoperable recurrences we prefer to give radiotherapy with high single doses, 10 Gy every second day up to 30 Gy. We have no positive experience with chemotherapy in malignant melanoma of the vulva.

10

Vaginal intraepithelial neoplasia

Vaginal intraepithelial neoplasia (VaIN) is a very rare disease. In our experience it is most frequently found in patients treated for intraepithelial neoplasia of the cervix. It may be detected from one up to 10–30 years after for example conization or hysterectomy for carcinoma in situ of the cervix. A few of these patients will later also develop intraepithelial neoplasia of the vulva (1, 2). A case report of such an occurrence of multiple separate intraepithelial lesions in the lower genital tract of a woman will be described later.

The etiology of VaIN is unknown. There are, however, reports in the literature which seem to indicate that it is a virus induced lesion. We have observed development of VaIN in papillomas of the vagina. Another etiological factor may be previous radiotherapy for cervical carcinoma. Such radiation induced lesions usually occur very late in the follow-up period after the primary treatment for cervical cancer, usually about 10 years or more after radiation therapy, and in some rare cases even after a period of up to 30 years.

In addition, individuals who have or have had vulvar neoplasia have an increased risk of developing a vaginal lesion.

Whenever a woman develops VaIN, a thorough search must be carried out for a recurrent neoplasm of the cervix. In the literature it has also been described that patients on chemotherapy and, especially, immunosuppressive therapy have a relatively high incidence of vaginal intraepithelial lesions (3, 4). We have not seen any such cases.

DIAGNOSIS

Preinvasive disease of the vagina gives no specific symptoms. There may be a complaint of a slight discharge, or more frequently of spotting or postcoital bleeding. By ordinary macroscopic inspection it is easy to overlook these often very small lesions. Usually, suspicion is aroused by a suspect smear after, for example, previous hysterectomy for carcinoma in situ of the cervix. If the intraepithelial neoplastic lesion of the cervix has been treated, either by destructive methods or conization, and no recurrence can be found in the cervix, a thorough colposcopic examination of the whole vagina should be performed. In some cases the lesion is papillomatous and can be seen even on macroscopic inspection. Benign papillomas and also VaIN are often multiple.

The colposcope does not add very much to the diagnosis of benign condylomas and papillomas. Their macroscopic appearance is characteristic. On colposcopy they appear as whitish, distinctly papillomatous excrescenses, irregulary scattered over the vagina and interspersed with normal epithelium. Their vascular pattern is hidden by the very thick hyperplastic squamous epithelium (Fig. 10.1). It should be remembered that condylomas of the vagina should never be treated without histological confirmation that the lesion is benign because in rare cases VaIN may develop from such papillomas.

Granulomatous polyps in the vaginal vault are readily diagnosed by macroscopic inspection and biopsy. Their colposcopic appearance is sometimes disturbing (Fig. 10.2).

The colposcopic patterns of VaIN are characteristic. They have an elevated, frequently papillomatous surface, because of the loose, richly vascularized epithelial connective tissue of the vagina. The proliferation of the vessels is more prominent than in cervical intraepithelial neoplasia. Therefore, an inexperienced colposcopist may suspect the lesion to be microinvasive or invasive. Examples of such patterns are shown in Figs. 10.3 and 10.4.

The ultimate diagnosis is made by histologic examination of a biopsy, and this should prefer-

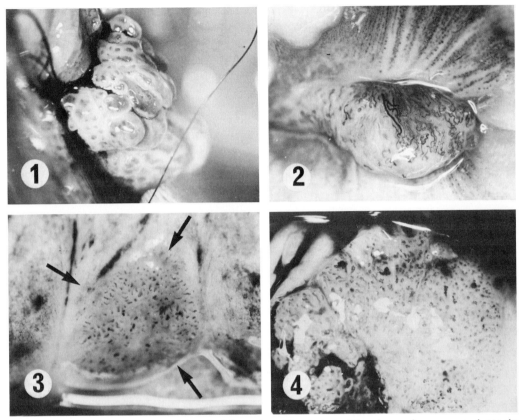

Figs. 10.1–10.4. (10.1) Papilloma (condyloma) of the vagina with a typical white colposcopic appearance due to the thick, acanthotic epithelium and with numerous dilated vessels within stromal papillae. (10.2) Granulation polyp at the vaginal vault after hysterectomy. Note the numerous curled vessels at the surface which explain the intense red color on macroscopic inspection. (10.3) CIN III at the vaginal vault after hysterectomy (arrows). Punctation vessels, dark color tone and slight elevation of the area. (10.4) Papillomatous type of vaginal CIN III.

ably be an excisional biopsy so that the whole lesion is removed and can be examined microscopically.

TREATMENT

In many cases the excisional biopsy is sufficient treatment. If there are multiple lesions and the most atypical of these have been removed, then laser vaporization can be used for those not excised. Laser therapy certainly has a great advantage in VaIN. Neither electrocoagulation nor cryosurgery can give such a precise destruction as the laser beam. The depth of the vaporization can easily be controlled.

DES INDUCED LESIONS OF THE VAGINA

Beginning in the mid-1950s, especially in the United States, DES (diethylstilboestrol) was used to prevent habitual abortion or abortion in other high risk pregnancies. It is now a well known fact that this medication induces vaginal adenosis in a large percentage of females born by mothers receiving DES during the first trimester of the pregnancy (5, 6). This method of trying to prevent habitual abortion never became popular in Scandinavia. At the Norwegian Radium Hospital the author has seen only two such cases during the last 20 years, and both had a benign vaginal adenosis. No single case of clear cell carcinoma of the cervix or vagina which can be related to DES exposure has been reported to the Cancer Registry. Therefore, we have no experience either with the clinical, cytologic or colposcopic diagnosis of such cases, or with the treatment.

MULTIPLE PREINVASIVE LESIONS OF THE LOWER GENITAL TRACT

Case report

E.B.H., born in 1911, was first treated for cervical intraepithelial neoplasia in another hospital by conization in 1966, when 55 years of age. She was followed-up by yearly gynecological examinations including cytologic smears. Six years later, in 1972, the smear became positive, indicating a new preinvasive squamous lesion. She was referred to the Norwegian Radium Hospital and, by colposcopy, a distinct vaginal intraepithelial neoplasia was found. This was excised with free margins. One year later a new lesion developed in the vulva. This was diagnosed as a microinvasive carcinoma. A radical vulvectomy with bilateral groin lymph-adenectomy was performed. One year later a new intraepithelial neoplastic lesion of the vagina was detected and resected. The margins were not free. It was found necessary to perform a total vaginectomy. This included resection of the lower one third of the urethra because of a distinct and separate lesion here, microscopically diagnosed as a microinvasive carcinoma. During the following five years no new lesions were observed in the vulvar region, but she ultimately died in 1979 of liver metastases 13 years after her first treatment for carcinoma in situ of the cervix.

During the last 10 years we have observed five similar cases with multiple squamous lesions of the cervix, the vagina and/or the vulvar region. It is difficult to explain such cases, but it seems that either there are some patients in whom the lower genital tract is predisposed to develop intraepithelial neoplasia, and, ultimately, invasive carcinoma. Another explanation may be that such lesions are caused by a virus that affects the whole lower genital tract.

11
Invasive epidermoid carcinoma of the vagina

STAGING

Stage 0. – Carcinoma in situ, intraepithelial carcinoma, vaginal intraepithelial neoplasia (VaIN). (See previous chapter).

Stage I. – The carcinoma is limited to the vaginal wall.

Stage II. – The carcinoma has involved the subvaginal tissue, but has not extended on to the pelvic wall.

Stage III. – The carcinoma has extended on to the pelvic wall.

Stage IV. – The carcinoma has extended beyond the true pelvis or has involved the mucosa of the bladder or rectum.

EPIDEMIOLOGY

Primary carcinoma of the vagina is a rare tumor. It was described first by Cruveilhier in 1826 (1). Because of the rarity of the tumor the number of cases reported by any single observer has been relatively small. Exact incidence figures were not available in these days. The different institutions related the number of vaginal carcinomas seen to the number of cervical cancer cases treated or to the total number of cancers of the female genital system. During the 10-year period 1971–80, 119 cases of primary vaginal carcinoma were reported to the Norwegian Cancer Registry. In the same period 4,309 cases of invasive cervical carcinoma and altogether 12,839 cases of malignancies of the female genital tract were registered. This means that the ratio between vaginal carcinoma and cervical carcinoma was 1:36 (2.8%) and that vaginal carcinoma comprised 0.9% of all genital carcinomas reported. The incidence rate of vaginal carcinoma in Norway is at present 0.5/100,000. There has been a slight decrease in this rate since the Cancer Registry started to publish their data in 1953. This decrease may, however, be due to a more precise clinical staging over the years. Today, carcinoma of the cervix is seldom falsely allotted to the group of vaginal carcinomas.

Epidermoid carcinoma of the vagina is rarely found in the younger age groups. The majority of the patients are postmenopausal. In two series published from the Norwegian Radium Hospital (2, 3) the mean age was 56 years and 58 years, respectively. The youngest patient was 24 years and the oldest 91 years of age. We have not found that marital status or number of pregnancies is related to vaginal carcinoma. It has been suggested that the disease is more frequently found among patients with vaginal prolapse. In our two series of 145 patients only two women had prolapse, and only one of these used a vaginal pessary.

PATHOLOGY

The most common type of primary malignancy of the vagina is epidermoid carcinoma. During the 20-year period 1956–75, 91 patients were admitted to the Norwegian Radium Hospital for primary therapy for vaginal malignancy (3).

The histopathological classification of the 91 cases is shown in Table 11.1. There were 67 squamous carcinomas, 10 malignant melanomas and 9 adenocarcinomas. The relative numbers of melanomas and adenocarcinomas are higher than in most series reported. In this chapter only the epidermoid carcinomas will be discussed. No grading of these lesions has been performed. A review of the available literature does not indicate that a histologic subclassification will influence treatment methods or results.

Three macroscopic growth patterns have been described: (1) A papillomatous cauliflower exo-

Table 11.1. Histopathological classification of primary vaginal malignancies.

Histology	Number
Squamous carcinoma.	67
Melanoma.	10
Adenocarcinoma.	9
Undifferentiated carcinoma.	2
Leiomyosarcoma.	1
Sarcoma.	1
Sarcoma botryoides.	1
Total	91

phytic tumor, (2) an ulcerating endophytic tumor, and (3) an indurated plaque-like lesion with little involvement of the surface epithelium.

As is the case in carcinoma of the cervix, the exophytic, papillomatous tumors seem to have a better prognosis than the other two categories.

The lymphatic drainage of the vagina has been extensively discussed by Plentl and Friedman (4). They divide the vagina into three parts: Upper third, middle third and lower third. The lymph flow from the upper and middle third is to the lateral pelvic wall and the periaortic region, while the lower third in addition drains to the groin lymph glands. Possibly, however one should rather divide the vagina into an anterior and a posterior part. It is of special interest to note that the posterior wall of the upper and middle third of the vagina more often drains to the same lymph nodes as the rectum and anus, that is, to the perirectal and the deep iliac lymph nodes. The anterior part of the vagina more often drains to the lymph nodes on the lateral pelvic wall. The secondary node groups would be the presacral, common iliac and the periaortic glands. From clinical studies reported in the literature and from our own investigations, there is no doubt that tumors in the lower third of the vagina may also metastasize to the inguinal lymph nodes. We have, however, also seen metastases to the groin from tumors located strictly to the upper third or to the upper and middle third. The reason for this is probably the rich network of lymph vessel anastomoses between all parts of the vagina. In two of our cases located to the upper third, metastases were found during the follow-up period in the supraclavicular region.

DIAGNOSIS

The presenting symptoms in epidermoid carcinoma of the vagina are similar to those of carcinoma of the cervix. In premenopausal patients, intermenstrual bleeding, spotting and postcoital bleeding with or without discharge are the usual complaints. Also in postmenopausal patients bleeding with or without discharge is the reason the patient consults a doctor. In different series bleeding symptoms are found in 50–80% of cases. In our own material, exactly 80% of the women had a history of irregular bleeding.

Discharge is the second most frequent symptom, and may sometimes be very profuse. Pain is a relatively late symptom, most frequently found in the later stages. In the earlier stages the pain is more vague and is described as a discomfort. In patients with an active sexual life, dyspareunia is not rare. When the tumor is located to the anterior wall, urinary symptoms may occur.

There is no reason to review the different statements about the duration of symptoms before diagnosis which have appeared in the literature. Because of the rarity of the disease most publications cover a long period of time and go back 20–40 years. There is no doubt that women today and in the future will be much more alert and will consult a doctor much earlier than described in the published series to date.

A thorough gynecologic examination is usually sufficient to disclose an invasive vaginal carcinoma. There is one point that should be emphasized, however. A lesion located to the posterior wall may be overlooked because the vaginal speculum is often inserted and removed by the doctor in a way that hides the lesion. When a self-retaining bivalved speculum is used, an anterior vaginal lesion may also be overlooked. After inspection of the cervix, it is of utmost importance that the speculum is slowly withdrawn from the vaginal fornix so that the total vaginal mucosa may be visualized.

COLPOSCOPY

When a macroscopic tumor or ulcer is found, it is usually unnecessary to take a cytologic smear or to perform colposcopy. A conchotome biopsy should be taken from the margin and another from the central part of the lesion. When the lesion is small or there is some doubt about its nature, colposcopy will help to pin-point the site of biopsy. It is not always easy to bring the lesion into focus because of tangential vision of the vaginal wall. Otherwise the diagnostic approach as described for the cervix (p. 72) may be applied. Evaluation of the vascular pattern, the surface contour, the color tone of the epithelium and the demarcation against normal tissue serve as guidelines. In Figs. 11.1 and 11.2 the typical colposcopical patterns of invasive epidermoid vaginal carcinoma are shown.

CYTOLOGY

For many years it was considered not necessary to follow-up patients who had been treated for carcinoma in situ or early invasive carcinoma of the cervix with hysterectomy. This is not so today. There is no doubt that these patients are at risk of developing vaginal lesions. A yearly or bi-yearly check with cytologic smears is therefore mandatory. This is in fact the only way to make an early diagnosis of a primary or secondary vaginal carcinoma. In some cases with positive cytology, colposcopy may be negative. The whole vagina should then be stained by iodine. Biopsies should be taken from iodine-negative areas. It should be remembered that early vaginal lesions are some-

times multifocal. Most invasive lesions are readily seen by macroscopic inspection. The dimensions and the location of the lesion should be described. If the lesion is well localized, every attempt should be made to excise it. In this way the histologic patterns of the lesion as well as the extent of stromal invasion can be accurately evaluated.

TREATMENT

Treatment of epidermoid carcinoma of the vagina has always been individualized. Guidelines for therapy are the location and the extent of the tumor. Two follow-up studies of vaginal carcinoma have been published from the Norwegian Radium Hospital. The first series comprised 78 patients treated in the period from the opening of the hospital in 1932 until 1945 (2). The second series was from the 20-year period 1956–75 and comprised 67 patients (3). As in other published reports it is difficult from our own studies to reach a definite conclusion as to the optimal treatment protocol, mainly because of the extreme individualization of treatment. The vast majority were treated with radiation, surgery being performed in only five cases from the first period and four from the last period.

Radiation treatment consisted of intravaginal, intrauterine or radium in needles applied for 4–9 days. Most of the patients in addition received external irradiation, usually to a pelvic field cover-

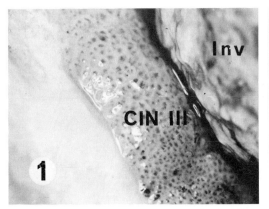 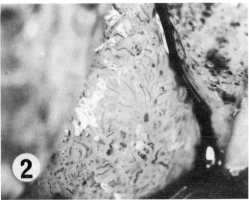

Figs. 11.1 and 11.2. (11.1) CIN III at the border of invasive vaginal carcinoma (Inv). The invasive part is not in focus, but the surface can be seen to be nodular. (11.2) Invasive carcinoma of the vagina with irregular atypical vessels and a papillomatous surface.

Table 11.2. Squamous carcinoma of the vagina, five year survival and stage distribution.

Stage	Number	Five year survivors
I	23	11
II	29	13
III	8	–
IV	7	2
Total	67	26

ing the total length of the vagina and the pelvic lymph nodes. During the first study period, external irradiation was given by 200 kV X-ray machines. From 1957 high-voltage irradiation has been preferred.

Out of the 78 cases treated in the years 1932–45, two patients were treated surgically by extirpation of the tumor prior to irradiation, and a third patient was treated with extirpation of the tumor and groin node dissection on one side prior to irradiation. All three survived for more than five years without signs of recurrence. In two other cases a radical operation was performed with extirpation of the uterus, adnexa and vagina. One of these patients died as early as two months after surgery, from metastases. The other patient lived without recurrence for more than five years after treatment.

Of the 67 patients treated during the years 1956–75, four were treated surgically. Surgical procedures included a partial anterior vaginal resection, two radical hysterectomies with bilateral transperitoneal pelvic lymphadenectomy and posterior exenteration, and one radical hysterectomy with a wide vaginal cuff including the tumor and pelvic lymphadenectomy.

In accordance with other studies it was found that the tumor was most often localized to the posterior vaginal wall. In almost 50% of the cases the posterior wall was involved, while only in approximately 20% was the anterior wall the main site of growth.

Comparing the two series it is obvious that there has been an improvement in the clinical material from the first to the second study period. During the years 1932–45, one out of five cases had clinical metastases to the inguinal nodes or involvement of the rectum or bladder, whilst Stage IV lesions were only found in one out of ten cases in the last study period. It is therefore not surprising that the 5-year survival rate improved from 22.7% to 38.8%. The introduction of high-

Table 11.3. Squamous cell carcinoma of the vagina, relationship between site of metastases and location of primary tumor.

Vaginal segment	Stage	Interval from presentation	Metastatic site
Inner third	I	8 months	supraclavicular*
	I	13 months	vertebral*
	II	16 months	vertebral*
	II	17 months	disseminated*§
	II	41 months	supraclavicular
Middle third	I	4 months	disseminated*§
	II	52 months	hepatic
Outer third	IV	present	pulmonary
	I	14 months	pulmonary
	II	103 months	inguinal, hepatic and vertebral
Middle and outer thirds	IV	present	pulmonary
	IV	present	inguinal
	I	14 months	vertebral*
Inner, middle and outer	IV	present	inguinal

*simultaneous local recurrence
§no more precise documentation

voltage external radiotherapy may possibly have contributed to this improvement. When discussing future treatment protocols it therefore seems appropriate only to give a more detailed report of the treatment and results of the series of 67 patients with squamous cell carcinoma seen in the department during the years 1956–75.

The stage of distribution and the related 5-year survival of these 67 women are shown in Table 11.2. No patient with extension to the bony pelvis or metastases at presentation survived for five years. No statistical difference in survival between Stages I and II was found.

The majority of the patients were treated with combined internal and external radiation. The result for this group was almost exactly the same as for the whole series of 67 cases, with 40% 5-year survivors. It is distressing to see that local recurrence occurred in as many as 55% of the patients treated with irradiation.

Metastatic spread was documented in 14 cases. The details of these are listed briefly in Table 11.3. In four cases metastases were detected at presentation. Inguinal and pulmonary metastases were associated with lesions involving the lower third of the vagina, and supraclavicular metastases were associated with lesions limited to the upper third.

FUTURE TREATMENT PROTOCOL

From the available literature it is obvious that the vast majority of patients with carcinoma of the vagina to date have been treated with a combination of intracavitary, interstitial and external irradiation. A relatively large series of surgically treated cases was presented by Herbst, Green and Ulfelder in 1970 (5). Their results compared well with those of irradiation only. The highest 5-year cure rate reported for all stages combined was 56.3% in a series of 71 patients treated by Prenpree et al. (6). It would appear from their analysis that the main modification of their treatment method appears to be the further extension of radium implantation to the vagina and parametrial regions in patients with involvement in these areas. In the more advanced lesions high dose total pelvic supervoltage irradiation was used with a pelvic wall boost to 50–55 Gy in Stages II and III.

Both the results presented by Herbst, Green and Ulfelder (5) and our own experience seem to indicate that in carefully selected cases excellent results can be achieved by surgery alone or surgery combined with irradiation. The difficulties of achieving optimal results in this disease are easily explained by the anatomical relationship between the vagina and the bladder and the urethra anteriorly and rectum posteriorly. Even if radiotherapy is well established in the management of vaginal carcinoma, recently, the improvement in the outcome of radiation treatment has been followed by a rise in morbidity.

Another important observation in the two series from the Norwegian Radium Hospital, as well as other series, is the predilection for metastases to the groin lymph nodes when the tumor involves the lower third of the vagina. These patients should therefore also receive treatment of these nodes.

Unfortunately we still have to use the expression "individualized treatment" when dealing with carcinoma of the vagina.

12
Carcinoma of the cervix

STAGING

Preinvasive carcinoma

Stage 0. – Carcinoma in situ, cervical intraepithelial neoplasia (CIN III).

Cases of Stage 0 should not be included in any
therapeutic statistics for invasive carcinoma.

Invasive carcinoma

Stage I. – Carcinoma strictly confined to the cervix (extension to the corpus should be disregarded).

Stage Ia. – Microinvasive carcinoma (early stromal invasion).

Stage Ib. – All other cases of Stage I.

Stage II. – The carcinoma extends beyond the
cervix, but has not extended on to the pelvic
wall. The carcinoma involves the vagina, but
not the lower third.

Stage IIa. – No obvious parametrial involvement.

Stage IIb. – Obvious parametrial involvement.

Stage III. – The carcinoma has extended on to
the pelvic wall. On rectal examination there is
no cancer-free space between the tumor and the
pelvic wall.

The tumor involves the lower third of the vagina.

All cases with a hydronephrosis or non-
functioning kidney should be included unless
they are known to be due to another cause.

Stage IIIa. – No extension on to the pelvic wall, but
involvement of the lower third of the vagina.

Stage IIIb. – Extension on to the pelvic wall
and/or hydronephrosis or non-functioning
kidney.

Stage IV. – The carcinoma has extended beyond
the true pelvis or has clinically involved the
mucosa of the bladder or rectum.

Stage IVa. – Spread of the growth to adjacent
organs (rectum or bladder).

Stage IVb. – Spread to distant organs.

Notes to the staging

Stage 0 comprises those cases with full thickness
involvement of the epithelium with atypical cells,
but with no signs of invasion into the stroma. The
term "Cervical Intraepithelial Neoplasia" (CIN)
is today used for the different degrees of dysplasia
and carcinoma in situ. CIN III is identical with
Stage 0.

In earlier years *Stage Ia* carcinoma was simply
defined as a tumor showing early stromal invasion
or a small cancerous tumor of a measureable size.
At the meeting in the Cancer Committee of FIGO
in Berlin September 1985, the following definition
was unanimously agreed upon: Carcinoma of the
cervix Stage Ia (microinvasive carcinoma) is a
histological diagnosis which should be made on
a large biopsy which removes the whole lesion,
preferably a cone biopsy.

Two groups should be recognized:

Stage Ia1 where there is only early stromal invasion in which invasive buds are present either
in continuity with an in situ lesion, or apparently
separated cells not more than one mm from the
nearest surface or crypt basement membrane.

Stage Ia2: Measurable lesions should be measured in two dimensions. The depth should be
measured from the base of the epithelium from
which it develops and should not exceed 5 mm,
and the largest diameter should not exceed 10 mm
on the section that shows the greatest extent.

When reporting Stage Ia lesions, the chosen
depth and diameter for including the cases in the
statistics should be given. Furthermore, the percentage of confluent lesions and cases with involvement of endothelial lined spaces (vessels)
should also be stated.

As a rule it is difficult, clinically, to estimate
whether a cancer of the cervix has extended to the
corpus or not. Extension to the corpus should
therefore be disregarded.

A patient with a growth fixed to the pelvic wall by a short and indurated, but not nodular, parametrium should be allotted to Stage IIb. It is impossible at clinical examination to decide whether a smooth and indurated parametrium is truly cancerous or only inflammatory. Therefore a case should be placed in Stage III only if the parametrium is nodular out on the pelvic wall, or the growth itself extends out on the pelvic well.

The presence of hydronephrosis or non-functioning kidney due to stenosis of the ureter by cancer, permits a case to be allotted to Stage III, even if according to the other findings the case should be allotted to Stage I or Stage II.

The presence of a bullous oedema as such, should not permit a case to be allotted to Stage IV. Ridges and furrows into the bladder wall should be interpreted as signs of submucous involvement of the bladder if they remain fixed to the growth at palposcopy (i.e. examination from the vagina or the rectum during cystoscopy). A cytological finding of malignant cells in washings from the urinary bladder requires further examination and a biopsy from the wall of the bladder.

EPIDEMIOLOGY

The earliest epidemiological study of cancer of the cervix cited in the literature was conducted in the middle of the nineteenth century by Rigoni-Stern (1) at the University of Padua in Italy. He investigated the frequency of marriage in relation to risk of both uterine and breast cancers. On the basis of mortality records he concluded that uterine cancers were found more frequently in married than in unmarried women, that cancer of the uterus was prevalent in women between the ages of 30 and 40, that the frequency of this cancer doubled in the following two age decades and then dropped off, that it was rare among unmarried women, and that it was almost absent in certain orders of nuns. In 1950, one century later, Gagnon (2) in a 20-year follow-up of a fully documented cohort of nuns verified the observation by Rigoni-Stern that carcinoma of the cervix was almost unknown in this cohort. In 1955 Towne (3) confirmed these findings in a study on carcinoma of the cervix in nulliparous and celibate women. At the Norwegian Radium Hospital during a 30-year period, from 1951 to 1980, only two verified cases of squamous cell carcinoma of the cervix were found in virgin females, one of which was a nun. During the same time period 9,673 patients with invasive carcinoma of the cervix were treated.

There is substantial evidence today that carcinoma of the cervix is a sexually transmittable disease. In 1973, Rotkin (4) reviewed all the epidemiological data at hand related to the occurrence of cervical cancer. He found that the following variables are significant in case control studies: First marriage under age 20 or 21, two or more marriages, first coitus before age 20, two or more sexual partners, divorces, separations, and unstable sexual relationships. Some of these factors are interrelated. The correlation with age at sexual initiation is even higher if the division is taken before and after age 17. Some variables, which in the past were suspected as being associated, are not related when a number of studies are considered. Such variables include coital frequency, mean age at menarche, contraceptive practices, and partner not circumcized.

Coppleson and Reid (5) have emphasized that women are at highest risk for initiation of cervical carcinoma during adolescence and after the first pregnancy and delivery. During these two periods of a woman's life the ectocervix is more or less covered by a transformation zone. Columnar epithelium is being transformed to squamous metaplastic epithelium. This is an active process and if a carcinogen is introduced into the vagina at this time, the metaplastic process may become atypical with eventual development of CIN. The use of the colposcope as a research tool has proven beyond doubt that cervical carcinoma always develops within the transformation zone and not from the original squamous epithelium laid down on the cervix during foetal life (6). This fact has now been accepted almost universally. In a monograph from 1966, however, Johannisson, Kolstad and Söderberg (7) have shown that at the periphery of CIN the vascular pattern of dysplasia may develop from pre-existing hairpin capillaries within stromal papillae of the original squamous epithelium.

The virus theory
The accepted concept that squamous cell carcinoma of the cervix is a sexually transmitted disease

has led to a large series of investigations to ascertain if there is one single carcinogen or different carcinogens that can trigger the development of CIN. Over the past two decades there has been an increased effort to evaluate the role of viruses in this respect. The major suspected viral etiological agent for many years was Herpes Simplex Virus Type 2 (HSV-2). An extensive review of the problem of HSV-2 and cervix cancer was published by Rapp and Jenkins in 1981 (8). In particular, sero-epidemiological data have in many studies demonstrated a significantly higher frequency of neutralizing antibodies to HSV-2 in cervical cancer patients than in controls, but, unfortunately, the data are inconsistent. In an unpublished study from the Norwegian Radium Hospital performed in cooperation with Rawls from Canada, we did not find a significantly higher frequency of antibodies in patients with carcinoma in situ or invasive cervical cancer as compared with patients with ovarian cancer or with benign gynecological disease. Our results were comparable to those reported from New Zealand (9).

In recent years female genital infection by Human Papilloma Virus (HPV) and their association with CIN and invasive cervical cancer has come into focus. We have not performed any studies on this question, but from our long experience with colposcopy and colpophotography, it has been found that condyloma acuminatum located to both the vulva and the cervix in some cases can develop into invasive cancer. This is, however, an infrequent occurrence.

Of more interest is the fact that sophisticated studies of the so-called flat or inverted papilloma seem to indicate that these lesions, which initially show a prominent koilocytosis with typical "balloon cells", may in a relatively high percentage be the forerunner of CIN lesions and ultimately invasive squamous cell carcinoma. Today about 35 types of HPV viruses are known; types 16, 18 and 31 in particular, have been connected with cervical cancer. An extensive review of this problem was published in 1984 by Syrjänen (10). It must be emphasized, however, that the ultimate proof is still lacking that HPV viruses are the main carcinogens which induce cervical cancer. Possibly also one or more co-carcinogens must be present, one of which may be HSV-2.

Incidence

Studies of the incidence of carcinoma of the cervix based on the data collected by cancer registries throughout the world show a striking variation in rates. Also within a single country there are variations between different ethnic groups and races. For example, in the United States the El Paso Latin-American females have a higher incidence than the black population. The Caucasian USA females have an incidence which is half that of the aforementioned groups. In Europe, Denmark has always shown a higher incidence of cervical carcinoma than other countries, both on the Continent and in Scandinavia. A low incidence is found in Wales in the United Kingdom and in Ireland. The lowest reported incidence of carcinoma of the cervix comes from Israel and from some Muslim countries.

In interpreting the reported figures one must be constantly aware of differences in reporting practices and the problem of the accurate identification of cancer of the cervix. The histopathologic interpretation of the biopsy specimen is also of great importance. Cases of in situ carcinoma of the cervix may be included in the statistics of some cancer registries. However, there is no doubt that there are great international differences, and it seems difficult to avoid the conclusion that there must be a substantial environmental component which may be operating differently in different countries.

In the Scandinavian countries compulsory notification of all cases of cancer was introduced in the early 1950s. The total number of invasive carcinoma of the cervix reported to the Norwegian Cancer Registry from 1955 to 1983 is shown in Fig. 12.1. With an increase in the population there has been a steady increase in the number of cases detected until 1974. From then on there has been a decrease, probably due to the widespread use of cytological smears for the detection of the precursors of invasive cervical carcinoma. In 1974 altogether 495 new invasive carcinomas were reported, and in 1984 this figure had been reduced to 337 cases, 60 of which were Stage Ia.

If we compare the age-adjusted incidence rate of cervical cancer in the Nordic countries, the decrease seen during the last few years in Norway is not as conspicuous as the decrease in the other

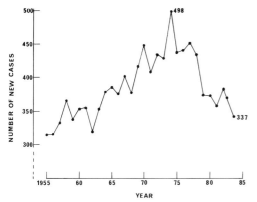

Fig. 12.1. Yearly number of new cases of invasive cervical cancer reported to the Cancer Registry of Norway (1955–84).

tenstiy in each country. In Iceland the screening has been more intense than in the other Nordic countries. It has covered the entire country and has been repeated every 2–3 years. The age coverage has also been wide, from 25 to 70 years. The changes in incidence trends have been greater in Iceland than in the other Nordic countries. Also in Finland and Sweden the mass-screenings cover the whole country. There are differences between administrative districts, but in general the program has covered a shorter age span, and the screening has been repeated at longer intervals than in Iceland. In Denmark about 40% of the female population has been covered by an organized screening program, and the relative changes in incidence are smaller than in Iceland, Finland or Sweden. In Norway there has been an organized program which has covered only one county. However, more and more females have been included either in small screening programs or they have been examined by smears taken by general practitioners, specialists or in out-patient departments of the local hospitals. Shown in Fig. 12.3 is the number of new cases of CIN grade III lesions reported to the Norwegian Cancer Registry throughout the period 1955–80. A gradual increase in the use of cytologic smears from the beginning of the 1960s has led to an increasing number of carcinoma of the cervix Stage 0 being detected and treated. The highest number reported was 937 in 1976. Most probably the decrease in invasive cervical cancer observed from

countries (see Fig. 12.2). Up to 1960 the incidence rate in Iceland, Finland, Norway and Sweden differed very little, while a definitely higher incidence was found in Denmark. From the early 1960s cytological screening started in all countries, and resulted in an increase in incidence rates the following years. After the peaks in the detection of new cases in these years, there has been a steady decrease in all countries (11). These changes should be correlated with the mass-screening in-

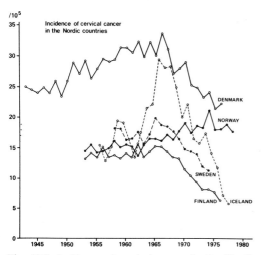

Fig. 12.2. Incidence of cervical cancer in the Nordic countries in the period 1945–78. Screening started at the beginning of the 1960s. From (11) and reproduced by courtesy of the editor (K. Magnus) and Hemisphere Publishing Corporation.

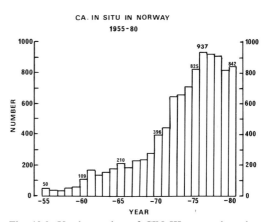

Fig. 12.3. Yearly number of CIN III reported to the Cancer Registry of Norway in the period 1955–80.

1974 onwards (Fig. 12.1) must be due to the relatively large number of CIN detected and treated.
It is now being discussed whether the capacity of
the cytopathological laboratories in the country
should be disposed of in a more rational manner
than to date. It is of special interest to find a
measure whereby those women who have never
had a smear can be persuaded to be included in
the screening program. Those who have had at
least two negative smears can be screened at intervals of 3–5 years. A computerized program for
the whole country has been suggested.

The Norwegian Cancer Registry has also studied geographical variations in cervical cancer incidence in Norway (12). The total annual age-adjusted incidence rate per 100,000 in the different
geographical regions is shown in Fig. 12.4. In all
regions except the northern part of Norway there
is a significantly lower incidence of cervical cancer
in rural, as compared to urban areas. In the northern region the incidence in rural areas is the same
as in urban areas, and markedly higher than that
of rural areas in the other regions. Diagnostic
factors can hardly explain these differences. A
possible explanation is that in the northern region,
it is claimed that the sexual activity of young
females is higher than in the rest of Norway as
judged by the high number of pregnancies in
young women and in non-married women.

In contrast to other types of cancer of the female genital tract, carcinoma of the cervix is a
disease which afflicts relatively young women, a
great proportion of whom are still of childbearing

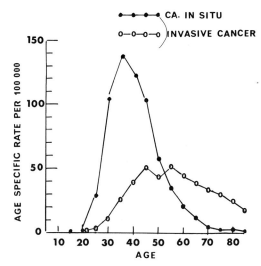

Fig. 12.5. Age specific incidence rates of carcinoma in
situ and invasive cervical cancer in Norway in the period
1972–76.

age. During the 5-year period 1972–76, altogether
2,212 cases of invasive carcinoma of the cervix
were reported to the Norwegian Cancer Registry.
Of these, 943 (42,6%) were premenopausal. The
highest age-specific incidence was found in the
40–55 years age group. The highest age specific
incidence rate for carcinoma of the cervix Stage
0 was found in the 30–34 years age group (Fig.
12.5). Today, approximately one third of all in
situ carcinomas are found in women below 35
years of age.

There is another traditional health statistic
which has been repeated in several series published from the Norwegian Radium Hospital,
namely that the mean age of the patients with
carcinoma of the cervix increases with increasing
stage of the disease (Fig. 12.6). There is a steady
increase in the mean age from about 41 years in
Stage 0 to 59 years in Stage IV. In the series
presented in Fig. 12.6 and also in an earlier series
it was found that the difference in mean age between Stage 0 and Stage Ia was 4–5 years, and
between Stage Ia and Ib also 4–5 years. This
indicates that the time from an in situ lesion becoming clinically invasive carcinoma, is on average, 8–10 years.

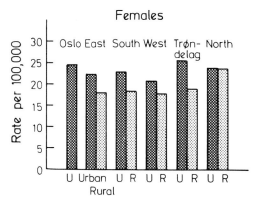

Fig. 12.4. Incidence of cervical cancer in urban and rural
areas in different geographical districts in Norway. From
(12).

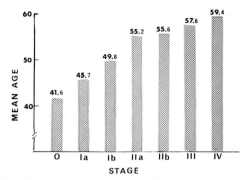

Fig. 12.6. Mean age of women with cervical cancer related to stage of the disease (3474 cases).

Mortality

During the last three decades death rates from cervical cancer have been decreasing in most developed countries. Low mortality rates have always been reported from Israel, Muslim countries, Italy, Ireland and Japan. High mortality rates have been found in developing countries, for example Chile, Venezuela, Puerto Rico and among the black population in the United States.

In Norway there has been a slight, but steady decrease in mortality for carcinoma of the cervix since 1915. This decrease, however, is only found in females below 55 years of age. We have not observed any increase in the mortality of cervical cancer in the later years in the youngest age groups as reported from other countries. The observed steady decrease in mortality cannot be caused by cytological screening alone, but also seems to be due to an earlier diagnosis of the disease and better treatment methods before screening started.

In Finland it is claimed that the decrease in incidence of cervical cancer after the screening started has now been followed by a significant decrease in mortality. This has also been shown in British Columbia where they have had an extensive screening progam since 1949. Experience from the Aberdeen area points in the same direction. It can be stated, therefore, that screening for cervical cancer is one means of reducing mortality from this disease.

DIAGNOSTIC CYTOPATHOLOGY

The method of exfoliative cytology was introduced at the Norwegian Radium Hospital in 1951. Throughout the 1950s the cytopathological laboratory established itself by studying the use of the method, mainly in the detection of female genital cancer, but also in the diagnosis of cancer at other sites, e.g. bronchial carcinoma. As early as 1956 a study of the transtubal spread of corpus cancer was published (13). In 1958 the radiation changes in carcinoma of the cervix as revealed by cytology and their role in determining prognosis were reported (14). In 1959 a mass screening for cervical cancer was started in one of the counties in Norway. It was decided to screen a defined population several times to get information about the value of such screening in detecting preinvasive carcinoma and preventing invasive carcinoma.

The screening program conducted by the Norwegian Cancer Society in Østfold County has had a great impact on the interest in the use of cy-

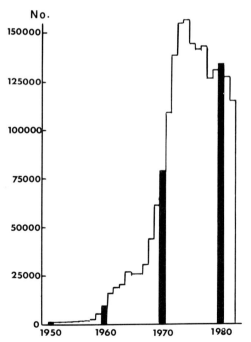

Fig. 12.7. Yearly number of cytologic smears examined at the Cytopathologic Laboratory of the Norwegian Radium Hospital.

tology in the detection of preclinical and invasive carcinoma of the cervix throughout the whole country. This interest is reflected in the work load of the cytopathological laboratory of the hospital. As can be seen in Fig. 12.6, ten years after the initiation of the screening program the number of cytological examinations performed in the Norwegian Radium Hospital had passed 110,000. In 1973 the figure was 160,000.

During the 1960s and 1970s a number of cytopathological laboratories were established throughout the country, and the number of cytologic smears examined in the Norwegian Radium Hospital decreased somewhat to around 120,000 a year. The total number of smears examined in the whole country is at present about half a million.

During the early years Ayre's spatula was always used as a sampling technique. Our experience, however, has shown that this spatula does not always sample enough material from the endocervix. Therefore another spatula was designed (see Fig. 12.8). The endocervical part of this spatula reaches high up into the cervical canal, and a high frequency of endocervical cells will always be found in the smear from this site. Furthermore, this end also covers the whole transformation zone on the cervix. In agreement with experience all over the world we have found a high specificity and sensitivity of this method for detecting preinvasive and invasive carcinoma of the cervix. The false positive rate is extremely low. The false negative rate of one single smear though, has been calculated to be about 20% when taking into account all the factors which are involved in the sampling, fixation, staining and interpretation of each smear. When the technique is therefore used as a routine test in healthy women, we recommend that two smears should be taken with relatively short intervals of about 6–12 months. When these two smears are both negative and there are no

symptoms or signs which are suspicious, the next smear can be taken after 2–3 years; later on the interval between each smear can be extended to 3–5 years. This recommendation takes into account both the cost and also the capacity of medical personnel and the cytopathological laboratories throughout the country.

Fine needle aspiration cytology

This method was introduced in the Gynecology Department in 1965. It is also called fine needle aspiration *biopsy* because the specimen, as a rule, contains sheets of cells when spread out on a slide (Fig. 12.9). The equipment used is that described by Franzén in 1960 (15). The instrumentarium is shown in Fig. 12.10. Aspiration specimens are generally accepted as a valuable tool in the diagnosis of palpable tumors and suspected metastases in many organs. We have used it for the primary diagnosis of pelvic tumors, as well as for the diagnosis of recurrences and metastases, in the pelvis, liver and lymph nodes.

In cervical cancer, aspiration biopsy is used mainly in connection with possible recurrences in the pelvic region, especially on the lateral pelvic wall. Aspiration of tumors on the pelvic wall is usually done through the vagina or, in some cases, also through the rectum. A guiding device is placed on the index finger, and the fine needle inserted directly into the tumor. The needle is placed in several parts of the tumor, and aspiration performed by producing a negative pressure in the syringe. This negative pressure must be released before the needle is withdrawn, otherwise blood is aspirated from the vagina. The vaginal route of aspiration is preferred because the wall of the vagina can be cleaned before insertion of the needle. Puncturing of the tumor via the rectum involves a certain, although minor risk of infection. Cystic tumors should not be punctured via the rectum. Aspiration cytology specimens of ovarian tumors presenting above the symphysis and metastases in the omentum or liver can be obtained through the abdominal wall. Suspect lymph nodes found in the groin, in the supraclavicular region or in the axilla, can also be punctured. In this way unnecessary surgical biopsies of the lymph nodes can be avoided. The risk of

|2cm|

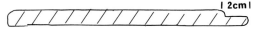

Fig. 12.8. Design of wooden spatula at present being used in the hospital. The tip reaches high up in the endocervix and also covers the transformation zone. The other end is used to take a sample from the vaginal fornix.

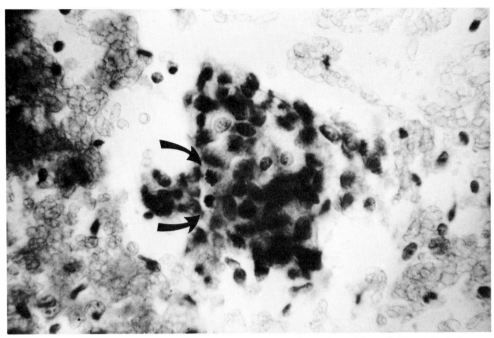

Fig. 12.9. Aspiration cytology specimen obtained from a metastasis on the pelvic wall. Two mitotic figures are clearly seen (arrows).

spread of tumor cells by fine needle aspiration is minimal.

In ovarian tumors it is frequently possible to differentiate between serous, mucinous and endometrioid tumors (16).

False positive aspiration smear diagnoses are extremely rare. A false negative diagnosis is usually due to the needle not entering into representative areas of the tumor.

In conclusion, a cytopathological aspiration smear may be of great help when tumor cells are found. A negative smear must not be accepted as the final truth. The smear should be repeated, or other diagnostic means should be taken into account.

Enzyme studies

The biochemical assay of 6-phosphogluconate dehydrogenase (6-PGD) in vaginal fluid was proposed by Bonham and Gibbs in 1962 as a screening test for the early detection of cervical cancer. The sensitivity and specificity of the test have been questioned by several authors. It was found that more work was needed to assess whether the test

might be useful in mass screening for uterine cancer. Three studies emanated from the Norwegian Radium Hospital between 1967 and 1970 (17, 18). The outcome of these studies was that the large variations in the results with the conditions under which the samples are handled, render measurement of 6-PGD in vaginal fluid an unsuitable method for mass screening of uterine cancer.

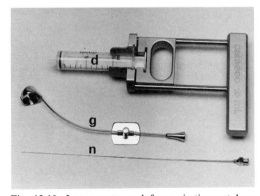

Fig. 12.10. Instruments used for aspiration cytology. Reproduced by courtesy of S. Franzén. d: disposable syringe, g: guiding device, n: long, fine needle.

COLPOSCOPY

In Norway, colposcopy was introduced by Koller in 1953, first as a research method, but later also as an important tool in the diagnosis and treatment of preclinical neoplasia of the lower genital tract. Koller was mainly interested in the vascular pattern of the mucosa of the cervix in benign disease, preinvasive and invasive carcinoma (19). Some years later the method of colpophotography developed by Koller made it possible to study the vascularization and oxygen tension of cancer of the cervix in great detail (20). Also the changes in the vascularization during external irradiation were investigated (21). The colpophotographic method made it possible to have an exact and extremely detailed documentation of the different patterns which can be studied in the cervix, especially concerning the vascular supply and the capillary bed. This resulted, in 1966, in a monograph on the cytologic, vascular and histologic patterns of dysplasia, carcinoma in situ and early invasive carcinoma of the cervix (7). During all these investigations a much clearer understanding of the underlying processes which lead to intraepithelial neoplasia and eventually to invasive carcinoma was achieved. This had a great impact on problems related to terminology and diagnostic criteria. Altogether 15 years of study culminated in 1972 in the publication of an *Atlas of Colposcopy* as a cooperative work between Stafl at the Medical College of Wisconsin in Milwaukee and Kolstad at the Norwegian Radium Hospital (22). Those who are interested in a more detailed and richly illustrated description of colposcopical pictures are referred to this work.

Diagnostic criteria

Through the years, we have used colposcopy as a tool in clinical practice and in research, and have found that an accurate diagnosis of cervical neoplasia can usually be made by reference to the following easily observable features: (1) Vascular pattern, (2) intercapillary distance, (3) surface pattern, (4) color tone and opacity, (5) clarity of demarcation, (6) aceto-white epithelium.

The vascular changes and the color tone cannot be properly examined without a green filter. With ordinary white or yellow light the contrast between the minute terminal vessels and the surrounding tissue is minimal and the picture vague. Evaluation of the arrangement and the distance between the capillaries is best performed by comparing the pathological area with that of the adjacent normal mucous membrane.

In some cases one of the above-mentioned criteria by itself can be sufficient to indicate a correct diagnosis. In other cases it is necessary to combine two or more. The whiteness and the demarcation after application of 3% acetic acid is also of great value.

Colposcopical classification

During the 1970s it became clear that the most important prerequisite for the further propagation of colposcopy was a standardized terminology to be used in textbooks and training courses. Through several international meetings it was agreed that colposcopic terms should not be the same as those used in cytology or histology. At the IIIrd World Congress for Cervical Pathology and Colposcopy in 1978 it was agreed that colposcopical findings could be divided into four groups after evaluation of the above-mentioned diagnostic features:

A. *Normal colposcopical findings*
1. Original squamous epithelium
2. Columnar epithelium
3. Transformation zone
B. *Abnormal colposcopical findings*
1. Atypical transformation zone
   (a) leukoplakia
   (b) aceto-white epithelium
   (c) mosaic
   (d) punctation
   (e) atypical vascular pattern
2. Suspect invasive carcinoma
C. *Indecisive colposcopical findings* (squamo-columnar junction not visible)
D. *Miscellaneous colposcopical findings* (inflammatory changes, atrophic changes, true erosion, condyloma, papilloma, etc.)

In the normal group no significant pathology is expected. In the group with abnormal findings, it is often possible, with experience, to predict the underlying histological picture. The final diagnosis must of course depend upon microscopic examination of biopsy specimens.

BIOPSY METHODS

Before deciding upon a therapeutic modality in preinvasive and invasive carcinoma of the cervix, it is absolutely necessary to have a representative biopsy. It should be remembered, however, that if the histopathological examination of the biopsy specimen differs from that of the cytological or colposcopical interpretation, further histopathological specimens may be necessary. For example, if the histological diagnosis is CIN grades II-III and the cytological and/or colposcopical examination reveals a picture suspicious of early invasive or invasive carcinoma, a new biopsy or a cone specimen may be necessary. One of the greatest advantages of colposcopy is that the areas from which a biopsy must be taken can be accurately identified. The atypical epithelium of CIN lesions are more easily loosened from the connective tissue than in normal squamous epithelium. Trauma of a relatively moderate degree, such as rubbing or squeezing by forceps or conchotomes, produces much greater damage than it does on normal epithelium. Carefully excised, well-preserved and rapidly fixed material will give the pathologist the best opportunity to make a correct diagnosis. Poor or delayed fixation of the biopsy leads to poor staining of both nuclei and cytoplasm and hence makes it difficult for the pathologist to give an opinion.

There are four main techniques commonly used for obtaining specimens from the cervix for histopathological examination: (1) punch biopsy, (2) excision biopsy, (3) curettage, (4) conization.

Punch biopsy
There are two biopsy punch instruments which we have found are useful in colposcopically directed biopsies from the cervix (Fig. 12.11). The Tischler biopsy punch has strong and sharp jaws, and does not easily slip off the relatively hard fibrous tissue of the cervix. The specimens are easy to orientate, but there are many clinicians who are of the opinion that the specimens taken are rather too large and may lead to difficulties with bleeding. This can easily be prevented by a vaginal pack. The ·

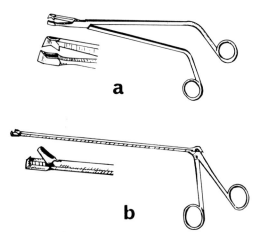

Fig. 12.11. a: Tischler conchotome, b: Kevorkian conchotome.

Kevorkian biopsy punch is also sharp, but the specimens taken with the jaw are so small that the pathologist may have difficulty in orienting the tissue in the paraffin block. For easy orientation of excised tissue for the pathology, the biopsy can be placed with the epithelium side up, on a small piece of marslene mesh or filter paper and placed in fixative. The tissue remains attached to the mesh plate in the fixative solution.

Excision biopsy
This type of biopsy is not often used on the cervix, except when a relatively large specimen is wanted. The specimen is excised with a scalpel and an effort is made to extend the excision into healthy tissue. As a rule it may be necessary to control bleeding by one or two sutures.

Curettage, endocervical and fractional
Endocervical curettage (ECC) has been criticized by many authors. It is claimed that if an endocervical curettage is necessary, it will, as a rule, in the next instant be necessary to perform a conization. We have found that ECC is indicated in all cases where cytology arouses suspicion of preinvasive or invasive carcinoma, and the colposcopical findings are indecisive. Several authors also recommend ECC in all patients for whom destructive methods of treatment of CIN are planned (electrocautery, cryosurgery, laser), even in cases where the squamocolumnar junction is fully vis-

ible. ECC provides histological documentation that the endocervix is free of disease prior to such destructive treatment. The very rare occurrence of a concomitant endocervical adenocarcinoma or adenosquamous carcinoma should not be forgotten.

To obtain adequate samples of tissue from the cervical canal it is of great importance that the instrument used is sharp and of proper size. We have obtained good results with the instruments shown in Fig. 12.12. The Novak curette is used when the cervical canal is relatively open, while the Kevorkian curette is used in cases with a narrow cervical canal. ECC can be performed without anesthesia, but many patients complain of cramp-like pain during the procedure.

The tissue sample from ECC is fragmented and therefore, in most cases, it is not possible to establish a definite histologic diagnosis. Because of the lack of orientation and, often, absence of cervical stroma, the histological findings can be divided into three groups:

1. *Negative* – Fragments of normal squamous and/or columnar epithelium are present. These patients should be followed-up cytologically. If cytology maintains a suspicion, conization should be performed if atypical squamous cells are found, and fractional curettage performed if there are atypical columnar cells.
2. *Suspicious* – Fragments of pathologic tissue are present. From these fragments it is not possible to differentiate between dysplasia, carcinoma in situ or microinvasive cancer and, therefore, diagnostic conization is indicated.
3. *Frank invasive cancer* – In the cases of frank endocervical cancer the suspicion of cancer is

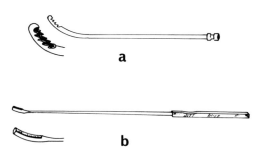

Fig. 12.12. a: Novak curette, b: Kevorkian curette.

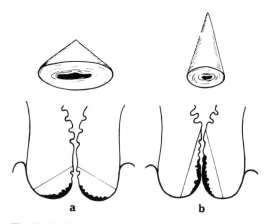

Fig. 12.13. Conization specimen adapted after the extent of the lesion on the ectocervix and the endocervix.

already obvious during clinical evaluation of the endocervical curettings. Usually, big pieces of tissue are obtained, often from an obvious crater, and in the histological preparation there is enough stroma to make a definite diagnosis of frank invasive cancer.

Diagnostic conization in such cases can thus be avoided. Cutting through the cancer will be against the principles of cancer therapy, and, also, after conization it may be necessary to delay either radical surgery or intracavitary radium treatment.

The value of fractional curettage has also been questioned by many authors. There should be no disagreement that fractional curettage is essential when cytology shows atypical adenomatous cells. It is also necessary in the pretreatment staging of endometrial carcinoma.

Conization

Only 10–15 years ago, in many parts of the medical world, the sequence of detection and treatment of CIN was as follows: cytology, conization, and hysterectomy. In some institutions random biopsies or biopsies after painting with Schiller's fluid were taken after suspicious cytology, followed by conization and hysterectomy. Cone biopsy was thus a diagnostic procedure. Today diagnostic conization is indicated only if: (1) the squamocolumnar junction cannot be visualized by colposcopy and invasive carcinoma has been ruled out by endocervical curettage, and (2) if the colposcopical picture is considered to be benign, biopsies and endocervical curettage are negative, but atypical squamous cells are repeatedly found in cytological smears, and (3) if there is cytologic, colposcopic or histologic suspicion of microinvasive cancer.

If the extent of the lesion on the ectocervix and in the endocervix can be seen, then this determines the size and length of the cone. In this way conization will be therapeutic. After careful evaluation of the localization and size of the lesion by colposcopy, it is wise to paint with Lugol's solution at the time of surgery to ensure that the incision on the vaginal portio can be made well outside the atypical area and the border of the transformation zone. Different techniques of conization are used in different institutions. Diathermy conization should be avoided because of difficulties with the histopathological interpretation of the specimen, especially as to the question whether the margins are free. Until the last five years, most surgeons preferred dissection of the cone specimen with a scalpel. The raw surface of the cervix can either be covered with Sturmdorf sutures or be left open. If it is left open, an injection in the wound with Vasopressin or local anesthesia containing adrenalin together with a pack in the vagina will prevent heavy bleeding. The most sophisticated, but also most expensive way of conization is by laser technique. There is no doubt that this technique is to be preferred if the institution has such an instrument. It can be performed on an outpatient basis. In many clinics conization with a scalpel will still be the main procedure in the years to come because of the cost of the laser. With proper technique and aftercare the reported frequency of serious complications is small, the total number being between 5 and 10%. It should be remembered, however, that large cones carry a risk of cervical incompetence and premature birth. This risk can be minimized by colposcopic determination of the necessary size of the cone.

13
Cervical intraepithelial neoplasia

TERMINOLOGY

A miscellany of terms have been used throughout the years to describe what the histologist considers may be the precursor of invasive squamous cell carcinoma of the cervix. The first description of such a lesion is probably that of Williams in 1886 (1). He called it cancerous squamous epithelium. Rubin in 1910 called it incipient carcinoma (2), and Reagan and Hamonic in 1956 introduced the term dysplasia (3) (dys = altered, plasia = development). In 1961 an international committee on histological terminology for lesions of the uterus and cervix (4) agreed upon the following definitions:

Carcinoma in situ. Only those cases should be classified as carcinoma in situ which, in the absence of invasion, show a surface lining epithelium in which, throughout its whole thickness, no differentiation takes place. The process may involve the lining of cervical glands without thereby creating a new group.

Dysplasia. All other disturbances of the squamous epithelial lining of the surface and glands should be classified as dysplasia. These may be characterized as of high or low degree, terms which are preferable to suspicious or non-suspicious, as the proposed terms describe the histological appearance and do not express an opinion.

In 1967 Richart (5) proposed his new nomenclature calling all disturbances of the squamous epithelial lining "Cervical Intraepithelial Neoplasia" (CIN). CIN I and II correspond to mild and moderate dysplasia, and CIN III corresponds to severe dysplasia and carcinoma in situ. This new nomenclature has become more and more popular through the years. The reason is the considerable evidence today that CIN I, II and III in many cases represent a continuum that ultimately may develop into invasive carcinoma. It is also of importance to remember that the lesser degrees of atypicality,

CIN I and II, may sometimes precede invasive carcinoma without passing through a detectable CIN III stage. Thus, lesions designated as mild and moderate dysplasia or CIN I and II are also significant lesions and the patients must be kept under surveillance. If the concept of CIN being a continuum is accepted, then to prevent the development of invasive cancer, it seems logical to treat not only CIN III, but also CIN I and II (Table 13.1).

Table 13.1. Pre-clinical cervical neoplasia

Dysplasia	Mild Moderate Severe	Cervical Intraepithelial *C.I.N. I–III* Neoplasia
Carcinoma in situ		

Ca. in situ = C.I.N. III = Ca. cervix St. 0

Early stromal invasion Microcarcinoma (< 5 × 10 mm)	Ca. cervix St. Ia

EPIDEMIOLOGY

Since 1952 carcinoma in situ has been a reportable disease in Norway. The lesser degrees of abnormalities, i.e. mild and moderate dysplasia (CIN I and II), have not been included in this registration system. We therefore only have exact data on the CIN III lesions.

As a result of the country-wide use of the smear technique, the incidence of reported women with carcinoma in situ has increased from approximately 50 per year in the 1950s up to approximately 900 a year in the late 1970s (Fig. 12.3, p. 67). The average age of the cases being detected is now 41.7 years. The age distribution of the preinvasive lesions compared to those with invasive lesions is shown in Fig. 12.5 (p. 68). Since smears are taken in younger and younger age groups, the average age in the near future will most probably be between 30 and 35 years.

The material of lesions of lesser grades, such as CIN I and II, in our hospital shows a tendency to be present in still younger age groups than CIN III.

SYMPTOMS AND SIGNS

It is a commonly held view that patients with carcinoma in situ have no symptoms. This is not true. On closer examination of a series of carcinoma of the cervix Stage 0 reported from the Norwegian Radium Hospital in 1966, as many as 41.7% of 422 cases complained of discharge and spotting or bleeding symptoms (6). Today, when most cases are detected by routine cytology, the frequency of such symptoms is much less. Postcoital bleeding is found in only a few percent.

It is also claimed that preinvasive lesions are characteristically free of any signs when examined by the naked eye. Again we cannot agree with this statement. In the same series of 422 cases detected before 1966, 60% showed a red patch (erythroplakia) on the ectocervix, and the examiner recorded as many as 16.5% having a so-called suspect erosion. In 4.5% a true leukoplakia was found. Once more it must be emphasized that this series was collected in the years before cytologic smears became a routine examination technique in the country.

CYTOLOGY

The technique used to obtain adequate cellular samples from the endo- and ectocervix has been described previously. There is no doubt that to detect CIN, smears should be taken even in women in the younger age groups, 20–29 years. In other countries teenagers are also included in cytologic screening programs. The yield in teenagers is low, however, and the question of cost-benefit arises.

COLPOSCOPY

When a suspect or positive smear is reported, it is mandatory that the lesion should be examined by colposcopy (7). Also in the evaluation of patients with erythroplakia or leukoplakia the colposcope is an invaluable tool. Thirty years of experience with this method have convinced us that the colposcope should occupy a central position in the evaluation and management of CIN. As a matter of fact, now we find it impossible to handle such cases without a proper colposcopic examination. We prefer a binocular colposcope with a magnification of $\times 16$ which provides a transition from macroscopic to microscopic vision. Use of the green filter is necessary for evaluation of the vascular changes (8).

The typical colposcopical appearances of the different degrees of epithelial abnormalities in preclinical neoplasia of the cervix are shown in Fig. 13.1–4. In many cases it is also possible to differentiate between the lesser degrees of CIN and CIN III.

When the lesion has been colposcopically identified as to the site, size and extent, directed biopsies should be taken from the most atypical part of the lesion. An expert colposcopist may take only one biopsy, but usually it is advisable to take two or more and also to perform an endocervical curettage even if it seems as if the cervical canal is free of CIN. After such a thorough diagnostic approach, it is possible to decide upon the proper treatment.

Colposcopy has of course its weaknesses, as have both cytopathology and histopathology. An experienced colposcopist will usually be able to make a correct diagnosis in 80–90% of the cases. It is especially in postmenopausal women, where the lesion is hiding high up in the endocervix, that the colposcopic picture must be registered as inconclusive.

DIAGNOSTIC CONIZATION

With the advent of colposcopy, the frequency of purely diagnostic cone biopsies has been markedly reduced. It has been limited mostly to the following cases:

1. Lesions extending into the canal outside the range of the colposcope.
2. Abnormal findings discovered on endocervical curettage.
3. Minimal, questionable or microinvasion suspected on colposcopically directed biopsy. The cone is made to rule out deeper invasion.

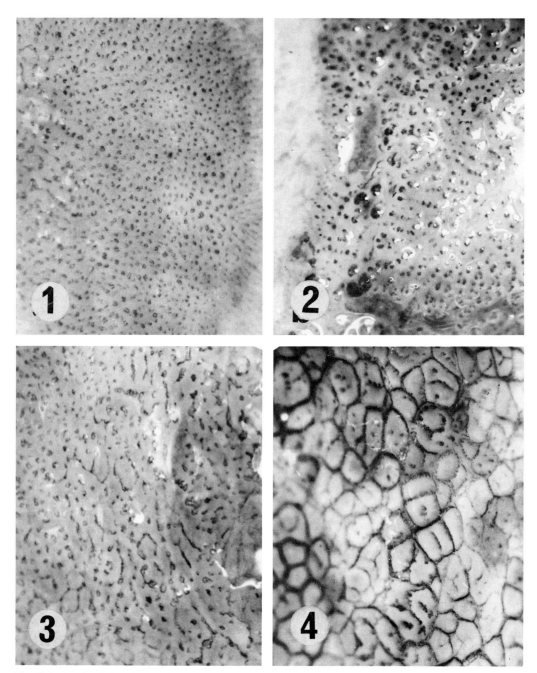

Fig. 13.1–13.4. (13.1) Regular and fine punctation pattern in CIN I–II. (13.2) Coarse and more irregular punctation in CIN III. (13.3) Punctation and mosaic pattern in CIN II. (13.4) Coarse mosaic with increased intercapillary distance in CIN III.

4. Repeated abnormal smears suggesting a significant lesion in the absence of a colposcopic lesion. If columnar epithelium occurs concentrically in the lower canal, the smear result is open to question and should be re-examined, and/or repeated.
5. Lesions where the smear indicates a greater likelihood of invasive disease than is indicated by the colposcopic findings, colposcopically directed biopsies and endocervical curettings.

In some instances a focal lesion may be so large that even multiple biopsies cannot assure a complete histologic diagnosis. In such cases, a cone biopsy may also be indicated.

TREATMENT

In the mid-1950s the colposcope came into use in the preoperative evaluation of carcinoma in situ, and the result was that treatment shifted from radical procedures towards conization, both as a diagnostic and therapeutic procedure. While conization in the first 5-year period (1950–54) was considered sufficient therapy in only 4.5% of the cases, in 1965–68 the same figure was 71.5% (7).

Today even conization is considered too radical, especially in young women. Therapeutic modalities such as cryosurgery, laser evaporation and laser conization are methods which are now used.

Destructive methods
Diathermy

This has been used infrequently in our hospital to treat small focal lesions of CIN I–II. It has never become popular as an outpatient procedure, however, because if sufficient depth of coagulation is to be obtained, the method is followed by considerable pain. We have never used the electrocoagulation diathermy therapy as recommended by Hollyock and Chanen (9). In their hands this method has given excellent results. It is necessary to perform electrocoagulation diathermy under anesthesia, which means that the patient must be hospitalized. The criteria for selection of patients for this therapy is the presence of a histologically confirmed CIN lesion, irrespective of the purported severity of the disease, where the anatomical extent of the atypical transformation zone is

in colposcopic range thereby facilitating exclusion of true invasive disease (10).

Cryosurgery

In the late 1960s and the beginning of the 1970s cryosurgery was introduced as a method of treating CIN in the United States (11). There are several reasons why this method has become so popular. With the increasing use of cytology in the last three decades, an increasing number of patients with CIN have been detected. Furthermore, the disease has also been shown to be relatively common in young women in the fertile years, often before their first pregnancy. Under such circumstances even conization will be a relatively radical procedure. There is always a risk of cervical insufficiency. The patients must be hospitalized, and even in the best hands a certain percentage of complications will be found after conization. The time needed, the cost and the complication rate have influenced the search for more conservative procedures like cryosurgery. Numerous reports in the literature have shown that with adequate pretreatment assessment of the patient, there is a success rate of cryosurgery which is close to 90% after a single treatment session.

At the Norwegian Radium Hospital we have used cryosurgery since 1973, first in a few selected cases of CIN I and II, but later also in cases of CIN III. We have found that the method is easy to apply. It is almost painless, and the complication rate is nil. Before treating a CIN lesion with cryosurgery we follow the same rules as have repeatedly been emphasized by experts in other countries (12). Cryosurgery can be used in all grades of CIN. It is not so much the grade of the lesion as the site and extent of it that must be assessed before the cryosurgical probe is applied. The method is of particular value in the treatment of young women, but the following prerequisites should be present:

1. The patient must be seen and assessed by a skilled colposcopist.
2. The entire lesion must be seen through the colposcope.
3. Invasive carcinoma must be excluded by biopsy or biopsies including endocervical curettage.

4. The skilled colposcopist must himself perform the treatment.
5. There must be adequate cytologic and colposcopic follow-up.

Once the gynecologist has treated a patient by cryosurgery, he has both a moral and ethical responsibility to ensure adequate and life-long follow-up. Many studies have shown that further disease can occur up to 20 years later, even if treated by a cone biopsy or hysterectomy. Such late "recurrences" are probably new virus-induced lesions developing in some high-risk patients.

Cryosurgery can be applied both two and three times, but in some cases it is necessary to perform cone biopsy to get rid of the total lesion, especially if it extends down into deep crypts. Lesions extending up into the endocervix should not be treated by cryosurgery even with probes especially designed for this type of treatment. Only focal lesions located to the ectocervix are, after careful colposcopic and histopathologic assessment, included in the cryosurgery series.

By this careful selection of patients for cryosurgery we have not seen a single case returning with invasive carcinoma. In the last five years, however, several such cases have been referred to us from other hospitals in the country. A careful evaluation of the clinical history and diagnostic methods used in these cases has shown that cryosurgery in all of them was applied without adequate pretreatment assessment. The follow-up cannot be claimed to have been adequate either. The time period between the cryosurgical treatment and the diagnosis of invasive cancer varied from 4 to 23 months.

The experience reported here is in agreement with similar reports from the United states. It is necessary to keep strict criteria for the selection of patients for this type of destructive treatment as well as for diathermy, electrocoagulation or laser treatment.

"Cold" coagulation

The use of the so-called cold coagulator designed by Semm has become increasingly popular in the United Kingdom (13). The criteria for selecting patients for this type of treatment are identical with those described above.

Laser treatment

Our experience with laser evaporation is relatively little. We have used it in some small ectocervical lesions and especially in cases with involvement of the vagina as well as primary vaginal neoplasia and condylomatous lesions of the vulvar region. In recent years, however, the laser equipment has been used for an outpatient conization in selected cases. Microsurgical conization of the cervix by carbon-dioxide laser was reported as early as 1979 by Dorsey and Diggs (14). The largest material from Scandinavia was published in 1983 (15). The author of this report claims that laser conization is an easy procedure to perform, and that it can be applied in almost all cases of CIN which in earlier years would have been treated by sharp knife conization. The complication rate is small and comprises mainly a few per cent with bleeding problems.

Cold knife conization

Also when deciding upon this therapeutic modality, it is absolutely necessary to have adequate cytologic, colposcopic and histologic assessment of the lesion. In addition, one must take into account the age of the patient, her wish for future pregnancies and other concurrent elements or gynecological symptoms. During colposcopy of fertile women, using a self-retaining speculum, it is possible to visualize at least 1.5 to 2 cm of the endocervical canal. By adapting the cone specimen according to the site and the extent of the lesion (as determined by colposcopy with a self-retaining speculum, punch biopsies, and, if indicated, endocervical curettage), it is possible in the majority of cases to eradicate the whole lesion.

It is possibly still too early to tell whether treatment by cold, heat or laser destruction is as safe as conization. In our own study of 1121 cases of carcinoma in situ followed for 5–25 years (Table 13.2) 795 were treated with conization and 238 with hysterectomy (16). In the conization group 2.4% of recurrent or new in situ lesions were found, and 0.9% developed invasive carcinoma. The corresponding figures for the hysterectomy group were 1.2% in situ recurrences and 2.1% invasive carcinomas, respectively. The most important observation in this large series in which a 100% long-term follow-up was achieved, was that the recurrences, especially of invasive carcinoma, often oc-

Table 13.2.

Treatment method	Total no. treated	Recurrent carcinoma in situ		Recurrent invasive carcinoma	
		No.	%	No.	%
Observation	8	0	0	2	25.0
Conization	795	19	2.4	7	0.9
Hysterectomy	238	3	1.2	5	2.1
Radium	55	0	0	1	1.8
Surgery + radiation	25	0	0	0	0
Total	1,121	22	2.0	15	1.3

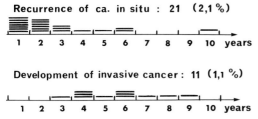

Recurrence of ca. in situ : 21 (2,1 %)

Development of invasive cancer : 11 (1,1 %)

Fig. 13.5. Observed recurrences in 998 cases of carcinoma in situ. From (16).

curred much later than five years after treatment (Fig. 13.5). It is therefore doubtful if the series published to date of CIN treated by heat, cold or laser are valid. First, the follow-up time is too short, secondly, few series are able to present more than approximately 70–80% of follow-up. An exception is the series of Chanen (10). He presented excellent long-term results treating dysplasia and carcinoma in situ with electrocoagulation diathermy. Richart et al. (12), in a multicenter study with cryosurgery, reported only 0.5% of recurrences in 2,839 cases. However, the drop out rate in follow-up was substantial, up to 80%. The author completely agrees with the conclusion:

The widespread application of these modalities (destructive methods) must be accompanied by a high degree of competence on the part of the clinician, a high level of understanding and skill on the part of the histologist and cytologist, and a rigorous method to ensure follow-up among those patients who are treated. If these criteria are not met, the morbidity and the mortality of the technique may outpace its utility.

Hysterectomy

Colposcopic assessment of CIN has demonstrated that hysterectomy with a wide vaginal cuff is rarely indicated. Several studies have shown an extension of CIN to the vagina in only 4–5% of the cases (6), and such extension is easily revealed by colposcopy or by painting with iodine solution. Our attitude is that hysterectomy is only indicated if there are additional reasons for this type of surgery, e.g. irregular or heavy bleedings, myomas or ovarian tumor. Hysterectomy may also be performed if the upper margin of the cone is not free. It is, however, possible to do a reconization in such cases. If hysterectomy is performed in a case with extension to the fornices, it is wise to paint the cervix and vagina with Lugol's solution and make the incision well outside the iodine negative area. Vaginal hysterectomy is to be preferred in such cases, but if abdominal hysterectomy is performed, one should even then start with the incision in the vagina. In some countries, hysterectomy is also preferred if the patient has many children and there is a clear wish for sterilization.

Radium irradiation

Although we recommend conservative measures in the treatment of the vast majority of the CIN lesions, there is a very small group of patients which in our series has been treated by radium irradiation, namely old women with either contraindications against every type of surgery, even conization, or those with a narrow vagina and a lesion high up in the endocervix, where cold knife conization will be very difficult. This last group of women may possibly today be treated with laser conization.

That CIN III is radiosensitive has been demonstrated by Bergsjø and Evans in a material from our hospital (17). By colpophotography and histologic examination of serial biopsies they found that both the colposcopic and histologic picture of carcinoma in situ disappeared during external high voltage irradiation. It should be stressed, however, that even in CIN lesions a full dose of irradiation should be given, otherwise recurrence may occur.

14
Microinvasive carcinoma of the cervix Stage Ia

In 1947 Mestwerdt (1) was the first to draw attention to a group of small carcinomas of the cervix which could only be classified by careful microscopic examination. Arbitrarily he suggested that if a lesion invaded into the stroma less than 5 mm, the case should be classified as "microcarcinoma". In 1951 (2) he reported on his experience with such lesions and recommended that they could safely be treated by less radical procedures compared to lesions of larger extent. Since that time, a heated discussion has been going on concerning the definition of such early carcinomas.

At a meeting in the Royal College of Obstetricians and Gynecologists in 1981 (3) an agreement was reached on a definition which takes into account both the depth and the horizontal spread of the lesion. This definition in September 1985 was adopted by the FIGO Cancer Committee (p. 64).

At the Norwegian Radium Hospital the depth of infiltration has always been taken into account when allotting a case to Stage Ia, and the limit for this infiltration has been set at 5 mm. Our experience with such cases has been published in 1969, 1979, 1982 and 1984 (4, 5, 6, 7).

EPIDEMIOLOGY

Carcinoma of the cervix Stage Ia is not reported to the Norwegian Cancer Registry as a separate group. It is therefore impossible to give any valid incidence rates of this lesion over the years. The material from the Norwegian Radium Hospital, however, clearly shows that microcarcinoma has become much more prevalent during the last two decades, certainly after the advent of exfoliative cytology. Fig. 14.1 shows the yearly number of new cases treated in the hospital during the years 1951–80. From 1960 on there was a constant and marked increase in the number of cases until a

peak of 82 cases was treated in 1978. The reduction in referral seen after this time is most probably due to the fact that such early cases are now also being treated in many other hospitals in the country, especially the three new regional hospitals.

The age distribution of Stage Ia carcinoma of the cervix peaks between 45 and 46 years, but the range extends from about 20 years to senescence. Microinvasive adenocarcinomas are detected at a later age than the squamous microcarcinomas.

DIAGNOSIS

The diagnosis of microinvasive carcinoma closely parallels the diagnosis of CIN. Cytology, colposcopy and histopathological examination of a cone biopsy form the triad on which the diagnosis should be made.

SYMPTOMS AND SIGNS

In our first series of Stage Ia lesions being studied (4), about two thirds of the patients had symptoms which could be classified as suspicious, such as discharge with spotting, metrorrhagia or contact bleeding. The relatively high frequency of such symptoms in this series as compared to other reports is undoubtedly due to the fact that the patients were not drawn by routine cytological check-ups or via mass screening programs.

The cervix looked entirely normal in 18.3% of the cases. A clinical diagnosis of "cervicitis" or cervical polyps was made in 7.9% and an innocent looking erosion was found in 34.8%. This means that macroscopic inspection of the cervix aroused suspicion of cancer in only 39% of the 164 early invasive squamous cell lesions.

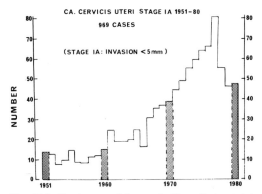

Fig. 14.1. Carcinoma of the cervix Stage Ia treated in the Norwegian Radium Hospital in the period 1951–80. See text.

Table 14.1. Cytologic findings in 375 patients with Stage Ia cervical carcinoma.

	Negative	CIN I–II	CIN III	Inv. Ca.
No.	11	159	87	118
Per cent	2.9	42.4	23.2	31.5

Some experts claim to be able to differentiate microinvasion both from intraepithelial carcinoma and frank invasion on the basis of exfoliated cells. Others refute this claim. At our own cytopathological laboratory an attempt has never been made to differentiate between microinvasion and frank invasion.

CYTOLOGY

Today the disease usually presents as an abnormal smear taken routinely or in connection with gynecological symptoms such as discharge or irregular bleeding. It is difficult to give an exact false negative rate for cytology in microcarcinoma of the cervix. The false negative rate of 2.9% found in one of our own studies (7) certainly must be a minimal figure (Table 14.1).

COLPOSCOPY

The same criteria for colposcopic evaluation of the lesions should be used as in CIN. There are no features which are specific for microinvasion. However, in an ectocervical lesion an extremely irregular punctation or mosaic may raise suspicion, as may small atypical vessels (Fig. 14.2). Furthermore, the microinvasive lesions have a

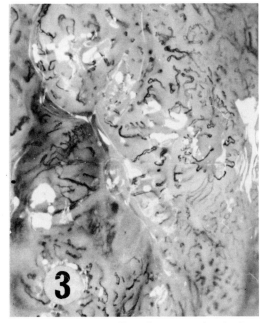

Fig. 14.2 and 14.3. (14,2) Extremely coarse and irregular mosaic with large intercapillary distance seen in microinvasive carcinoma of the cervix. (14.3) Irregular, atypical vessels and slightly nodular surface indicating microinvasion.

more irregular and elevated surface contour than their intraepithelial counterpart (Fig. 14.3). Colposcopic diagnosis in 283 patients (7) is shown in Table 14.2.

BIOPSY

Punch biopsies directed by colposcopy and supplemented with endocervical curettage are generally the first approach to histological diagnosis. Such biopsies are, however, inadequate for assessing the depth of invasion, the extent of the lesion or the presence of vessel invasion, which may be of importance in deciding the management. It is especially difficult to assess the microscopic picture of endocervical curettings.

Whenever a question of microcarcinoma arises, we prefer to perform a cold knife cone. In recent years laser conization has come into use. It should be remembered that Stage Ia lesions extend up into or develop more frequently in the endocervix than CIN lesions (Fig. 14.4).

When a cone specimen is sent to the histopathologist, the clinician should report on the colposcopic findings and suggest which part (quadrant) of the cervix is most likely to be the seat of microinvasive or invasive changes. The advantage of this is that the histopathologist can reduce the number of sections necessary to reach the correct diagnosis.

TREATMENT

As early as 1951, Mestwerdt (2) pointed to the fact that microinvasive carcinoma of the cervix invading less than 5 mm could relatively safely be treated in a less radical way than invasive lesions of greater extent. In his experience, and through a review of the literature, he concluded that such small tumors did not seem to metastasize. During

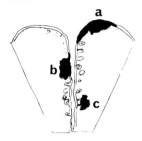

Microcarcinoma

a: ectocervical
b: endocervical
e: developing from crypt

Fig. 14.4. Different locations of microcarcinoma in the cervix.

the last decade a large number of studies of Stage Ia carcinoma of the cervix have appeared in the literature. Stormy discussions are still going on concerning both definition and treatment of this condition. The accepted invasion into the stroma for allotting a case to Stage Ia varies from 1 mm up to 5 mm and even 7 mm (8). Some Austrian and German authors prefer to measure the volume of the tumor in a cone specimen (9, 10). They set the limit for allotting a case to Stage Ia at 500 mm³.

Another factor which may influence the prognosis for the patients with microcarcinoma of the cervix is the occurrence of tumor cells in vascular spaces. The frequency of such tumor cells being found in a cone or hysterectomy specimen varies in different reports, and there are great differences of opinion about their true significance.

A third parameter which has been brought into focus is so-called confluency of carcinomatous cells. Such confluency should indicate a more radical treatment because, according to some authors, the chance for metastases should be greater. However, confluency is difficult to define, and the term is not accepted by many histopathologists.

A review of the world literature has revealed a bewildering variety of opinion about the treatment of Stage Ia carcinoma of the cervix. *On one point, however, there is general agreement. The prognosis for these patients is extremely good whatever type of treatment is chosen. It may be correct to state that to date, treatment has been too radical.*

Table 14.2. Colposcopic findings in 283 patients with Stage Ia carcinoma of the cervix

	Indecisive	CIN II–III	Micro-carcinoma	Inv. Ca.
No.	39	109	98	37
Per cent	13.8	38.5	34.6	13.1

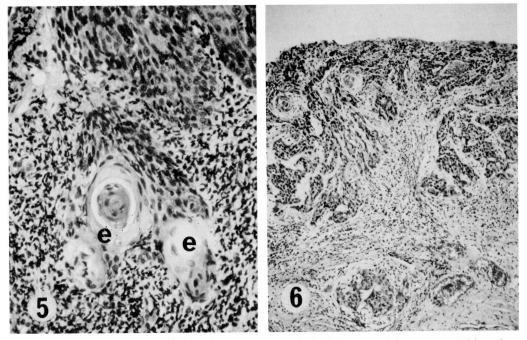

Fig. 14.5 and 14.6. (14.5) Early stromal invasion represented by bud of atypical epithelium surrounded by a dense lymphocytic infiltration. Eosinophilic epithelium with cornification and pearl formation (e). (14.6) Confluent lesion with foci of cells forming a measureable microcarcinoma. From (6) and reproduced by courtesy of W. B. Saunders Company, Ltd.

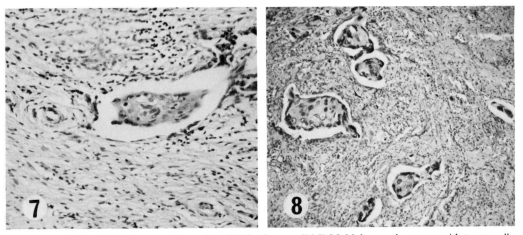

Figs. 14.7 and 14.8. (14.7) Tumor cells in endothelial lined space. (14.8) Multiple vascular spaces with tumor cells. Metastases were found in pelvic lymph nodes.

More and more authors have become sufficiently reconciled to the real nature of microinvasive carcinoma as to treat it conservatively.

OWN STUDIES

The first report on our experience with carcinoma of the cervix Stage Ia was published in 1969 (4). The study included 177 cases, 164 of which were squamous cell carcinomas and 13 adenocarcinomas. Treatment varied greatly, but could be classified into three groups: (1) pelvic lymph nodes not treated, (2) pelvic lymph nodes removed, and (3) pelvic lymph nodes irradiated. In four cases metastases to the pelvic wall were detected during follow-up. However, two of these probably should have been classified as Stage Ib, because there was not enough material to evaluate the true extent of invasion. The risk of spread in Stage Ia was found to be so small that routine treatment of the pelvic lymph nodes should not be necessary. The potential for spread in true microinvasive carcinoma with a depth of infiltration less than 5 mm is probably approximately 1–2%.

A second review of our material of microcarcinoma of the cervix was published in 1979 and 1982 (5, 6). In the latter paper, emphasis was placed on definition and treatment problems. During the total period 1951–75 altogether 367 patients were allotted to clinical Stage Ia. From this material, 122 cases were selected in which, during the primary operation, all the pathological tissue was regarded as completely removed.

Altogether 42 patients showed a histological pattern classified as carcinoma in situ with minimal stromal infiltration (Fig. 14.5). Stromal invasion with confluence of small foci of cells forming a minute invasive carcinoma, characterized by interlacing cords of neoplastic epithelium, was found in 80 patients (Fig. 14.6). The contour of the infiltrating nests and clusters appeared irregular and surrounded by a loose, edematous stroma. In most cases, there was a moderate lymphocytic infiltration of the invaded tissue. In some cases there was a more marked inflammatory reaction.

Unquestionable invasion in vessels was found in eight cases (Fig. 14.7 and 14.8). Five of these showed infiltration into the stroma of less than 3 mm. Questionable vessel invasion was found in six patients.

No patient was lost to follow-up. The follow-up time varied from 5 to 25 years (Table 14.3). Altogether eight recurrences were found, four of which were located to the vagina, cervix or the bladder (central recurrences), and four to the pelvic wall (lateral recurrences). It should be noted that five of the eight recurrences occurred after the conventional 5-year period of follow-up. In one patient a large pelvic lymph node metastasis was detected thirteen years after primary treatment which consisted of conization only. The 5-year survival rate in the series was 98%.

Of the four patients with central recurrences, the margin of the operation specimen was not free in three. The fourth patient showed unquestionable invasion in lymph vessels, and the recurrence in this case was located to the outer part of the vagina.

Of the four patients with recurrences on the pelvic wall, three had vessel invasion. The fourth case had an adenomatous lesion which could not be seen to involve capillary-like spaces. Out of 114 cases without clear evidence of vessel invasion only the patient with cervical adenocarcinoma developed metastases on the pelvic wall, whereas three of eight patients with vessel invasion did so (Table 14.4).

Our results seem to prove that recurrences on the pelvic wall may appear after many years. Three of four such metastases developed later than five years after follow-up, the last one after 13 years.

Only one patient died from cervical carcinoma during the first five years of follow-up. Three more patients have later died from their disease.

Most probably, the patients with late recurrences had only minute lymphatic metastases at the time of primary treatment, possibly consisting of a few tumor cells. Such metastases may well remain undiagnosed even if careful histological examination of every lymph node in the pelvis is carried out. It is therefore not suprising that extremely few cases with microinvasive carcinoma reported in the literature and treated with lymphadenectomy have shown any signs of metastases.

A third study on microinvasive carcinoma of the cervix was published in 1985 (7). A new treat-

Table 14.3. Recurrences and deaths in relation to time of follow-up

Duration of follow-up	Total No.	Recurrences		Died of cancer	Died of other causes
		Vagina/cervix or bladder	Pelvic wall		
Up to 5 years	122	2	1	1	1
Up to 10 years	120	2	2	2	1
Up to 15 years	58	–	1	–	1
Up to 20 years	18	–	–	–	–
Up to 25 years	7	–	–	–	–

Table 14.4. Correlation between tumor involvement of vessels and recurrence

Involvement of endothelial lined spaces (vessels)	Total No.	Recurrence	
		Vagina/cervix/bladder	Pelvic wall
None	108	2	1 (0.9%)
Possible	6	–	–
Certain	8	2	3 (37.5%)
Total No.	122	4	4

ment protocol was set up in the early 1970s on the basis of the two previous studies. It was stated that the diagnosis should always be made on a cone specimen. This should be followed by a so-called modified extended hysterectomy with removal of part of the parametria and preservation of the ovaries in the younger age groups. Instead of hysterectomy, postmenopausal patients might receive radium irradiation. If involvement of vessels was found, radical hysterectomy with pelvic lymph node dissection should be the treatment of choice. In older patients the pelvic lymph nodes could also be treated by external radiotherapy without lymphadenectomy.

Altogether 561 cases of microinvasive carcinoma of the cervix were treated in the years 1971–80. Histological diagnoses are shown in Table 14.5. Squamous cell carcinoma was found in 533 cases. Age distribution is illustrated in Fig. 14.9. The majority of the patients were between 30 and 50 years of age. The youngest was 21 and the oldest 79 years of age. Mean age was 45.7 years.

TREATMENT

During the review of the material many diversions from the treatment protocol mentioned above

Table 14.5. Distribution by histological diagnosis. Microcarcinoma of the cervix (stage Ia). 561 cases 1971–80.

Squamous cell carcinoma	533
Adenocarcinoma	20
Adenosquamous carcinoma	7
Clear cell carcinoma*	1
Total	561

* No history of DES-exposure.

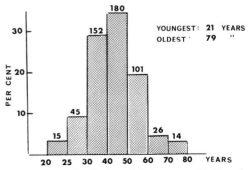

Fig. 14.9. Age distribution of 533 women with Stage Ia squamous cell carcinoma of the cervix.

were found (Table 14.6). This was to a great extent due to the fact that the majority of the patients were referred from other hospitals when a diagnosis of microcarcinoma was made, mostly on a cone specimen, but also after simple hysterectomy. The diagnosis was made on a cone specimen in 438 of 533 cases with squamous cell carcinoma.

Involved margins

The surgical specimens were all examined for the presence of carcinomatous tissue in the margins (Table 14.7). It is important to note that as many as 27.5% of the cone specimens showed involved margins. This is a much higher figure than that found in series of CIN treated by conization. Even those patients in which conization followed a thorough colposcopic examination showed as many as 13.8% of involved margins. This probably reflects the fact that microcarcinoma is a more extensive lesion than CIN and often extends relatively high up in the endocervix.

In the series treated by simple hysterectomy, margins were involved in 4.7%, and in the extended hysterectomy series in 1.8%.

Table 14.6. Treatment methods. 533 patients with squamous cell carcinoma.

Treatment	Number
Conisation	31
Simple hysterectomy	25
Extended hysterectomy	51
Conisation +	
simple hysterectomy	62
extended hysterectomy	199
radical hysterectomy and	
lymphadenectomy	42
intracavitary radium	100
external high voltage radiation	4
Intracavitary radium	19
Total No.	533

Table 14.7. Involved margins of the surgical specimen

Cone		Hysterectomy		Extended hysterectomy	
No.	Per cent	No.	Per cent	No.	Per cent
114/415	27.5	3/64	4.7	3/171	1.8

Table 14.8. Depth of infiltration, recurrences and deaths 533 microinvasive squamous cell carcinomas.

	Depth of infiltration			
	<1 mm	1–2.9 mm	3–5 mm	Total
No.	198	168	167	533
Per cent	37.1	31.5	31.3	100
Recurrence	3	4	3	10
Ca. deaths	1*	1	3	5

* Ca. vulvae.

Table 14.9. Radical hysterectomy with pelvic lymphadenectomy 42 patients

30 patients had capillary-space involvement

12 patients were operated with extended Wertheim because of findings at clinical and/or colposcopic examination

2 of the 42 patients had lymph node metastases, one in the parametrium and one in the obturator region. Both had lymph vessel involvement.

Depth of infiltration

Depth of infiltration in relation to recurrence and death is shown in Table 14.8. The one patient with a depth of infiltration less than 1 mm who died from cancer, was treated for vulvar carcinoma two years after conization for microcarcinoma of the cervix. Whether she died from spread of her cervical or vulvar malignancy is uncertain. There seems to be an increasing risk of recurrence and death with increasing depth of infiltration.

Vessel involvement

Radical hysterectomy and pelvic lymphadenectomy was performed in 42 patients (Table 14.9). The indications for this procedure were, vessel involvement in 30 patients, and in 12 patients a Stage Ib lesion was suspected because of findings at clinical examination, colposcopy or because of an abundance of endocervical curettings. Two of these 42 patients had lymph node metastases, one in the parametrium and one in the obturator region. Both had vessel involvement in the cone specimen. They are both living and well.

In the total series of 561 cases, 50 showed vessel involvement. Thirty-seven of these were treated

Table 14.10. Surgical complications.

42 Wertheim operations	1 vesico-vaginal fistula 1 uretero-vaginal fistula 2 lymph cysts 1 lymphedema 1 transitional lesion of the femoral nerve
250 extended hysterectomies	1 intestinal obstruction 5 pelvic infections 1 ureteral stenosis
89 hysterectomies	2 pelvic infections

Table 14.11. Radiation complications

119 intracavitary radium	1 rectal stenosis 1 bladder ulceration
4 external irradiation	1 rectal stenosis

Complications after radiotherapy are shown in Table 14.11. After intracavitary radium applications in 119 patients, one patient developed rectal stenosis which had to be treated by transitory colostomy. Another patient developed a bladder ulceration with complicating infection. The ulceration healed spontaneously after one year. Four patients received external radiation, and one of these also had a rectal stenosis. It was, however, not necessary to perform colostomy or resection.

with pelvic lymphadenectomy and four with external radiotherapy. These forty-one patients have suffered no recurrences. For some unknown reason the remaining nine patients were not treated according to the protocol, and lymphadenectomy was not performed. It is remarkable that three of these nine cases developed metastases and died from their disease.

Follow-up
Table 14.12 gives the treatment method in the total series, both of squamous cell carcinoma and adenocarcinoma, correlated with central (local) recurrences, pelvic wall metastases, distant metastases and deaths. Of the ten patients with local recurrences in the cervix or vagina, five had involvement of the margins of the surgical specimen. One patient had multiple condylomatous lesions, which possibly had not been completely removed. Of the lateral (pelvic wall) recurrences three out of four had vessel involvement and should have been treated with pelvic lymphadenectomy. The two patients with distant metastases also had vessel involvement. One of these had an adenocarcinoma and massive involvement of vessels. She was treated with Wertheim-Meigs operation, but

Complications
Surgical complications are shown in Table 14.10. It is quite obvious that radical hysterectomy with lymphadenectomy carries the highest risk.

In the series of 250 extended hysterectomies, one intestinal obstruction was treated by relaparotomy with division of adhesions. Five patients developed pelvic infections, and one patient had a urethral stenosis with slight reduction of the function of the kidney.

Simple hysterectomy in 89 cases was only followed by two cases of pelvic infections.

Table 14.12. Treatment and recurrence site.

Treatment	Total No.	Local rec.	Pelvic wall rec.	Distant met.	Deaths
Conization	34	3	–	–	1
Hysterectomy	94	2	–	–	–
Ext. hyst.	261	4	3	1	4
Wertheim-Meigs	46	1	–	1***	1
Radium*	126	–	–	–	–
Total No.	561	10**	3	2	6

* External high voltage irradiation: 4 patients.
** Not free margins 5 patients.
*** Adenocarcinoma, lung metastases.

there were no metastases to the lymph nodes. Six years after surgery massive lung metastases were found and she died six months later.

CONCLUSION

The three series of Stage Ia carcinoma of the cervix presented from our hospital since 1969 confirm numerous reports in the respect that this group of lesions has a very good prognosis. Only about 1–2% of patients will die from their disease.

The treatment protocol set up in the early 1970s seems adequate. The importance of having a cone specimen that is thoroughly scrutinized for the occurrence of vessel invasion before final therapy is chosen, should be especially stressed.

On the other hand, it may be questioned whether our treatment policy is too radical for patients without vessel involvement. It seems obvious that infiltration under 1 mm where the lesion has been completely removed by conization, does not call for further therapy. Also lesions invading up to 3 mm can be safely treated by conization provided there are ample free margins and no signs of vessel invasion. Simple hysterectomy should possibly be recommended for lesions between 3 and 5 mm, with free margins on the cone. If the margins are involved, one cannot be sure that there is a deeper lesion left behind and extended hysterectomy is recommended. A last modification would be that when conization has removed the whole lesion and this shows vessel invasion, it is probably unnecessary to perform radical hysterectomy. Simple hysterectomy with lymph node dissection should be adequate treatment. In this way, some of the complications which are known to occur after radical hysterectomy, can be avoided.

MICROINVASIVE ADENOCARCINOMA

In the total series of 561 cases, there were 28 (4.99%) adenocarcinomas, four of which were classified as adenosquamous carcinoma and one as a clear cell carcinoma. This last case had no history of DES-exposure.

Ten of the 28 cases were detected by routine smear, the others had clinical symptoms as discharge, bleeding or other symptoms that led to a gynecological examination. Colposcopy was in seven cases negative, five cases were believed to have a CIN grade II–III lesion, in four cases a diagnosis of microinvasive carcinoma was made, and in two cases frank invasive carcinoma was suspected.

Treatment methods were the same as described for the 533 squamous cell carcinomas. Four of the patients were treated with radical hysterectomy and pelvic lymphadenectomy, one of which had massive involvement of endothelial lined spaces. She had no lymph node metastases, but as mentioned previously returned with massive lung metastases 6 years after treatment. We possibly could have detected the metastases earlier if we had done serial CEA determinations. She had a slightly elevated CEA, 5.8 μg/l at primary operation, and 15000 μg/l when the lung metastases were detected.

15

Vascularization, oxygen tension and radiocurability in cancer of the cervix

In 1961 Gray (1) wrote:

Of all molecules that have thus far been observed to exercise a marked influence on radiosensitivity by their presence during the period of irradiation, oxygen remains at the center of interest to the radiotherapist for a number of reasons, such as: (1) oxygen is a normal physiological variable, (2) oxygen affects radiosensitivty to a greater extent than any other agent tested thus far, (3) there are reasons for believing that hypoxic or anoxic foci militate against the curability of some tumors, and (4) oxygen is subject to experimental control in man as well as in animal.

At that time Gray and his group, as well as many other investigators, had shown that hypoxia and anoxia protect against ionizing radiation. This had been shown in studies on plants, insects, bacteria and mammalian tissue. In general, it has been found that to produce a specified effect in the absence of oxygen comparable to that in air, the radiation dose must be increased by a factor of about 2.5–3.0. Increase in tissue oxygen tension (pO_2) from 0 to 10 mm sharply enhances the effect of ionizing radiation.

Although several theories have been suggested to explain the oxygen effect, there seems to be general agreement that oxygen must be available at the very moment of irradiation to exert its effect, and that only a certain part of the radiosensitivity of a specific biological system is oxygen dependent. It seems, in particular, that the so-called indirect action by free radicals can be modified by oxygen. Thus, hypoxic tumor cells may well be destroyed by X-rays if the dose is sufficiently large. This probably often occurs in intracavitary radium treatment of cervix cancer.

The widespread interest in the oxygen effect brought about a series of investigations in the Department of Gynecology of the Norwegian Radium Hospital. Attempts were made to assess to what extent the oxygen tension affects the radiocurability of cervix cancer.

The following methods were used:

1. The vascularization of the normal uterine cervix and that of intraepithelial neoplasia and invasive cervix cancer was studied by the colpophotographic method of Koller (2).
2. Blood oxygen tension was determined by a spectrophotometric method (3) in capillary blood samples taken from the normal mucous membrane as well as from preinvasive and invasive cancer of the cervix.
3. Tissue oxygen tension measurements were performed with polarographic microelectrodes after the method of Cater et al. (3).
4. The pretreatment assessment of vascularization and oxygen tension was correlated with the outcome of radiotherapy by a careful follow-up of a series of patients (3).

In addition, a study on the effect of anemia on the result of radiotherapy has been published (4). In a selected series of patients the effect of vasodilator drugs and of the breathing of a mixture of carbondioxide and oxygen was also investigated (5, 6). Since it has been postulated that fractionated radiation treatment induces an increase in the vascularity of cervical cancer, this problem was also taken up. Detailed description of the results of many of the above problems have been given in monographs: Koller in 1963 (2), Kolstad in 1964 (3) and Bergsjø in 1968 (7). Only a relatively brief summary of many of the observations made during these years can be given here. Detailed descriptions of the methods and results will be found in the three monographs and in a series of publications in international journals (4, 5, 6, 7, 8, 9, 10).

Before describing the results it is necessary to

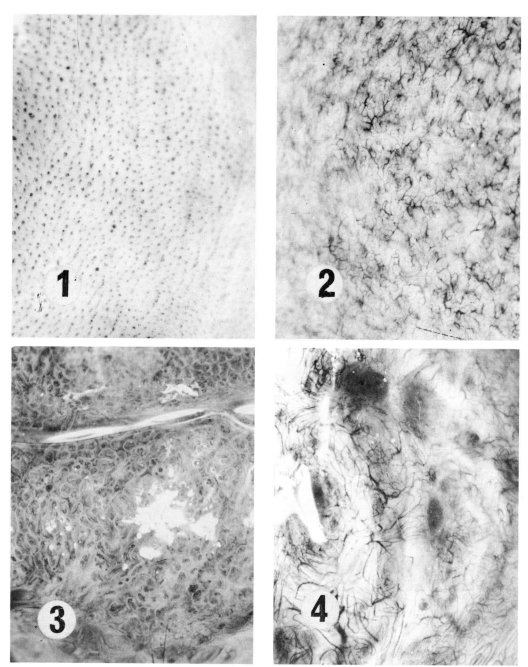

Figs. 15.1–15.4. (15.1) Hairpin capillaries in normal squamous epithelium. (15.2) Network type of capillaries. (15.3) Villi of columnar epithelium containing dense network of curled capillaries. (15.4) Branching type of capillaries in transformation zone. Note treelike branching with an ultimate fine network.

Table 15.1. Mean tissue oxygen tension and stage of the disease

Study group	No. of cases	No. of observations	Mean PO₂ ± S_mean	Range of PO₂
Controls	48	116	40.5 ± 2.18	4–79
Adjacent to invasive cancer	35	80	31.6 ± 2.39	11–63
Stage 0	33	87	26.2 ± 2.33	8–69
Stage I	16	70	17.4 ± 2.19	2–38
Stage II	19	86	18.6 ± 3.03	0–50

clarify a few controversial points. First the term "vascularization" or, as used in the present context, "vascularity", should be defined. An abundance of large vessels in a tumor may give an impression of rich (increased) vascularization. However, the oxygenation of parts of the tumor may nevertheless be insufficient. It is not so much the larger vessels as the status of the capillary bed which determines the oxygen tension of the tissue. The factor of greatest significance is the intercapillary distance (3). In the following, the term "vascularization" will therefore be used with reference to the capillary bed and the oxygenation of the tissue.

VASCULARITY AND INTERCAPILLARY DISTANCE IN THE NORMAL CERVIX

Koller demonstrated that the normal squamous epithelium of the cervix is characterized by two basic types of capillaries: (1) hairpin-like capillaries of a fine caliber, with a regular distribution and often arranged in rows (Fig. 15.1), and (2) a fine network of capillaries running more or less parallel to the surface, sometimes with larger subpapillary vessels also visible (Fig. 15.2). The hairpin capillaries are found to be spaced with fair regularity at an average distance of about 100 μ, with a range of approximately 50–250 μ. The network pattern has a mesh size of approximately the same size or somewhat smaller.

Koller found the vascularization of cervical columnar epithelium to be excellent with an extremely fine meshwork of capillaries within each "grape" or "villous" of columnar epithelium (Fig. 15.3). The branching type of vessels often revealed in transformation zones demonstrated a regular branching pattern and a terminal network with meshes of normal size (Fig. 15.4).

VASCULARIZATION AND INTERCAPILLARY DISTANCE IN INTRAEPITHELIAL NEOPLASIA AND INVASIVE CARCINOMA OF THE CERVIX

The majority of the cases of intraepithelial neoplasia studied were characterized by two basic types of vascular pattern: (1) hairpin-like, dilated, and often irregular so-called punctation vessels (Fig. 15.5), and (2) mosaic-like superficial vessels delineating relatively large circular, ovoid or polygonal fields (Fig. 15.6). In cases of microcarcinoma of the cervix these two patterns were found less frequently, the vessels being more irregular, atypical, delineating large avascular fields. A striking observation was that even CIN lesions showed a marked increase in the intercapillary distance. In frank invasive carcinoma the vascular pattern was found to be strikingly irregular. In some cases the growth of the vascular tree seemed to keep up with tumor growth, while in other cases atypical vessels with a great increase in intercapillary distance and subsequent necrotic foci were observed (Fig. 15.7). It was demonstrated that an association exists between a large intercapillary distance and an advanced stage of the disease.

Tissue oxygen tension measurements were performed with a platinum microelectrode of 0.05 mm measuring surface (Fig. 15.8). The electrode was inserted into the surperficial part of the tumor by the guidance of the colposcope. The relatively large intercapillary distance of the more advanced lesions frequently made it possible to place the tip of the electrode between the visible capillaries. The electrode was inserted in different locations both in the tumor surface and in the adjacent mucous membrane, care always being taken to get readings from the most avascular part of the tumors.

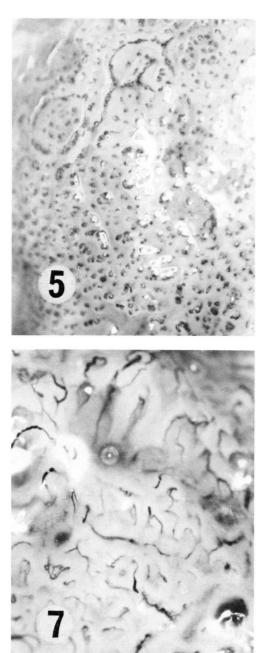
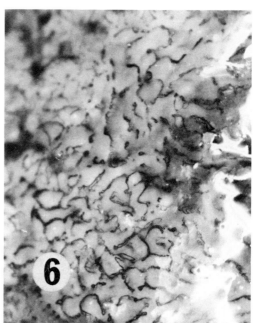

Figs. 15.5–15.7 (15.5) Coarse punctation and some mosaic vessels with increased intercapillary distance in CIN III. (15.6) Irregular mosaic vessels with increased intercapillary distance in CIN III. (15.7) Atypical, extremely irregular vessels in invasive cancer. Decreased vascularity due to large avascular areas.

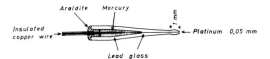

Fig. 15.8. Design of platinum oxygen cathode.

Altogether 582 polarographic readings were available for analysis. In 169 cases continuous recordings before, during and after inhalation of pure oxygen at atmospheric pressure were made. In Table 15.1 the material of single readings in the controls, the preinvasive and invasive lesions is demonstrated. The observed difference between the readings in intraepithelial neoplasia and the invasive carcinomas was highly significant.

The values presented in Table 15.1 were based on the calculated mean pO_2 in each single case. In many tumors a large scatter of polarographic readings was observed. Thus, the mean values do not give a complete picture of the oxygenation of the tumors. Of greatest significance for the evaluation of a possible relationship between oxygen tension and radiotherapy, are the anoxic or hypoxic foci that can be demonstrated. In Fig. 15.9 the lowest tissue oxygen tension values ob-

served in each case are plotted for the different groups of lesions. It can readily be seen that it was easier to find avascular hypoxic areas in the more advanced stages of the disease. Of the controls 4.2% showed readings below 10 mm pO_2. The corresponding figure for the Stage 0 lesions was 28.0% and for the invasive carcinoma Stages I and II 42.5% and 68.4% respectively. As many as 13 of the 19 Stage II squamous cell carcinomas had an observed lowest value in the range 0–10 mm Hg.

The influence of atmospheric oxygen breathing upon tissue oxygen tension was studied by continuous polarographic records or by a series of measurements before, during and after oxygen inhalation. In the controls, rapid and steep increase to a new plateau was found after a latency phase of only 20–30 seconds following the application of the oxygen mask (Fig. 15.10). In the Stage 0 lesions the slope of the rising part of the curve was slightly more oblique, and the steady state was reached somewhat later. Furthermore, the plateau was as a rule lower than in the controls. (Fig. 15.11).

The differences between the invasive cancers and the controls were still more apparent, often

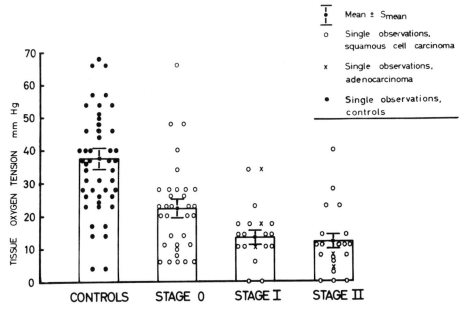

Fig. 15.9. Lowest observed tissue oxygen tension in 48 controls, 39 Stage 0, 19 Stage I and 21 Stage II carcinoma of the cervix.

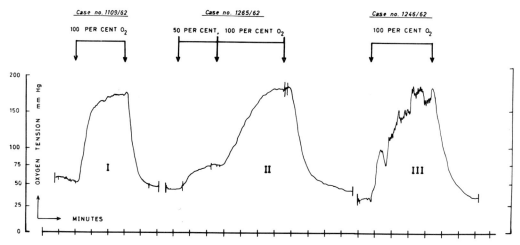

Fig. 15.10. Variation in polarographic measured tissue oxygen tension in the normal squamous epithelium during oxygen breathing.

with a long period of latency; the increase in the oxygen tension was slow and small, indicating either a long diffusion path from the nearest functioning capillary to the electrode, or insufficient circulation in the distorted vessels with local decrease in the rate of blood flow. In many cases no increase in pO_2 was found (Fig. 15.12).

FOLLOW-UP STUDY

In the series of patients studied by colpophotography, measurements of the largest intercapillary distance and the lowest observed tumor pO_2 were

followed for five years. At the follow-up examinations, care was taken to detect local recurrence within the irradiated area of the pelvis.

In the normal squamous epithelium of the cervix an intercapillary distance > 250 μ was not encountered. Arbitrarily, it was decided that if avascular areas with a diameter of 400 μ or more were observed, the chance of recurrence should be greater than in cases with an intercapillary distance below this range. Table 15.2 shows the number of cases followed for five years and grouped according to an intercapillary distance less than or more than 400 μ. There was a signifi-

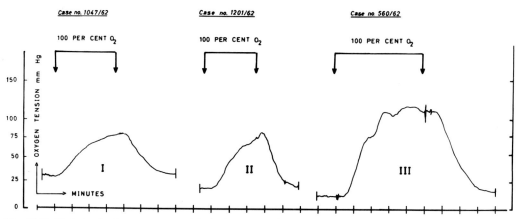

Fig. 15.11. Variation in tissue oxygen tension during oxygen breathing in three cases of CIN III.

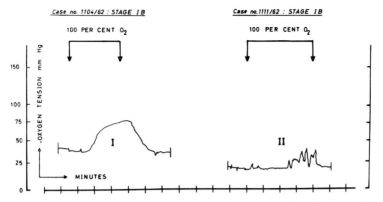

Fig. 15.12. Variation in oxygen tension during oxygen breathing in two cases of invasive cervical cancer.

cant increase in the frequency of local recurrences in those cases with an intercapillary distance more than 400 μ.

Table 15.3 shows the number of recurrences in a total series of 31 cases which arbitrarily were divided into those with a $pO_2 < 10$ mm, 10–19 mm, and 20–40 mm pO_2.

Thus, the evidence in the literature that many tumors have an abnormal circulation leaving some cancer cells hypoxic and radioresistant, has been confirmed in our studies.

CLINICAL TRIAL WITH ATMOSPHERIC OXYGEN BREATHING DURING RADIOTHERAPY OF CANCER OF THE CERVIX

The observations that inhalation of pure oxygen at atmospheric pressure resulted in increased oxygenation of some hypoxic areas in a substantial number of Stages I and II carcinomas of the cervix initiated a study with oxygen breathing during radiotherapy.

A material of Stage II lesions was divided into three groups by random numbers:

1. A control group comprising 106 cases,
2. 53 patients receiving oxygen inhalation during radium irradiation only, and
3. 49 patients receiving oxygen during both radium and external irradiation.

The histological diagnosis was squamous cell carcinoma of varying differentiation in 200 cases and in 8 cases adenocarcinoma. Therapy consisted of a combination of intracavitary radium treatment after a modified Paris method, and external fractionated irradiation to pelvic fields.

The results of this study after a follow-up of between 3 and 5 years after treatment have been published in detail (10). In Table 15.4 the most important data are reproduced. In the control series 59.4% were alive without signs of disease in the course of the follow-up period, while of the patients who received oxygen breathing during both radium and external irradiation 67.3% were

Table 15.2. Largest measured intercapillary distance and recurrence of cervix cancer Stages I–IV

Intercapillary distance	Stage I			Stage II			Stage III & IV		
	No. of cases	Recurrence No.	%	No. of cases	Recurrence No.	%	No. of cases	Recurrence No.	%
< 400 μ	32	2	6.3	18	5	27.8	4	2	(50)
≧ 400 μ	16	5	31.2	28	14	50.0	7	7	(100)
Total	48	7	14.6	46	19	41.3	11	9	81.9

Table 15.3. Lowest observed tumor pO_2 and local recurrence

pO_2 mm Hg	No. of cases	No. of recurrences
0–9	10	6
10–19	14	3
20–40	7	1
Total	31	10

alive. A statistical analysis of the results, however, showed that the difference was not statistically significant at the 5% level.

We have followed, with great interest, the results of hyperbaric oxygen and radiotherapy set up by the Medical Research Council in Great Britain. The report in 1978 (11) seems to show that patients with carcinoma of the head and neck and carcinoma of the cervix may benefit from such therapy. It is interesting to note that especially those cases with Stage III carcinoma of the cervix and at an age below 55 years seem to show the best results.

In connection with our studies of atmospheric oxygen breathing, we have also studied the influence of administration of vasodilator drugs and of breathing a carbondioxide mixture and pure oxygen (5, 6). Three vasodilator drugs were used, but both colpophotographic studies and polarographic measurements showed such a small increase both in vascularization and oxygen tension that these studies were not continued.

THE INFLUENCE OF ANEMIA ON THE RESULTS OF RADIOTHERAPY IN CARCINOMA OF THE CERVIX

Most radiotherapists have the clinical impression that the radiation response of cancer in anemic patients is diminished. A study on this program was published from the Norwegian Radium Hospital in 1965 (4).

A significantly lower survival rate in anemic patients was demonstrated. It was also found that there was a higher incidence of persistent local cancer in the cervix after radiation in anemic patients with Stages II or III carcinoma. The poor prognosis of the anemic patient may be due to tumor anoxia resulting in diminished radiation response. The prognosis of the anemic patient is likely to be improved by transfusion prior to radium treatment.

RADIATION-INDUCED CHANGES IN VASCULARITY AND OXYGEN TENSION OF CERVICAL CARCINOMA

It has been postulated that one of the benefits of fractionated radiotherapy is that hypoxic radioresistant cells, during radiotherapy, can be effectively recruited into the oxic compartment of tumors by reoxygenation following removal of well-oxygenated cells (12). The reduction in size of the tumor during radiotherapy may also lead to a reduction in the intracapillary distance which also

Table 15.4. Atmospheric oxygen breathing and recurrences and deaths after a follow-up period of 3–5 years

Treatment group	Total No.	Dead with local recurrence No.	%	Dead from distant metastases No.	%	Dead from intercurrent disease No.	%	Alive with local recurrence No.	%	Alive with distant metastases No.	%	Alive without signs of active disease No.	%
Control series air breathing	106	32	30.2	5	4.7	2	1.9	3	2.9	1	0.9	63	59.4
Oxygen breathing during radium irradiation only	53	15	28.3	1	1.9	3	5.6	1	1.9	0	0	33	62.3
Oxygen breathing during radium and external irradiation	49	11	22.4	3	6.1	1	2.1	0	0	1	2.1	33	67.3
Total	208	58	27.9	9	4.3	6	2.9	4	1.9	2	1.0	129	62.0

influences the oxygenation of the tumor cells. It was decided to investigate patients with carcinoma of the uterine cervix Stage II (7). Clinically the Stage II patients represent a well-defined homogeneous group of cancers with particular regard to size, surface contours and vascular patterns. The main tool of investigation was colpophotography, but in a smaller group of patients oxygen tension measurements were also made with a Clark microelectrode.

The results indicate that, in general, the tumors may get an increasingly better blood supply during the fractionated radiation therapy and hence better oxygenation. This favors the theory that fractionation is beneficial by gradually increasing the radiosensitivity of the tumor in relation to that of normal tissue.

RADIOSENSITIZERS

Studies on radiosensitizers such as hydroxurea and misonidazole have been performed in many countries. A Scandinavian multicenter study on the value of misonidazole as a sensitizer in cervical cancer Stages IIb, III and IVa was published in 1982.

The Norwegian Radium Hospital took part in this study, which lasted from April 1979 to January 1982. Three hundred and forty-one patients were included in this double blind trial. Life table analysis showed no significant difference in survival between the control and the treatment group in any of the stages.

16

Clinical features and special examinations in carcinoma of the cervix Stages Ib–IV

CLINICAL FEATURES

It has already been mentioned that the mean age of patients with carcinoma of the cervix increases with increasing stage of the disease.

When the tumor becomes so large that it can be diagnosed macroscopically, a common symptom, especially of an ectocervical or exophytic tumor, is bleeding. If the neoplasm is necrotic, it may be followed by a foul-smelling vaginal discharge.

As the tumor progresses laterally into the parametrial tissues, it eventually impinges upon the ureters and the various structures located on the pelvic side wall. Involvement of lymphatic channels ultimately leads to occlusion, causing an intractable edema in the lower extremities. Involvement of the ureters leads to progressive luminal narrowing, which eventually causes uremia in the end stages of the disease.

Invasion of nerves and bone produces an excruciating pain that frequently is more severe when the patient is lying in bed at night than when she is up and about during the day (1).

All patients with cervical carcinoma should be carefully questioned about pain, its character and localization. If by clinical, neurological and roentgenological examination other causes can be ruled out, the pain must be considered to be due to cancer. Pain in the lower abdomen, the suprapubic area or the groins ("dysmenorrhea pain") is not necessarily serious. Pain in the lower back irradiating to the buttocks, the thighs, or the legs often worse at night time, is of great prognostic import, both as an initial and a recurrence symptom.

The macroscopic appearance of the tumor may also be of prognostic significance. The exophytic, cauliflower type of tumor which frequently has a colposcopic vascular pattern described by Koller and Bergsjø as complete loops (Fig. 16.1), has a much better prognosis than an endophytic, and,

especially, an endocervical tumor with a barrel-shaped cervix. If the clinical examination and colposcopy show many areas with necrosis, radiotherapy frequently fails (Fig. 16.2). Even if an endocervical lesion is classified as a Stage I carcinoma, it is well known that the frequency of metastases on the pelvic wall is much higher than in an exophytic, cauliflower lesion. Sometimes, however, the exophytic lesion, even in Stage Ib, is of such size that it almost fills up the whole vagina, and these cases also have a very poor prognosis whatever type of treatment is tried.

ADDITIONAL EXAMINATIONS

The staging of carcinoma of the cervix should be performed by an experienced examiner and under anesthesia. In addition to palpation and inspection, the following examinations should be carried out: Colposcopy, endocervical curettage, cystoscopy, intravenous urography and X-ray examinations of the lungs and skeleton. It is our experience that proctoscopy is of no use as a routine examination. Only when the clinical examination with palpation and inspection indicate that the rectum may be involved, should proctoscopy be performed. In clinical Stage I, cystoscopy could probably be omitted, too.

In addition to urography, venography was a routine examination for many years in the Norwegian Radium Hospital. In 1964 a study of 241 cases of cervical carcinoma in which both urography and venography had been performed was published (2). In Table 16.1 distribution by stages and roentgenological findings in this material is presented. With the advancing stage of the disease, the frequency of positive findings by urography and venography increases dramatically.

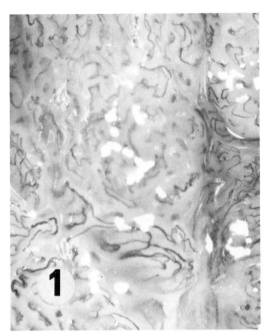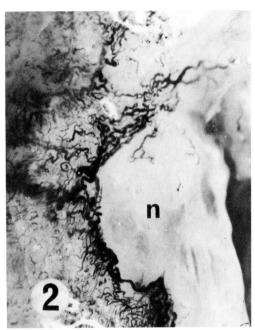

Figs. 16.1 and 16.2. (16.1) Squamous cell carcinoma of the cervix with complete loops vascular pattern indicating good radiosensitivity and good prognosis. (16.2) Invasive carcinoma of the cervix (endocervical) with large areas of necrosis (n). The tumor never went to healing after intracavitary and external irradiation.

ISOTOPE NEPHROGRAPHY

The rules for staging carcinoma of the cervix include the one that intravenous pyelograms should be performed in all cases. Throughout the years we have tried to follow this recommendation, but unfortunately more and more patients who are admitted have some allergic disease. Since the injection of iodine containing contrast may be of some hazard to such patients, we have introduced isotope nephrography as an alternative to intravenous pyelography.

It has been reported repeatedly that there is a significantly poorer prognosis in patients with ureteric involvement demonstrated either by urography or nephrography. To evaluate the sensitivity of isotope nephrography, this investigation was performed before radical hysterectomy with pelvic lymph node dissection in 90 cases of Stage Ib cervical carcinoma (3). It was found that isotope nephrography gives excellent information concerning the function of the renal pelvis and the ureter. The method is probably even more sensitive than urography. Impaired nephrography was

Table 16.1. Distribution by stages and roentgenological findings in 241 patients with carcinoma of the cervix Stage I–IV

Stage	Total No.	Positive urography	Positive venography	Positive urography + venography	Per cent positive findings
Stage I	97	1	1	0	2.3
Stage II	101	3	7	5	14.9
Stage III	33	9	1	4	42.5
Stage IV	10	2	4	2	80.0
Total	241	15	13	11	16.2

found to improve or become normal during external irradiation therapy. This could indicate successful treatment of lymph node metastases. However, the conclusion of the study was that isotope nephrography alone gives limited information in cases of early carcinoma of the cervix.

VENOGRAPHY

In the earlier years of our studies venography seemed to give reliable and important additional information about lymph node metastases, especially in the later stages of the disease (2). We have now surveyed approximately 1000 venograms in cervical carcinoma. This study has not been published. The method is both time-consuming and expensive, and gives very little additional information which will influence the treatment of the patient even in the later stages of the disease. In Fig. 16.3 a positive venogram in Stage III carcinoma of the cervix is shown. Such a finding is of very grave prognostic importance. However, we have concluded that routine venograms are not

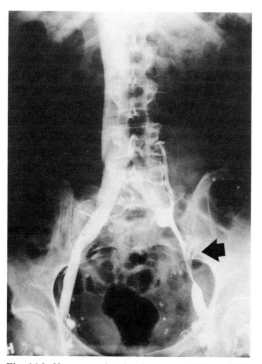

Fig. 16.3. Venogram showing large constriction of left iliac vein due to lymph node metastases.

indicated in carcinoma of the cervix irrespective of the stage of the disease. More information can be obtained by lymphography and/or computer tomography. Nevertheless, venography is a useful examination that can be applied both in the later stages of the disease and when recurrences occur. It is an easy and safe method if the patient is not allergic to iodine, and, at the same time as the venograms are obtained, urograms will follow. In expert hands injection into the femoral veins is an easy procedure.

LYMPHOGRAPHY

When lymphography was introduced in the diagnosis of metastases from carcinoma of the uterine cervix, the method was received with varying degrees of enthusiasm. Some authors reported a high accuracy, and it was stated that lymphography as a routine was not only justified, but necessary. Other investigators have emphasized the limitation of the diagnostic possibilities, and it has also been stated that lymphography is unreliable and probably unwarranted as a routine examination (4). In the Norwegian Radium Hospital lymphography was introduced as a routine method in 1969. We found that the reasons for differences in diagnostic accuracy might be due to several factors, such as the experience of the radiologist, quality of the radiograms, and selection of patients, especially with regard to clinical stage. Kolbenstvedt (5) stated that the most important reason for the differences in regard to the value of lymphography in carcinoma of the cervix, is probably the method used in making the final assessment. Possible reference systems for determining lymphographic accuracy are:

1. The course of the illness and the combined results of clinical and other radiologic examinations.
2. Aspiration biopsy.
3. Operation with either lymph node biopsy or lymphadenectomy.
4. Autopsy.

Kolbenstvedt critically analyzed these different reference systems. He pointed out that the first system claimed that if the lymphographic diag-

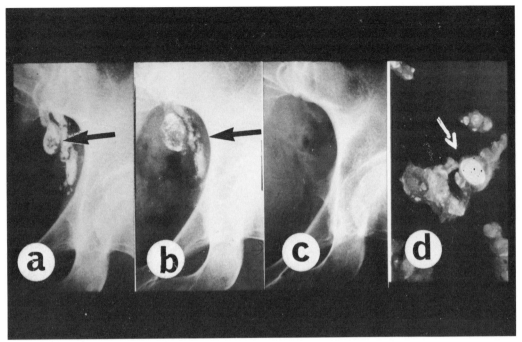

Fig. 16.4. Lymphogram showing nodal defect increasing in size from examination before (a) and six weeks after (b) intracavitary radium. In (c) the nodes have been removed, and (d) shows radiogram of the specimen. Arrow points to the node which is almost completely filled up with cancer cells. From (6) and by courtesy of Academic Press Inc.

nosis was positive, and the patient later died from metastases, then the finding is assumed to be correct, although the actual spread might be in another region of nodes of normal appearance.

Lymph node fine needle aspiration cytology or biopsy may provide cytologic or histologic confir-· mation of a positive or dubious lymphographic finding. If the cytologic or histologic findings are negative, however, the question arises whether representative material has been obtained. Autopsy allows the most thorough examination of all nodes. The period of time between lymphography and autopsy will, however, vary considerably, and might well allow for additional lymph node metastases to occur.

The safest reference system is undoubtedly operation with lymphadenectomy and histologic examination of all removed nodes. A complete dissection of all the lymph nodes of interest may yield an exact histologic and lymphographic correlation (5).

By close cooperation between the Gynecology Department, the Department of Diagnostic Radi-

ology and the Department of Pathology, it has been possible to study: different problems related to the method for lymphographic and histologic correlation, the problems of foot lymphography in the demonstration of the regional lymph nodes in carcinoma of the uterine cervix, the possibility of performing a complete lymph node dissection under intraoperative lymphographic control, the normal lymphographic variations of lumbar, iliac and inguinal lymph vessels, the projection difference index in lymphographic diagnosis of lymph node metastases and the problem of lymphography in the diagnosis of metastases from carcinoma of the uterine cervix. The leader of the team from 1970 to 1975 was Kolbenstvedt, and his observations and results have been published in a series of papers (5, 6, 7, 8, 9, 10).

A total of 300 patients with carcinoma of the uterine cervix, 275 with Stage I and 25 with Stage II, were treated by intracavitary radium irradiation followed six weeks later by radical hysterectomy and pelvic lymphadenectomy. Lymphography was performed during the first hospitaliz-

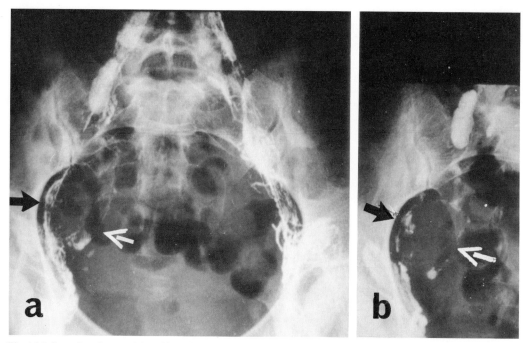

Fig. 16.5. Lymphangiogram (a) and lymphogram (b) showing non-opacification of metastatic lymph node. A totally infiltrated node in the right external region may be indirectly diagnosed by deviation of lymph vessels (arrows). From (6) and by courtesy of Academic Press Inc.

ation period, and new radiograms were taken immediately before the operation. As an aid to obtain complete lymphadenectomy, one or more radiograms were also taken during the operation.

In the first paper a method for lymphographic and histologic correlation was published (5). Thereafter the question of whether foot lymphography will reveal all nodes of interest was studied. In our opinion, the answer is yes. In our series a total of 9,187 lymph nodes were removed, of which 97 (1.1%) contained no contrast medium. All solitary metastases found were situated in regions ordinarily opacified. Of 209 lymph nodes containing metastases, 32 (15.3%) showed little or no contrast medium.

The normal anatomic variations of the lymph vessels and the nodes are numerous. Knowledge of these variations is necessary if false diagnosis is to be avoided (8).

Wiljasalo's (11) claim in 1965, that a so-called projection difference index can be made, based on the hypothesis that normal nodes are flat while metastatic nodes are globular or grape-like, was investigated in a material of 220 removed lymph nodes. The transverse diameters were measured on films exposed in four projections. As a rule the metastatic lymph nodes deviated from the globular or grape-like shape and serious doubt is therefore expressed about the diagnostic value of the projection difference index.

Of great importance is the diagnostic accuracy of lymphography. In our total series of 300 patients with carcinoma of the cervix Stages I (275) and II (25), the detection rate was not sufficiently high to be solely relied upon in the choice of treatment. Combined with the findings at operation, however, lymphography was considered of value. It was always an aim to remove nodes classified as positive or uncertain.

It should be emphasized that this conclusion is based on lymphography in early stages of carcinoma of the cervix, and that it is not automatically valid for more advanced stages of the disease.

Accuracy depended on the size of the metastases and had little to do with the number of nodes involved. The new appearance or increase in size

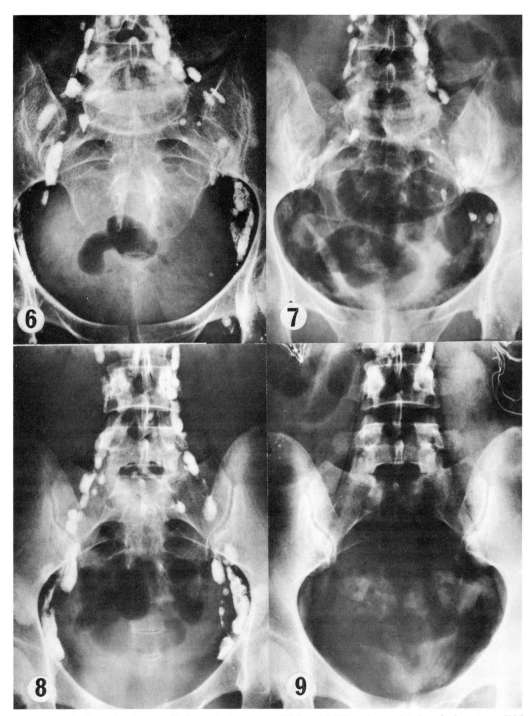

Fig. 16.6–16.9. Example of non-radical lymphadenectomy (16.6 and 16.7), and complete lymphadenectomy (16.8 and 16.9). From (7) and by courtesy of Academic Press Inc.

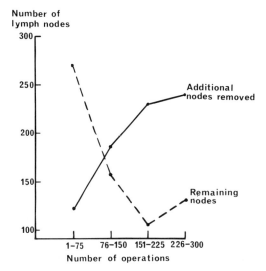

Fig. 16.10. Influence of intraoperative lymphographic control of lymph node dissection in 300 consecutive cases. From (7) and by courtesy of Academic Press Inc.

of a nodal defect during a 6-week period after intracavitary radium treatment before surgery, was the most reliable indication of metastases (Fig. 16.4). It was found that more than half of the patients with nodal defects >1 cm had metastases, while irregular defects <1 cm were generally non-metastatic.

Differentiation between filling and retention defects was difficult in most pelvic nodes, and a great importance attributed to such a distinction could not be confirmed. In this series, mainly consisting of Stage Ib carcinoma, complete obstruction with formation of collaterals was rare. Greater accuracy may be expected in more advanced stages of carcinoma of the cervix. Also in Stage Ib, however, empty node areas with deviation of lymph vessels are most reliable signs of metastases (Fig. 16.5).

As a conclusion to this extensive study it may be said that in the early stages of carcinoma of the cervix where radical surgery is planned, lymphography may help in removing all the lymph nodes (Fig. 16.6–9). This is made possible by intraoperative radiograms. During the study there was a decrease in the number of remaining lymph nodes from 3.4 to 1.6 per patient (Fig. 16.10).

A special importance is that after 10 years of follow-up, we have found that the survival rate of 197 patients with 0–3 remaining nodes was 85%, as compared to 74% for those with more than 4 remaining nodes. Pelvic recurrences occurred in 7.3% in those with 0–3 remaining nodes, and in 18% in those with >4 remaining nodes.

It has been claimed that lymphography will be of great value for the planning of treatment in carcinoma of the cervix Stages II, III and IV. We would, however, warn against this.

LYMPHOSCINTIGRAPHY

This isotope technique for visualizing the lymph nodes in the pelvis has become popular in some centers in Europe. Comparison between lymphoscintigraphy and lymphography was performed by zum Winkel and Müller in 1965 (12). There was a good correlation between the two methods. Several authors have used different isotopes to visualize the lymph nodes, and the method has been used to achieve a complete removal of the pelvic lymph nodes (13).

In our own unit, 24 patients with cervical cancer Stage Ib, operated in 1981, participated in an investigation with pelvic lymphoscintigraphy using the isotope ^{99}technecium colloid (14). Histologic examination showed that four of the patients had lymph node metastases. No difference in the lymphoscintigrams was found between the patients with pelvic metastases and those without. The removed involved lymph nodes did not contain less radioactive colloid than the normal nodes. Lymphoscintigraphy gives information about the localization of the lymph nodes which is of interest both during surgery and in determining the size of the radiation field. Complete removal of the pelvic lymph nodes can be achieved, but it is necessary to use an appropriate detector during operation to localize the nodes.

17

Radiotherapy in the treatment of carcinoma of the cervix.
The Oslo method

In 1903, Margareth Cleaves of New York City used radium for treatment of cancer of the cervix for the first time. Abbé was the first who reported the cure of a patient with cancer of the cervix by radium treatment alone. His first case was published in 1913 and showed a complete clinical regression for eight years (1).

Today there are four basic methods of intracavitary treatment of carcinoma of the cervix. In 1914, Forsell and Heyman defined the essential philosophy of radium treatment, now this is described as the "Stockholm method". Kottmeier further developed this method into an individualized, intracavitary, high intensive, intermittent type of radium treatment.

In Paris at the Institut du Radium, Regaud and Lacassagne developed the so-called "Paris method". This type of treatment can be described as an intracavitary, low intensive, protracted treatment with small amounts of radium.

Meredith and Tod derived the "Manchester method" from the Paris method during the 1930s. They wanted to base the intracavitary treatment on physical calculations, and they defined two points where a predetermined dosage should be delivered. These points of reference in the pelvis, points A and B, are defined as follows: Point A is located 2 cm proximal to the external os and 2 cm lateral to this point. Point B is defined as 2 cm proximal to the external os and 5 cm lateral to this point. This means that point A is located approximately in the parametrium where the ureter passes close to the cervix. Point B is located approximately in the region where we find the three chains of the external iliac glands, in the obturator fossa and along the external iliac vessels.

During the last decades a fourth approach to intracavitary radiation has been made by the introduction of rapid dose remote afterloading techniques with either caesium or cobalt sources. Recently also trials with the neutron emitting Californium 252 have been started.

Radiation treatment of cancer of the cervix aims to destroy tumor tissue without impairing the normal function of the surrounding tissue. The radiation dose therefore must be adjusted to the tolerance of the normal tissue.

As the radiation dose from an intracavitary radiation source decreases rapidly towards the pelvic walls, it is not possible to give a tumoricidal dose at point B by increasing the intracavitary dose. The result would be necrosis of the cervix and the medial parametrial tissue and an injury to the upper part of the vagina, the bladder and the rectum. The primary tumor in the cervix and the medial part of the parametrium can be destroyed by intracavitary radiation alone. Spread to the lateral part of the parametria and to the lymph nodes on the pelvic wall can be sterilized by an additional dose of external radiation. This was achieved in earlier days by giving a so-called four field technique with conventional 170–220 kV machines. Today high-voltage machines are used, preferably linear accelerators. Different combinations of intracavitary and external irradiation may give an adequate dose distribution both to the primary tumor and throughout the pelvis.

The Oslo method of treatment of carcinoma of the cervix follows the philosophy described here (2). Until the last decade intracavitary radium was the standard primary treatment. This intracavitary treatment is a modification of the Paris method and consists of two applications, one intrauterine and one intravaginal. The intrauterine applicator carries 20 or 30 mg radium, depending on the length of the uterine cavity. The intravaginal applicator bears 30 mg radium. The duration of each application is 120 hours (5 days) to produce between 6,000 and 7,000 rad (60–70 Gy) to point A (Fig. 17.1).

The intrauterine applicators are straight or slightly angulated cylinders measuring 6×80 mm (active length 68 mm) and 6×58 mm (active length 45 mm) for 30 and 20 mg radium, respectively. The filter equals 1.5 mm Pt.

The vaginal radium is applied in 10 mg tubes of platinum covered with steel with an active length of 13.5 mm and a filter equal to 1 mm Pt. The three vaginal tubes are usually placed on the shallow bell-shaped end of an applicator moulded by hand from a dental impression compound to fit the individual cervix and tumor. The tubes are placed sagittally with 20–40 mm separating the lateral tubes depending upon the size of the tumor (Fig. 17.2).

In the last decade, the Cathetron, an afterloading machine with cobalt sources has been introduced. We cannot give any details about this treatment, nor the results to date, because radium has been the main source for our intracavitary radiotherapy. It is well known that one of the essential advantages with radium is its long half life of more than 1,600 years. This means that almost no adjustment of treatment time has to be made because of radiation decay. The most important gamma radiation from radium comes from radium C and is equivalent to 2 MeV roentgen rays. This, unfortunately, makes radiation protection an important problem.

The Oslo system of intracavitary radiation is well tolerated, although the patients are confined

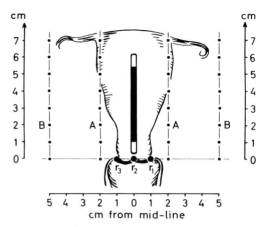

Fig. 17.2. Geometry of the intrauterine and vaginal applicators. r_1, r_2, r_3; sagitally placed platinum tubes with radium on the end of an individually made dental mold.

to bed for two periods of five days. Complications requiring interruption of the radium insertions are exceptional. With regard to radiation hygiene, constant dosimetry has revealed that the personnel in charge of the radium applications are kept well below the permissible tolerance limits of radiation. But it is obvious that from the radiation hygiene point of view an afterloading system is much better. However, high-intensity afterloading treatment may cause more complications especially from the small bowels. We have been slow, therefore, in taking part in the development of such a high intensity intracavitary treatment, but afterloading with high intensity sources undoubtedly has some definite advantages for the patients. They will receive treatment over a few minutes and can be up and about between the fractions given. The cure rate for afterloading treatment with high intensity sources equals that of radium irradiation (3).

The first results from the Norwegian Radium Hospital concerning radiotherapy of cervical cancer were published in 1937 (4). At that time intracavitary treatment was followed by a four field technique with external X-ray treatment. Since 1956 external radiation has been given by high-voltage machines. Today we prefer the flexible linear accelerators.

It is well known that radiation damage to the surrounding normal tissue is the limiting factor

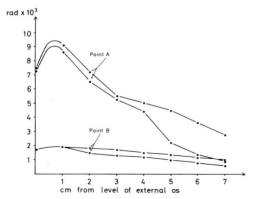

Fig. 17.1. Dose distribution by intracavitary radium irradiation after the Oslo method (2).

in radiation therapy of malignant disease. The normal structures in question in cancer of the cervix are the rectum, bladder and small bowel. In 1965 we reviewed the cases of cancer of the cervix treated in our unit from two different time periods with special regard to radiation complications (5). During the first period, external irradiation was given with conventional radiotherapy machines, and during the latter period the patients received X-rays from a 31 MeV betatron machine.

The radium system was unchanged during these two periods. The contribution from external irradiation increased from approximately 20 Gy to 30 Gy at mid-pelvis from the first to the second period. The radiation lesions were graded according to Kottmeier and Gray (6). Slight subjective discomfort (Grade 1) was not recorded. Grade 2 comprised necrosis, ulcerations and protracted bleeding, and Grade 3 comprised fistulas, stenosis requiring colostomy, or death from radiation complications. During the first period, when conventional external radiotherapy was given, 2.5% Grade 2 lesions and 1% Grade 3 lesions were observed, and during the second period, 5.9% Grade 2 lesions and 1.1% Grade 3 lesions. A consistent correlation was found between dose/time versus complications/survival. It was concluded that late radiation complications were relatively infrequent with the Oslo method of combined intracavitary radium and external radiotherapy.

It is quite obvious, however, that in the future afterloading technique will be our brachyradiotherapy of choice. Both patients and personnel will benefit from this charge.

18
Combined treatment of carcinoma of the cervix Stage Ib

In 1954 Joe Vincent Meigs stated, "There is not, nor should there be, any attempt to make the surgical treatment rival radium and X-ray treatment. The two methods are partners in the attack of the disease, for unquestionably some patients will be cured by the one method and not by the other" (1). Since the 1930s, the chiefs of the Department of Gynecologic Oncology at the Norwegian Radium Hospital have all been well trained in surgery. The first chiefs received their training in radiotherapy through visits to Sweden and France. It may seem strange that the Paris method of radium treatment was chosen. It must be appreciated, however, that the distances from the different regions in Norway to this central institution in Oslo are so great that it would be difficult to apply the Stockholm method to all patients. The Stockholm method would necessitate the patient travelling a very long distance two or three times before radium treatment was completed. The distance from the northern part of Norway to Oslo can be compared to the distance between Oslo and Rome in Italy. This was certainly one of the main factors in the choice of the Paris method.

As to the surgical treatment of cervical carcinoma, it must also be appreciated that those who have been responsible for the treatment principles have all been gynecologists with a long training in surgery. Therefore, from the very beginning in 1932, combined radiological-surgical treatment of carcinoma of the cervix became popular.

The first report about treatment of carcinoma of the cervix in our unit appeared in 1941 (2). The 5-year survival rate for 142 patients in all stages was 36%. In the eighteenth *Annual Report* (3), the 5-year crude survival rate for all stages was 68.6% and corrected survival rate 73.7%. The main reason for this large difference is of course that the disease is now discovered at an earlier stage. The

increase in survival rate is demonstrated in Fig. 18.1.

The combined radiological-surgical treatment, which started in the 1940s, comprised full radiation treatment followed 6–8 weeks later by what was called prophylactic simple hysterectomy. Schjøtt-Rivers published his results in 73 Stage I cases and 43 Stage II cases in 1951 (4). His successor as chief of the Gynecologic Oncology Department, Dahle, after visiting Meigs in Boston, introduced combined radiological-surgical treatment consisting of primary radium irradiation followed 6–8 weeks later by radical hysterectomy with lymphadenectomy. His philosophy was close to that published by Schlink in 1960 (5) and Stallworthy in 1964 (6). Both the so-called prophylactic simple hysterectomy series (4) and the series published by Dahle (7) were highly selective. The results, however, were encouraging. Koller (8) in 1964 pointed to the fact that the most important problem in the treatment of early stages of carcinoma of the cervix was the spread to the lymph nodes.

In a consecutive and non-selective number of cases, all patients were given intracavitary radium and eight weeks later readmitted for further evaluation and therapy. If gynecological examination including cytologic smears, biopsies and endocervical curettage did not show any signs of residual tumor growth in the cervix, extraperitoneal pelvic lymphadenectomy was performed. If any clinical, cytologic or histologic signs of residual tumor growth were found, an extended Wertheim operation was the treatment of choice. Patients with histologically proven lymph node metastases received additional external high-voltage treatment to a pelvic field. During the years 1958–61 a total of 196 extraperitoneal lymphadenectomies were performed. In the course of the follow-up in this series, however, it was discovered that about 12%

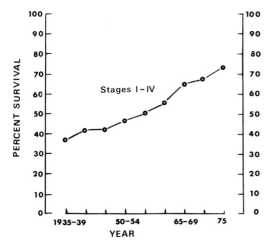

Fig. 18.1. Treatment results in carcinoma of the cervix in the years 1935–75.

of the patients developed local recurrence in the cervix. The diagnostic procedures with smears, biopsies and endocervical curettage thus seemed unsatisfactory with regard to detecting tumor foci deep in the cervix. As a consequence of this, and as experience with the extended Wertheim operation increased, more and more radical operations were performed.

Since 1962 the standard treatment of cervical cancer Stage Ib has been preoperative radium treatment followed 6 weeks later by radical hysterectomy and transperitoneal lymphadenectomy. Only patients regarded as poor operative risks and patients in the older age groups are excluded and treated by radium and external high-voltage irradiation.

The so-called extended Wertheim series reached 498 cases in 1965. An evaluation of the extraperitoneal lymphadenectomy series and the extended Wertheim series was presented in 1968 (9). In particular, the problems of lymph node metastases were scrutinized. In the total series of 694 patients, 20% of metastases were found to the lymph nodes in the pelvis. Eight weeks after intracavitary radium treatment, so-called residual tumor in the cervix was found higher in the patients with adenocarcinoma compared to those with squamous cell carcinoma. Altogether 16% had histologically proven residual tumor, although it must be stressed that we have no proof that these residual tumor cells were viable at the time of surgery.

It was quite obvious, nevertheless, that the occurrence of metastases was of the highest prognostic significance. In Fig. 18.2 and 18.3 it can be seen that if no residual tumor was found in the cervix at operation, the 5-year survival rate was 92.4%. So-called residual tumor alone did not seem to influence the survival rate very much, but metastases did so appreciably. The combination of residual tumor in the cervix and metastases carried the poorest prognosis.

Altogether 694 cases were followed for 2–8 years. It is of interest to note the causes of death. Table 18.1 shows that altogether 5.9% died of distant metastases, 3.5% of extensive pelvic spread at time of operation, 1.4% of intercurrent disease, and there were two patients who died postoperatively, one of lung embolism and one of intestinal obstruction. This means that about 10% of the deaths could be classified as "inevitable". The crude survival rate in this series was 83.5% and the corrected survival rate 88%.

Since these earlier reports we have reviewed our treatment results several times (10, 11, 12). We have paid attention not only to the ultimate treatment results, but also to complications. Especial

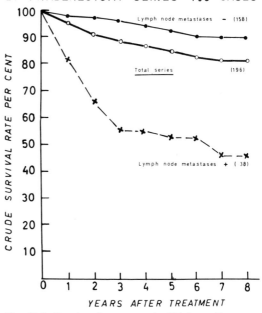

Fig. 18.2. Results of treatment in 196 Stage Ib cases treated by intracavitary radium followed 8 weeks later by extraperitoneal lymphadenectomy (9). See text.

EXTENDED WERTHEIM SERIES 498 CASES

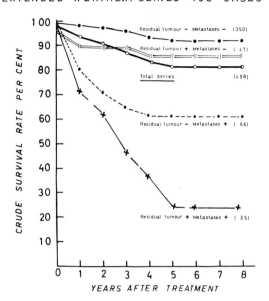

Fig. 18.3. Results of treatment related to the occurrence of lymph node metastases and residual tumor in 498 cases of Stage Ib cases undergoing radium irradiation followed 8 weeks later by radical hysterectomy and lymphadenectomy (9).

Table 18.1. "Inevitable" deaths in cancer of the cervix Stage Ib treated with a combination of radium and extended Wertheim operation (498 cases) or radium and extraperitonel lymphadenectomy (196 cases), – 694 patients followed 2–8 years

Cause of death	No. of patients	Per cent
Distant metastases	41	5.9
Extensive pelvic spread at operation	24	3.5
Postoperative deaths	2	0.3
Intercurrent disease	10	1.4
Total	77	11.1

attention has been paid to the problem of lymph node metastases, urologic complications and the occurrence of lymphedema.

In 1973 a series of 537 patients with Stage Ib carcinoma of the cervix treated by combined radium and Wertheim hysterectomy with lymphadenectomy was published (10). The overall 5-year survival rate was 88.3%. The finding of positive pelvic lymph nodes was the most significant prognostic factor. The 5-year survival was 62.9% for those patients with node involvement as compared with 92.9% for those in whom lymphatic extension was not appreciated. The significance of location and number of positive node groups was pointed out. If positive nodes were found above the common iliac bifurcation, 67% died from cancer as compared to 39% of those in whom positive node groups were found below the common iliac bifurcation. The old statement that the younger patients have a poorer prognosis in cervical cancer than the older patients could not be confirmed. The incidence of significant urologic complications was 2.8%. It was concluded that preoperative radium will reduce the need for extensive parametrial dissection, with subsequent bladder denervation, for complete skeletonization of the lower ureter and for removal of a large vaginal cuff. A third survey of urinary and gastrointestinal complications was made in 1983 (11). Complications from the urinary and gastrointestinal tract in this series was 20 out of 612 (3.3%). Especially those with lymph node metastases who receive postoperative irradiation against a pelvic field are apt to develop complications.

It may be justified to conclude that the number

Table 18.2. Significance of location and number of positive node groups

Node groups	Total No.	Dead of cancer No.	Per cent
Above common iliac bifurcation	15	10	66.6
Below common iliac bifurcation	61	24	39.3
One group	45	19	42.2
Two groups	21	7	33.3
More than two groups	10	8	80.0

and severity of the complications after combined treatment must be considered acceptable when considering that the patient has a deadly disease.

One complication that has not received much attention in the literature is the occurrence of lymphedema and lymphocysts. We published our experience in this field in 1978 (12). About 5% suffer from severe lymphedema after radical hysterectomy with lymphadenectomy. Whether the addition of external irradiation influences this complication is uncertain, but there is no doubt that if a patient who has undergone radical hysterectomy with pelvic lymphadenectomy gets a streptococcus inflammation with lymphangitis, severe lymphedema may develop which may be absolutely intractable. We have tried to treat lymphedema in such patients with a lymphovenous shunt. This means that we implant one of the lymph nodes in the inguinal region into the greater saphenous or the femoral vein. In approximately 25–30% a relief of lymphedema will be achieved.

RADICAL HYSTERECTOMY AND PELVIC LYMPHADENECTOMY

The technique of radical surgery for carcinoma of the cervix varies from clinic to clinic and even from surgeon to surgeon within the same unit. This special operation has been the focus of attention of gynecologic oncologists far back to the turn of this century, when Clark in 1895 (13) and Wertheim in 1900 (14) published their results on radical hysterectomy. Okabayashi presented his modifications in 1921 (15), while Meigs introduced obligatory lymphadenectomy in 1951 (1). One year earlier, Schlink (5) had recommended radical hysterectomy for cervical cancer after a full course of intracavitary radium irradiation, a method that was adopted by Stallworthy (6) and by Dahle at the Norwegian Radium Hospital (7).

As pointed out by Gusberg (16), the operation technique is essentially an anatomic dissection of the pelvis, the manner of the dissection varying from surgeon to surgeon. Some prefer to do an "en bloc" dissection and strive to remove the uterus with the parametriae and the lymph nodes in one piece. Others prefer to remove the uterus first, before plucking the nodes along the vessels and on the pelvic floor by sharp dissection with scis-

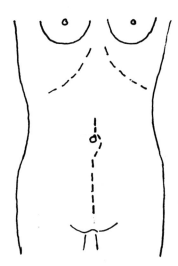

Fig. 18.4. Incision line for radical hysterectomy.

sors. Still others prefer to do the lymphadenectomy first before removing the uterus with the three retinaculae which include the parametriae, the sacrouterine ligaments and the pillars of the bladder.

It is this last procedure that the author of this book follows. In removing the bundles of fat tissue containing the lymph vessels and nodes, a combination of sharp and blunt dissection has been found very satisfactory, reducing bleeding and operation time.

Three clearly defined lymph node groups—the common iliac, the external iliac and the obturator nodes—are loosened by an initial dissection with scissors. With ring forceps and the fingers, and when the correct dissection plane has been found, the bundles can easily be stripped off the vessels and the pelvic floor with very little bleeding. The internal iliac (hypogastric) and the presacral nodes usually have to be plucked away, preferably after the other lymph nodes and the uterus have been removed, i.e. at the end of the operation when the operation field is completely dry. After the vessels and the pelvic floor have been freed of fat tissue and lymph nodes, the uterus with the retinaculae and the ureter are clearly defined, and the parametriae, the bladder pillars and the sacrouterine ligaments can be dissected free and removed as radically as necessary in accordance with the extent of the tumor.

The steps of the operation are as follows (see Figs. 18.4–18.28):

1. A long abdominal incision is made extending from the symphysis to about 3–4 cm above the umbilicus (Fig. 18.4). It is not necessary to clamp the small bleeders in the abdominal wall except for the two superficial epigastric arteries which are found in the lowermost angle of the incision. All other vessels stop oozing as soon as the abdominal retractor is inserted. We prefer the Wachenfeldt retractor because it allows excellent access to all pelvic structures and also to the common iliac and the periaortic region up to about L3–4.

2. After the retractor has been inserted, the lymph node areas in the pelvis and along the aorta are carefully palpated. This is then followed by an exploration of the total abdominal cavity as described in Chapter 38, p. 187 (Fig. 38.1).

If no extension of the tumor is found outside the pelvis, and if there are no massive or firmly fixed palpable nodes in the pelvis, the operation can start. It has to be borne in mind that even although cancer involved nodes firmly fixed to the iliac vessels can usually be removed by sharp dissection without any bleeding problems, our experience in a large series of such cases is that removal is of no benefit to the patient. It is better to close the abdomen and to give external irradiation. Whatever procedure is chosen, the patient will die from her disease, but surgical removal of fixed lymph nodes carries more and severe complications.

3. The intestines are now packed away. We prefer one single large pack which keeps the intestines well out of the operation field. The sigmoid colon will be stretched upwards and slightly to the left. Two long, slightly curved, slender clamps are placed close to the side walls of the uterus and include the broad ligament down to the origin of the ascending branches of the uterine arteries. When this has been done the assistant can pull the uterus forwards towards the symphysis. The infundibulopelvic and the round ligaments are stretched and clearly defined (Fig. 18.5).

4. Using one long chromic catgut or mercilene suture, the infundibulopelvic and round ligaments are stitch-ligated (Fig. 18.6 and 18.7). The ligaments are cut through and the peritoneum incised between them and upwards on the medial side of the ovarian vessels. A "stocking-protected" S-shaped large speculum is inserted to keep the sigmoid colon away, and the common iliac artery appears in the upper part of operation field (Fig. 18.8).

5. To facilitate the removal of fat and lymph nodes, three "dry spaces" are opened up. The first is located medially between the peritoneum with the attached ureter and the iliac vessels (the pararectal space); the second space is found between the pelvic wall and the vessels, while the third, the perivesical or Latzko's fossa, is located on the lateral side of the bladder and cervix, close to the anterior pelvic wall and medial to the obliterated umbilical artery (Fig. 18.9).

In dissecting these three spaces, where bleeding should not occur if the correct dissecting planes are found, the author prefers to use long, thin, blunt scissors and the second and third fingers of the left hand. One should avoid using the edges of the scissors (Fig. 18.10). At the point where the blunt tip of the scissors is located in Fig. 18.10, two small vessels will be found between the psoas muscle and the iliac artery and vein. With experience it is possible to feel these two vessels, and to avoid bleeding small clips should be applied. During the whole operation, it is wise to use metal clips instead of ligatures on most of the bleeders located deep in the pelvis. The lateral dry space should be opened up to the sacroiliac joint, deep down to the pelvic floor, so that the obturator nerve is clearly in sight.

6. The tissue bundles which are to be removed from the vessels and pelvic floor are now well defined. With ring forceps the bundle lying anterior to the bifurcation is grasped, lifted up, and cut distally (Fig. 18.11). The common iliac nodes are then dissected with the second and third fingers of the right hand underneath the bundle and the thumb on the anterior side. With finger dissection it is possible to get up to about the third or fourth lumbar vertebra lateral to the aorta, and then to "milk" the fat tissue with the lymph vessels and nodes away without using scissors. If bleeding occurs, it will usually be slight. It is best just to pack the area and to let the assistant make

compression with the S-shaped speculum. "Blind" clamping will lead to profuse bleeding and should be absolutely avoided.

7. The cut end of the bundle, the proximal part of the external node group, is now grasped with the ring forceps, lifted up, and by dissection with the scissors freed from the bifurcation of the arteries and from the underlying external iliac vein (Fig. 18.12). When the dissecting plane is clear, it is possible by finger dissection to strip the whole group of external iliac nodes down to the inguinal canal. The last node, which is easily palpable, is the large lateral lacunar node. When it has been located, it should be lifted away, together with the tissue bundle, from the vessels and positioned against the anterior abdominal wall. This is simple to do when the vessels are pushed down with a small gauze sponge (Fig. 18.13).

8. The third group of nodes which must be removed is the medial external or the obturator group. The uppermost part of this tissue bundle is grasped at a point deep lateral to the lower part of the common iliac vessels where it was separated from the common iliac nodes. *This is a crucial point.* It is necessary to be careful so that none of the three short veins which pass into the pelvic wall are torn. Bleeding from these veins is difficult to control (see Fig. 18.25). It is advisable to lift up the tissue anterior to these veins and to let it fall off the ring forceps. This manoeuver should be repeated until the veins can be clearly seen. The bundle of fat and lymph nodes can then be grasped and pushed distally and medially under the vessels. The ring forceps is moved over to the medial side, and the whole obturator node group is stripped by finger dissection distally and forwards towards the inguinal canal (Fig. 18.14). The end of this bundle is easy to determine because the node of Cloquet lying on the medial side of the vessels in the inguinal canal has a characteristic almond shape.

Sometimes the obturator vessels do not follow the course of the nerve, but originate at the lower part of the external iliac vessels and thus cross over the nerve. This anomaly may be detected by the dissecting fingers. If the vessels are torn, it is best to rapidly remove the fat tissue with nodes before they are clamped. The bleeding is usually

not troublesome, and the bleeders are easily seen when all fat tissue has been removed.

9. The iliac vessels have now been dissected completely free. To locate the uterine artery, it is helpful to clamp the obliterated umbilical artery and to stretch it upwards. The hypogastric and uterine arteries come into view, and a clamp is placed exactly in the angle between the umbilical and the uterine arteries (Fig. 18.15). The arteries are cut and ligated. The superior vesical artery will also be cut and ligated with this technique, but we have never had any trouble with an insufficient blood supply to the bladder.

10. The uterus is pulled over to the contralateral side, and the ureter is isolated where it enters the ureteral tunnel. The attachment to the peritoneum is still intact all the way down. With a long, slender clamp, the tunnel is opened up and the part of the parametrium which passes over the ureter to the uterus is identified. During this dissection, care should be taken to avoid damaging the vessel-containing sheath of the ureter. The isolated part of the parametrium and the uterine veins are freed bit by bit down on the pelvic floor with a long slender clamp, cut and ligated. There are always several uterine veins. In this way the ureter is freed to the point where it enters the bladder (Fig. 18.16).

11. The uterus is pulled upwards, the bladder peritoneum incised, and the bladder pushed as far down on the anterior vaginal wall as necessary (Fig. 18.17).

12. The bladder pillars are dissected free by passing a long, slender clamp through the tissue just in the angle where the ureter enters the bladder wall (Fig. 18.18).

Another clamp is passed through just anterior to the ureter to dissect free the bladder pillar's extension onto the cervix. The pillar and part of the parametrium in this location can now be cut completely free from the side wall of the bladder and the ureter (Fig. 18.19).

13. When exactly the same type of dissection has been performed on the other side, the uterus is pulled towards the symphysis, and the recto-vaginal space is opened (Fig. 18.20). The dissection

continues, cutting taking place through the perito-neum over the sacrouterine ligaments. With a fin-ger on each side of the ligament, and the ureter pushed laterally, a solid clamp is now placed on each ligament. The clamp can be pushed far down on the pelvic floor, care being taken not to inter-fere with the anterior rectal wall (Fig. 18.21). The ligaments are cut, and can be stitch-ligated at this point in time or after the uterus has been removed.

14. The uterus is once more pulled proximally and the anterior vaginal wall opened (Fig. 18.22). The ureters are then completely freed from the cervix and vagina, and it is a simple matter to continue the incision in the vagina also on the posterior side. The uterus can then be removed along with an ample part of the vagina. The ureter will have no attachment to the peritoneum for a length of 4–6 cm, but the vessel-containing sheath should be intact.

15. The vagina is closed with a continuous suture. The author prefers to stitch-ligate the sacrouterine ligaments at this point and to use the solid chro-mic-catgut stitch to draw the corners of the vagina up to the ligaments (Fig. 18.23).

16. The whole operation field should now be completely dry, and dissection of the deep internal iliac and presacral glands is simplified (Fig. 18.24). At the same time, all the node areas should be explored for remaining nodes. Areas where nodes are usually difficult to dissect during the initial lymphadenectomy are deep down on the medial side of the hypogastric vessels and underneath the common iliac vein (Fig. 18.25).

17. The bladder and the rectal peritoneum are now sutured down to the vaginal wall (Fig. 18.26). No attempt is made to peritonealize the lateral pelvic walls. We have never had any difficulty with for example intestinal obstruction by having omitted to attempt to make some sort of a roof of peritoneum over the vessels and the pelvic floor.

The abdomen is closed after suction drains have been placed to each side of the pelvic floor. These are kept for 3–5 days depending upon the amount of fluid that is obtained.

An example of the specimens removed by the technique described here is shown in Fig. 18.27 and 18.28.

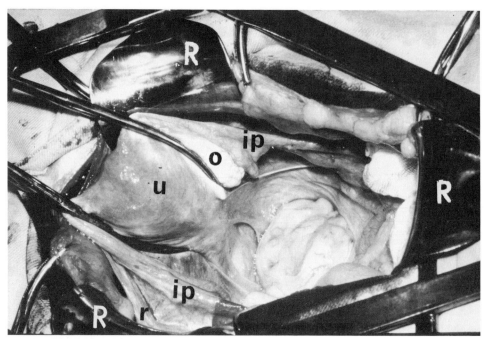

Fig. 18.5. Clamps on both sides of uterus (u). The intestines packed away, R: Wachenfeldt retractor, ip: infundibulo-pelvic ligaments, r: round ligament, o: ovary.

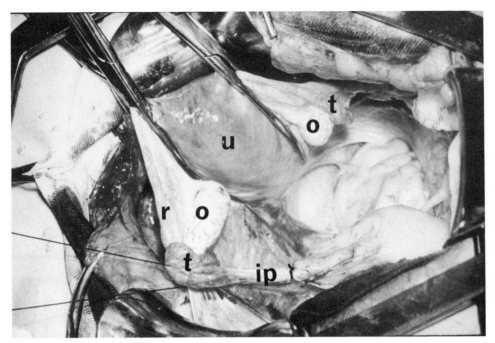

Fig. 18.6. Stitch-ligation of infundibulopelvic ligament (ip). r: round ligament; o: ovaries, t: tubes, u: uterus.

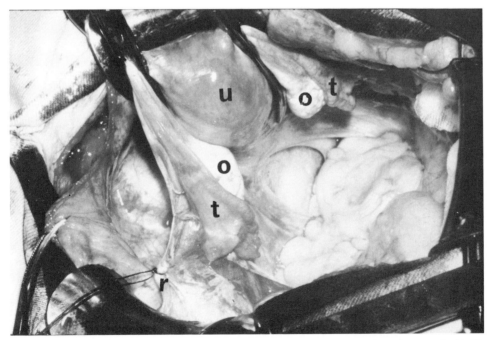

Fig. 18.7. The round ligament (r) has been stitch-ligated and the peritoneum opened up down to the bladder. u: uterus, t: tubes, o: ovaries.

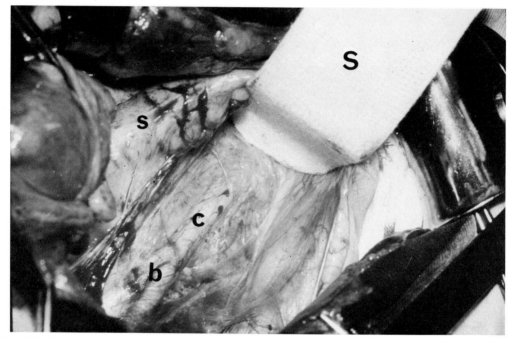

Fig. 18.8. The peritoneum has been incised upwards medially to the infundibulopelvic ligament and a large S-shaped speculum covered by a gauze "stocking" (S) is pulling the sigmoid colon (s) away from the operation field. b: bifurcation of common iliac artery (c).

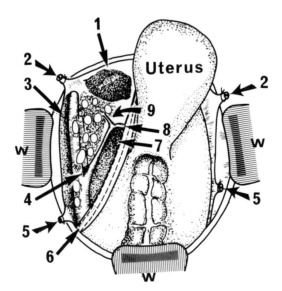

Fig. 18.9. Opening of three dry lateral spaces: 1: paravesical space, 3: space between iliac vessels and pelvic wall, and 7: pararectal space. 2: round ligaments, 4: bifurcation of iliac vessels, 5: infundibulopelvic ligaments, 6: ureter, 8: uterine artery, 9: obliterated umbilical artery, w: Wachenfeldt retractor.

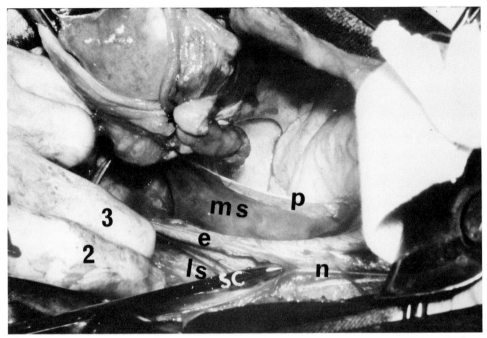

Fig. 18.10. Opening of the lateral dry space (ls) with blunt scissors (sc) and the second (2) and third (3) fingers of the left hand. p: peritoneum with attached ureter, ms: medial dry space, e: external iliac artery, n: genitofemoral nerve.

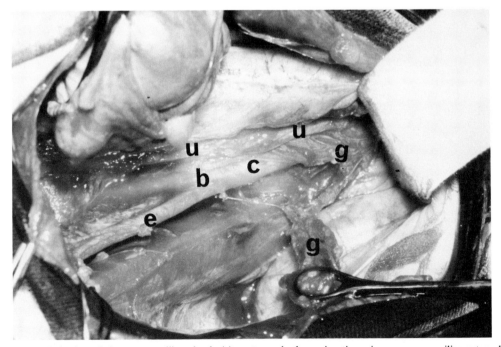

Fig. 18.11. Stripping of the common iliac glands (g) up towards the periaortic region. c: common iliac artery, b: bifurcation, e: external iliac artery, u: ureter.

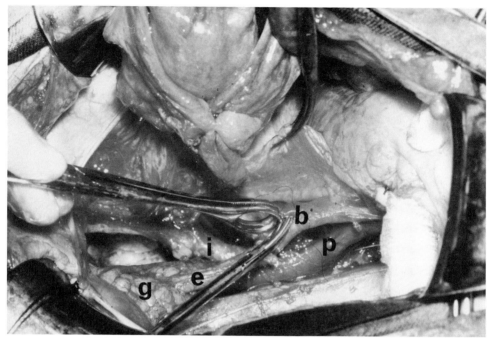

Fig. 18.12. Cutting loose the external iliac group from the bifurcation and the underlying external iliac vein using ring forceps and scissors. b: bifurcation, e: external iliac artery, i: internal iliac artery, g: lower part of bundle with external iliac glands, p: psoas muscle.

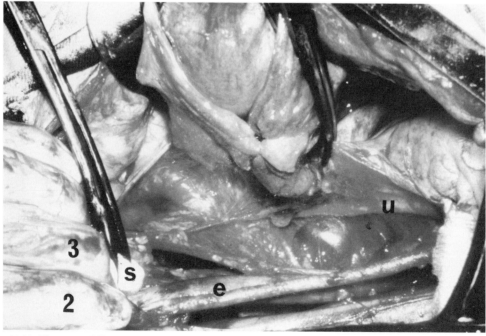

Fig. 18.13. The external iliac vessels have been stripped (e) and the lateral lacunar gland is pressed up against the abdominal wall by the second (2) and third (3) fingers of the left hand. The vessels are pushed down with a small gauze sponge (s), u: ureter.

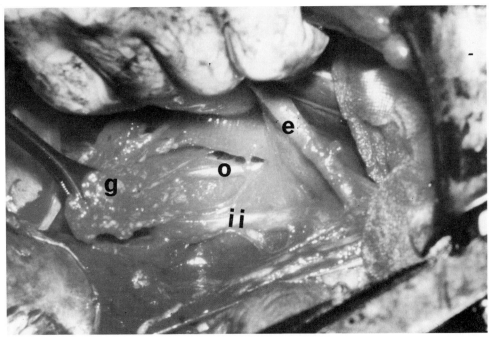

Fig. 18.14. The obturator glands ((g) here shown on the right pelvic floor) have been picked up on the lateral side of the external iliac vessels (e), pushed underneath the vessels, and will now be stripped from the obturator nerve (o) and the pelvic floor. ii: internal iliac artery.

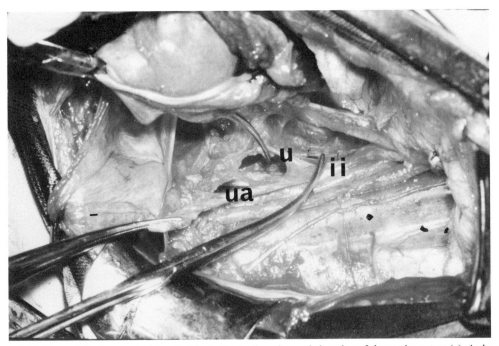

Fig. 18.15. The umbilical artery (ua) is raised to facilitate dissection and clamping of the uterine artery (u). A clamp is put on the angle of these two vessels exactly at the point where they emerge from the internal iliac artery (ii).

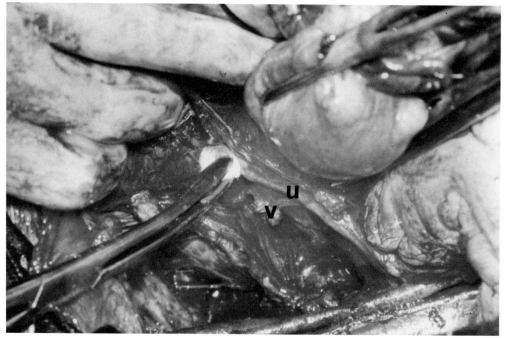

Fig. 18.16. The veins (v) and the part of the parametrium passing over the ureter (u) on the lateral side have been clamped, cut through and ligated.

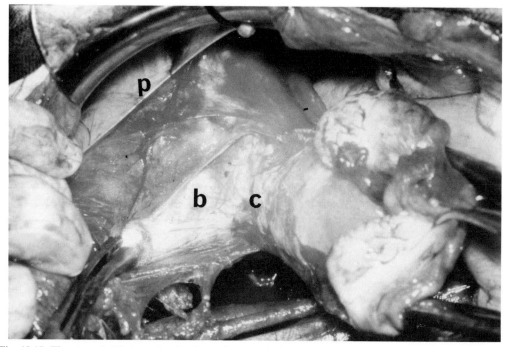

Fig. 18.17. The uterus is lifted proximally, the peritoneum (p) incised and the bladder (b) dissected free from the cervix (c) and the vagina.

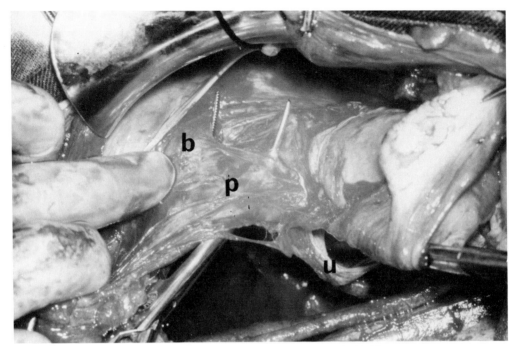

Fig. 18.18. The bladder pillar (p) is dissected free from the ureter (u) and the bladder.

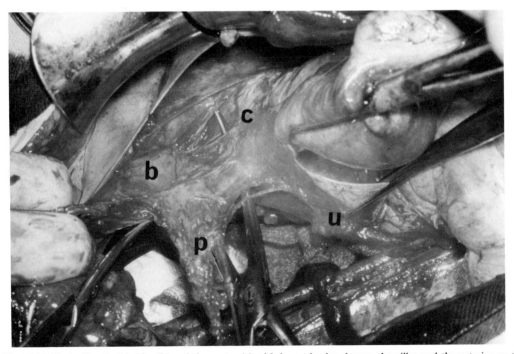

Fig. 18.19. Protecting the bladder (b) and the ureter (u) with long, slender clamps, the pillar and the anterior part of the parametrium (p) are cut away from the lateral and anterior bladder wall.

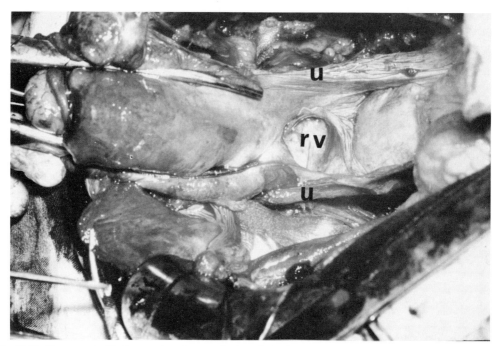

Fig. 18.20. The uterus is lifted up against the symphysis and the dry rectovaginal space opened (rv) u: ureter.

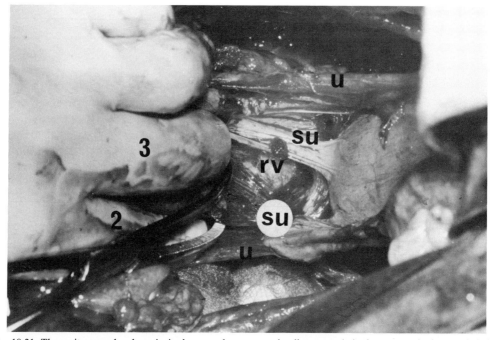

Fig. 18.21. The peritoneum has been incised across the sacrouterine ligaments (su), the rectovaginal space (rv), has been opened up down on the posterior vaginal wall, and a strong clamp is being placed on the left sacrouterine ligament. The ureter is protected by the second (2) finger of the left hand, while the third (3) finger is placed on the medial side of the ligament, u: ureter.

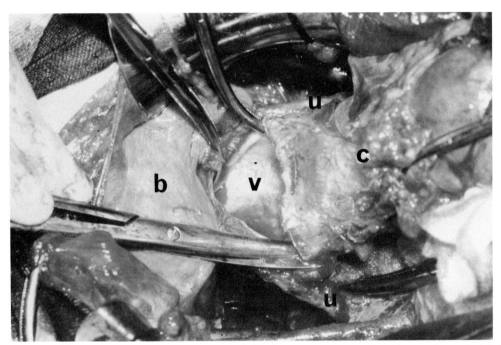

Fig. 18.22. The uterus is lifted proximally, the bladder (b) has been dissected free from the anterior vaginal wall, and the vagina (v) is opened. Using scissors, both ureters (u) are dissected free from the vagina and the cervix, leaving 4–6 cm free from the peritoneum, but with intact vascular sheath. c: cervix.

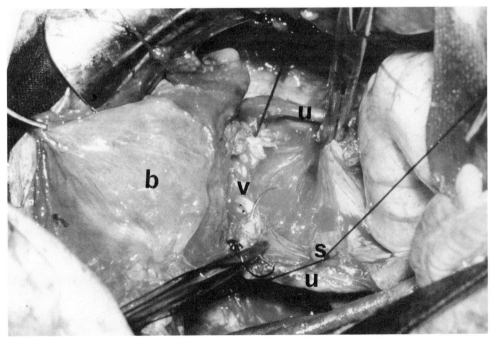

Fig. 18.23. The uterus has been removed, the vagina (v) closed by a continuous suture, and the sacrouterine ligaments (s) stitch-ligated and sutured down to the vagina. b: bladder, u: ureter.

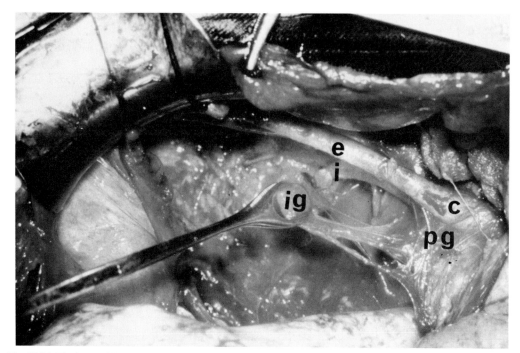

Fig. 18.24. The internal iliac glands (ig) and the presacral glands (pg) are removed. c: common iliac, e: external iliac and i: internal iliac artery.

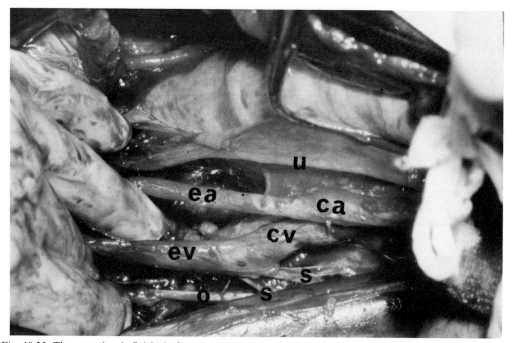

Fig. 18.25. The operation is finished after all lymph node areas have been explored once more. The ureter, the vessels and the obturator nerve are clearly identified. u: ureter, ca: common iliac artery, ea: external iliac artery, cv: common iliac vein, ev: external iliac vein, s: lateral sacral veins, o: obturator nerve.

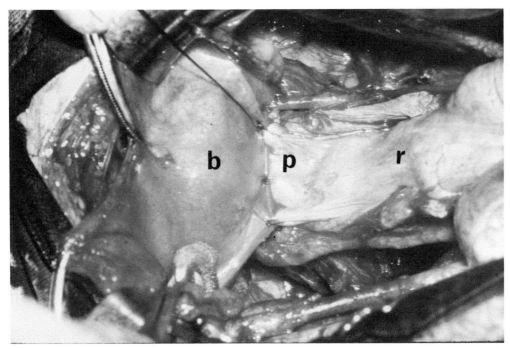

Fig. 18.26. The peritoneum (p) is sutured down to the vagina. No attempt is made to peritonealize the lateral pelvic walls. b: bladder, r: rectum.

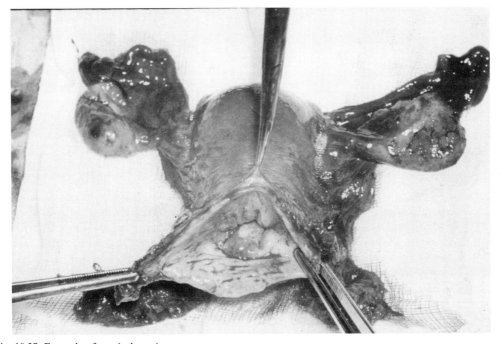

Fig. 18.27. Example of surgical specimen.

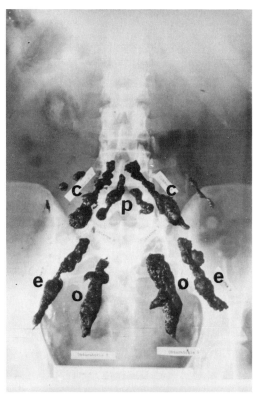

Fig. 18.28. Example of lymph node specimens placed on the preoperative lymphogram. e: external iliac, o: obturator, c: common iliac and p: presacral groups.

SURGERY, RADIOTHERAPY, OR COMBINED TREATMENT?

"There is not, nor should there be, any attempt to make surgical treatment rival radium and X-ray treatment. The two methods are partners in the attack on the disease, for unquestionably some patients will be cured by the one method and not by the other" (Meigs 1954 (1)).

In the later stages of cervical cancer there seems to be general agreement that radiotherapy is to be preferred. In Stages Ib and IIa, however, the results obtained with expert surgery are the same as with expert radiotherapy, or in our experience with combined treatment. There is one important aspect that we see today, however. More and more young women are admitted with relatively small Stage Ib or Stage IIa tumors. They can easily be cured by primary surgery and it is possible to preserve ovarian function. This latter factor should not be forgotten. For some years we have

been mostly interested in the so-called 5-year results of our treatment. But today we should also think of the hormonal status and the future sexual life of patients undergoing treatment for cervical cancer. Ovarian metastases are so infrequent that, especially in the early stages, it is unnecessary to remove the ovaries. Transposition to the lateral colonic gutters should be performed routinely so that eventual postoperative external irradiation because of lymph node metastases will not interfere with their function.

In the larger Stage Ib and IIa tumors we still feel more secure when we sterilize the tumor with intracavitary radiation before surgery. The risk of cutting through the edge of the tumor will definitely be reduced by this combined method. Primary surgery in these cases must only be undertaken by skilled gynecologic oncologists. And it is our philosophy that to get this skill, centralization of treatment is absolutely necessary.

19

Histologic classification, grading and prognosis in Stage Ib cervical carcinoma

The variety of growth patterns in cervical carcinoma has intrigued investigators for many years. As early as 1923, Martzloff published a paper about the relative malignancy of cancer of the cervix uteri as indicated by the predominant cancer cell type (1). Three years later, in 1926, Broders (2) discussed carcinoma-grading and practical applications. More recently, such cellular and morphological characteristics as keratinization, cellular size, and degree of differentiation have been invoked as affecting the overall survival in this disease. Large cell epithelial carcinomas, particularly those with keratine formation, have been depicted as less aggressive than the non-keratinizing, anaplastic carcinomas (3) (Fig. 19.1, 19.2 and 19.3).

The assumption that small cell carcinomas are more aggressive has never been statistically supported. The hypothesis was studied in 245 Ib cases uniformly treated during the years 1970–73. To evaluate prognosis two parameters were selected: lymph node metastases and crude survival rate (4).

All 245 consecutively and identically treated patients with Stage Ib lesions received two 5-day radium courses according to the modified Paris method. Radical hysterectomy and pelvic lymphadenectomy followed six weeks later. Lymphogram comparison films at the time of surgery helped to assure a thorough dissection from the aorta to the inguinal ligaments. Those women who had one or more metastatic lymph nodes

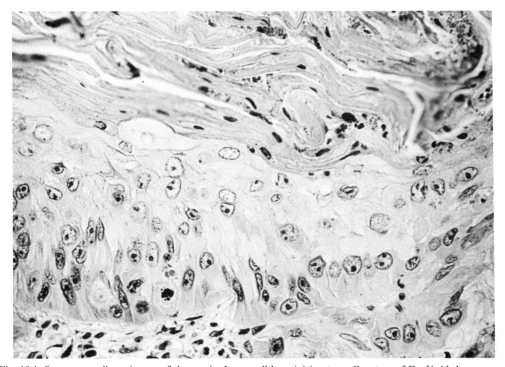

Fig. 19.1. Squamous cell carcinoma of the cervix. Large cell keratinizing type. Courtesy of Dr. V. Abeler.

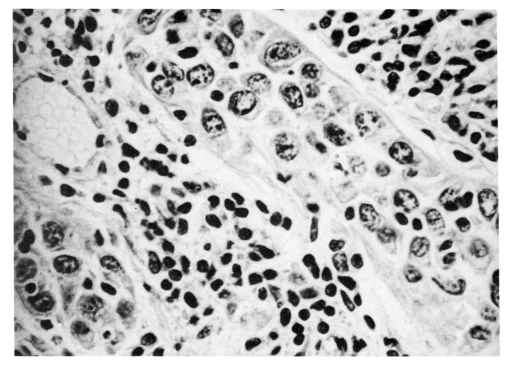

Fig. 19.2. Large cell non-keratizing type. Courtesy of Dr. V. Abeler.

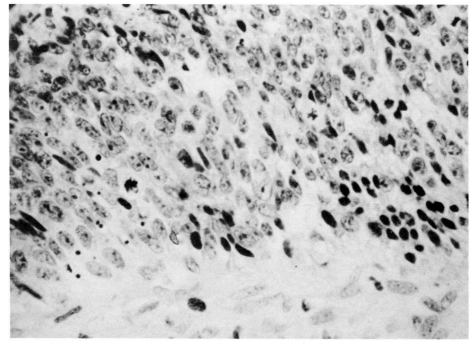

Fig. 19.3. Small cell carcinoma of the cervix.

Table 19.1.

Histologic group	Number	Percentage
Large cell keratinizing carcinomas	54	22
Large cell nonkeratinizing carcinomas	139	57
Small cell carcinomas	15	6
Adenocarcinomas	37	15
Total	245	100

Table 19.2. Lymph node metastases in relation to histologic tumor type

Histologic group	Metastases	
	Number/total number in group	Percentage
Large cell keratinizing carcinomas	13/54	25
Large cell nonkeratinizing carcinomas	35/139	25
Small cell carcinomas	4/15	27
Adenocarcinomas	9/37	24
All cases	61/245	25

Table 19.3. 2-Year Tumor-Free Survival Rate

Group	Number/total number in group	Percentage
Large cell keratinizing carcinomas	47/54	87
Large cell nonkeratinizing carcinomas	123/139	88
Small cell carcinomas	12/15	80
Adenocarcinomas	32/37	86
All cases	214/245	87

received postoperative radiation therapy consisting of a tumor dose to the whole pelvis of 40 Gy, shielding of the central field of 20 Gy. It is calculated that the preoperative radium irradiation added approximately 10 Gy to the lymph node areas.

A pathologist and a gynecologist together reviewed all the primary biopsies. In those patients who had multiple specimens, the one which most clearly reflected any predominating histologic features was selected. A radiologist and a pathologist together studied all lymph nodes removed. Step-sectioning techniques, frequently revealing micrometastases, demonstrated a 25% incidence of lymph node spread. The pa-

tients were divided into four histologic groups: those with adenocarcinomas, large cell keratinizing carcinomas, non-keratinizing large cell carcinomas, and small cell carcinomas. Special stains were used when necessary. To classify the epithelial malignancies, criteria initially proposed by Wentz and Reagan (3) and currently accepted by WHO (5) were used.

In Table 19.1 the frequency of occurrence of the different cell types is shown and in Table 19.2 the occurrence of lymph node metastases in the different groups. The 2-year tumor free survival rate is shown in Table 19.3. We did not find any significant difference in survival rate between the different histologic groups.

It must of course be emphasized that this study has been based on biopsies prior to treatment. It is well known that many tumors show a heterogeneity throughout the lesion. It is therefore not certain that the biopsies which have been examined represent the major part of the tumor. Biopsies merely represent a random sample of a biologic event. Nevertheless, as a result of this study we have concluded that histologic grading according to Martzloff, Broders, Wentz and Reagan has no demonstrable relationship to the frequency of lymph node metastases and to the survival. It must be admitted, however, that the studies by the German and Austrian investigators (6) where surgery has been the primary treatment and where the whole tumor has been subjected to an extremely thorough examination, seems to substantiate the existence of a relationship between the histologic pattern of the primary tumor and the result of treatment. Stendahl, too, has found a good correlation between the combined value of eight histological parameters and prognosis (7) In particular the occurrence of vessel invasion indicated a poor prognosis. This is in agreement with our own observations in different types of genital cancer.

20

Simple hysterectomy in the presence of invasive cervical cancer

It is accepted that invasive cervical cancer should be treated either by radical surgery, radiotherapy or a combination of both. However, it does happen that patients with invasive cervical cancer are treated by simple hysterectomy, either because of negligence with preoperative evaluation or because an emergency situation has occurred. All workers in the field agree that simple hysterectomy is an inadequate form of treatment. Various authors have reported series treated inadequately in the first instance, and have offered suggestions for improvements both in diagnostic accuracy and salvage. Some recommend early repeat surgery, and others propose radiotherapy as a reasonable alternative to radical surgery for optimum salvage. In 1973 Andras, Fletcher and Rutledge (1) presented a series of 148 cases in which

they reported that in the early stages of the disease, the prognosis may be as good as in those treated more conventionally provided radiotherapy was given immediately after hysterectomy. The most obvious way to reduce the number of patients inadequately treated is to improve the standard of preoperative assessment.

During the years 1956–69, 74 cases of invasive cervical carcinoma treated by simple hysterectomy were referred to the Norwegian Radium Hospital. Of these, 48 had at the time of the survey been observed for at least ten years. During the same period, 4,492 patients with invasive cervical cancer received all their treatment in the hospital (2).

As many as 28 of these 74 women presented with, what may be called, a "cancer suspicious

Table 20.1. Findings at operation and time of referral

Patient group	Observation time	
	5 years	10 years
1. Free operative borders ("Stage I")	48	29
2. Not free borders, referred within 6 months	16	12
3. Not free borders, referred after 6 months	10	7
Total	74	48

Table 20.2. Results of follow-up at 5 years

Patient group*	Alive		Alive with disease	Dead of cancer	Dead of intercurrent disease	Lost to follow-up
	No.	Per cent				
1.	37/48	77.1	3	4	2	2
2.	6/16	37.5	–	10	–	–
3.	2/10	20.2	–	8	–	–
Total	45/74	60.8	3	22	2	2

* Group 1: Stage Ib, free operative borders.
  Group 2: Tumor transected, irradiated within 6 months after surgery.
  Group 3: Tumor transected, irradiated later than 6 months after surgery.

history" of metrorrhagia. Another three were operated with simple hysterectomy after a positive diagnosis of invasive cancer had already been made at biopsy.

Only cases with proven histological evidence of invasion have been considered, and all cases of microinvasion (Stage Ia) are excluded. For ease of comparison the cases were divided into three groups (Table 20.1). Group 1 corresponds to clinical Stage Ib, Group 2 represents those with known gross disease cut through at operation and referred within six months of the original surgery, whilst Group 3 are those with tumor transected at operation, but whose follow-up treatment was delayed more than six months.

All patients were treated with a combination of intravaginal radium and external radiotherapy.

The 5-year survival rate is shown in Table 20.2. Group 1, i.e. those with free operative borders, showed a relatively high 5-year survival rate, 77.1%. In those with transected tumors receiving radiotherapy within six months the 5-year survival rate was 37.5%, and in those who received radiotherapy later than six months after primary operation, the 5-year survival rate was only 20%.

The obvious conclusion of our study was that it is still necessary to improve the standard of preoperative assessment in all women being operated for supposed benign conditions. All cases should be fully screened preoperatively using cytology, colposcopy, biopsy of any suspicious lesion, and, if indicated, cervical or fractionated curettage. If in spite of these measures an occasional case of invasive cancer is overlooked, immediate postoperative megavoltage radiotherapy should be given so as to ensure the best chance of cure.

21

Radiotherapy versus combined treatment in carcinoma of the cervix Stage IIa

A RANDOMIZED CLINICAL STUDY

It has always been questioned whether surgery alone, combined treatment, or radiotherapy should be preferred in the early stages of cervical carcinoma. Since the Norwegian Radium Hospital has a relatively large number of cases in the early stages of the disease, the author decided in 1968 that a controlled clinical trial should be conducted with the aim of seeing if radiotherapy alone was better or equivalent to combined treatment in the early Stage IIa lesions of the cervix. Only those with a relatively minor extension to the vagina and with no other signs of extension of their disease were included in the material. The study we can present comprises 119 patients with squamous cell cancer of the cervix Stage IIa (1). All of them were initially treated with intracavitary radium in accordance with the aforementioned Paris method. Following randomization they were subjected either to radical surgery with pelvic lymphadenectomy, or to high-voltage external irradiation with 40 Gy to a pelvic field. All patients who entered the trial were considered well suited for surgery and had tumors which engaged the upper third of the vagina only. There were 62 patients in the surgery group and 57 in the radiation group, the mean ages being 48 and 47 years respectively.

The study was conducted over the 10-year period 1968–77, and the principles of the treatment remained the same throughout the whole period.

Patients in the surgery group were operated approximately six weeks after intracavitary treatment. From 1970 intraoperative lymphographic control ensured an adequate lymph node dissection. All patients were consecutive, and the outcome of lymphography did not influence the choice of treatment. If lymph node metastases were found at operation, postoperative pelvic irradiation was started about two weeks later giving a dose to the pelvic wall of 40 Gy, shielding of the central field, 20 Gy.

RESULTS

In the combined radiation/surgery group the 5-year survival was 83% compared to 76% in the group of patients who received radiotherapy only. This difference is statistically significant.

Twenty out of the 62 operated patients (32%) had metastases to the pelvic lymph nodes, and the 5-year survival rate for these patients was 60%, whereas the 5-year survival rate for patients without metastases was 97%.

There were three serious complications in the radiotherapy group. In the combined treatment group four patients developed fistulas. In the radiotherapy group a high death and recurrence rate was observed within the first year of treatment. Five patients in this group (9%) developed vaginal recurrence, and it can be questioned whether these tumors ever went to primary healing. Only one patient in the combined treatment group developed a vaginal recurrence; it appeared in a patient with microscopically free resection borders of the specimen, but with metastases to the pelvic lymph nodes.

This material is of course selected, because it consists of relatively small Stage II tumors. It may be concluded that with the treatment protocol used, the 5-year survival is favorably influenced by the addition of radical surgery to intracavitary irradiation. This is in agreement with statistics which have appeared in the *Annual Report* (2).

Neither primary surgery nor radiotherapy can control disease outside the pelvis. In both treatment groups the proportion of distant and pelvic recurrences was the same, 6 out of 11 recurrences in the combined treatment group and 7 out of 13 in the radiotherapy group. The number of distant metastases in the whole material was 13 out of 119 (11%).

A similar proportion of so-called residual tumors was found in the hysterectomy specimens after intracavitary irradiation as in Stage Ib lesions. Of 62 specimens, residual tumor was observed in 10 (16%). Not all these residual tumors may be considered viable, but the presence of so-called residual tumor in the hysterectomy specimen has a negative prognostic significance. The metastasis rate in this group of patients was 50%. In the combined treatment group radioresistant tumors accounted for 4 out of 6 distant recurrences.

Comparing complication rates in the two groups is an easy task if only severe complications are included. The combination of radium insertions and a full course of external irradiation was given to all five patients in this series who developed fistulas. Four of these belonged to the combined treatment group, and all had postoperative irradiation due to metastases in the pelvic lymph nodes. To date, ten patients belonging to the combined treatment group with metastases

to the pelvic lymph nodes have survived for more than five years. In this small group of patients, severe urinary tract complications were high, 3 out of 10. In the entire combined treatment group 6% of the patients developed serious urinary tract complications. This is higher than the complications which we experienced in Stage Ib lesions treated with radium and radical surgery.

Lymphedema is a complication usually associated with surgery and was seen in 5 of the 62 operated patients. Three of these patients developed severe discomfort and were operated with lymphovenous shunts, with acceptable results in two. It is probable that our high frequency of lymphedema is due to the very thorough lymphadenectomy carried out in all our patients. In patients treated solely by radiotherapy, lymphedema is almost pathognomonic of recurrent pelvic wall disease.

It may be concluded that the 5-year survival rate in the combined treatment group of early Stage IIa lesions is significantly higher than when radiotherapy alone is applied. We are therefore now more apt to offer combined radiological-surgical treatment to patients with Stage IIa lesions, which are good operative risks.

22

Carcinoma of the cervix Stages II, III and IV

Through the years the more advanced stages of cervical carcinoma have always been treated with radiotherapy only.

As mentioned previously, standard treatment for Stages II, III and IV has been intracavitary radium followed by external irradiation. Since 1957 external radiotherapy has been given by high-voltage machines. Today we prefer the linear accelerator, which is a flexible radiotherapy machine. We have machines delivering 4.3, 6, 8 and 15 MeV. Selection of patients for the different machines depends simply upon the anatomical situation, so that obese patients are usually treated on the 15 MeV machine.

In 1970 it was decided that the larger tumors in Stages IIb, III and IV should initially be treated with external radiotherapy to shrink the tumor, so that the anatomical situation became more suitable for intracavitary radium treatment. This led to better results in the Stage II lesions, while neither the introduction of high-voltage machines, nor the treatment schedule with 30 Gy external radiotherapy followed by intracavitary radiation and thereafter 20 Gy external radiotherapy with the central part of the field shielded, seemed to influence the treatment results in Stage III. Therefore, in 1975, it was decided that the periaortic region should also be included in the external radiation field (1). In many of the advanced cases it was not possible to apply the radium sources, so that in Stage IIb approximately 3–5% received external radiation only. In Stage III it was found that 33% could be treated by external radiation only; the percentage for Stage IV was 45%.

The treatment results in Stages I, II and III before periaortic irradiation was introduced are shown in Fig. 22.1. In the eighteenth volume of the *Annual Report* (2), the results obtained in 1973–75, inclusive, are presented. The crude survival rate for a total of 1,120 cases including Stage

I was 68.6%, the corrected survival rate 73.7%. In Stage II the 5-year survival rate was 60.6% in 310 cases; of 155 cases in Stage III, 31.6% survived for 5 years, and out of 54 patients in Stage IV 13% survived 5 years.

A paper on the value and complications of periaortic irradiation in Stages IIb, III and IV was published in 1983 (1). Our studies on the value of lymphography in predicting metastases to the pelvic wall had convinced us that it was not safe to select cases for periaortic irradiation on the basis of lymphography (3). Since our studies had also convinced us that a complete dissection of all the lymph nodes in the pelvis is difficult, even with the use of preoperative lymphograms, we did not believe that a complete lymphadenectomy in the periaortic region could be achieved without considerable experience and the use of intraoper-

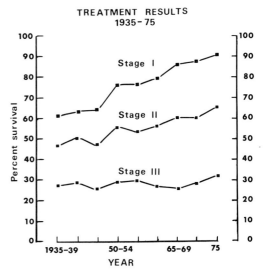

Fig. 22.1. Treatment results for carcinoma of the cervix Stages I–III in the period 1935–75.

Table 22.1. Distribution by stages and withdrawn patients in 163 Stage IIb–IV cases treated with periaortic irradiation during the years 1975–77.

Stage	No. of cases	No. withdrawn	No. evaluable
IIb	73	2	71
III	77	8	69
IV	13	2	11
Total	163	12	151

Table 22.2. Number and percentage of patients ≥ 60 years

Stage	Total No.	≥ 60 years	
		No.	Per cent
IIb	71	22	31
III	69	30	43
IV	11	6	55
Withdrawn	12	9	75
Total	163	67	41

ative control of the completeness of the dissection. The risk of immediate surgical complications and complications following postoperative irradiation in patients with positive nodes presumably must be high.

PERIAORTIC IRRADIATION IN CERVICAL CANCER

During the years 1975–77, altogether 163 cases with Stages IIb, III and IV were treated. Only 13 had Stage IV lesions (Table 22.1). Twelve patients had to be withdrawn because of inability to tolerate the extended irradiation fields. They had complicating diseases and were older than the rest of the patients in the study. Thus, 151 patients were finally available for evaluation, all of whom were observed for 3–5 years.

The patients belonged to an older age group than the earlier stages of disease, and it was found that the percentage of patients over 60 years of

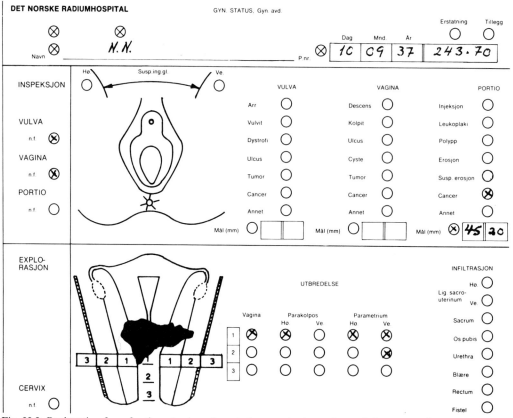

Fig. 22.2. Registration form for the extension of cervical cancer in the vagina and the parametriae.

Table 22.3. Treatment for Stage IIb, III and IV carcinoma of the cervix

Daily dose, 5 times a week	1.67 Gy (167 rads)
Weekly dose	8.35 Gy (835 rads)
Total dose external irradiation	50.0 Gy (5000 rads)

Radium insertions after 30 Gy (3000 rads), central shielding of the last 20 Gy of external irradiation. Radium dose: Point A: 50–70 Gy. Point B: 8–15 Gy.

age increased with increasing disease stage (Table 22.2).

Approximately 90% of the patients had tumors of the squamous cell group, while 5% had pure adenocarcinoma. There were two patients with adenosquamous carcinoma and four unclassified cases.

TREATMENT SCHEDULE

Before actual treatment was begun a work-up was performed including gynecologic examination under anesthesia. The size of the tumor was recorded. In Stage IIb lesions were also recorded if the tumor extended more than half way out to the pelvic wall, and if it was bilateral. Bilaterality was also recorded in Stage III lesions (Figs. 22.2). Other standard examinations included cystoscopy, chest X-ray, urography, venography, lymphangiography, whole blood count, and renal and liver function tests. When indicated, sigmoidoscopy was also performed.

The details of the radiological treatment are shown in Table 22.3. External irradiation 30 Gy was given through anterior and posterior portals using a so-called "chimney field" (Fig. 22.3). The patient was then examined to determine if it was possible to apply radium. After intracavitary radiation, external radiotherapy was continued to a total dose of 50 Gy. During the last 20 Gy of external radiation the central part of the pelvis including the bladder and rectum was shielded.

During the study it was clear that we could not follow the above treatment schedule in all cases, especially in patients with Stage III or Stage IV disease, since an adequate insertion of radium was not possible. In patients with Stage IIb disease, as many as 97% were treated according to the planned schedule, while the figures for patients with Stage III and Stage IV disease were 67% and

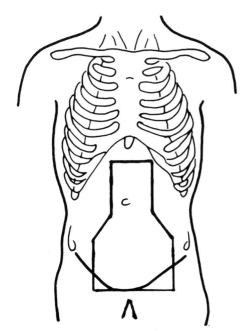
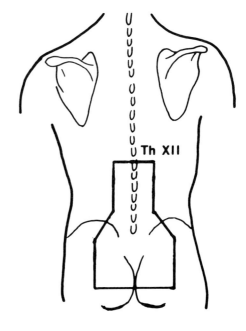

Fig. 22.3. Pelvic and periaortic irradiation field ("chimney field") for patients with Stage IIb–IV carcinoma of the cervix. From (1) and reproduced by courtesy of Raven Press, New York.

Table 22.4. Treatment given in 151 cases available for evaluation

| | Stage | | | | | |
| | IIb | | III | | IV | |
Treatment	No.	%	No.	%	No.	%
After schedule	69	97	46	67	6	55
External radiation only, 50 Gy	2	3	19	27	1	9
External radiation, pelvic dose 60 Gy, periaortic 50 Gy	0	0	4	6	4	36

55%, respectively. In some patients with very large Stage III and Stage IV tumors the dose to the pelvis was increased to 60 Gy (Table 22.4).

RESULTS

Only patients whose treatment followed the standard schedule achieved a reasonable 3–5 year survival rate of 54%. When external radiation could not be combined with intracavitary radium, only 4 out of 22 patients survived during the period of observation. None of the patients with large tumors which received a pelvic dose of 60 Gy survived.

Table 22.5. Parametrial extension in 71 cases of Stage IIb and 64 cases of Stage III carcinoma of the cervix.

| | | Survival rate | |
Extension of tumor	Total No.	No.	%
Stage IIb:			
Medial half	22	15	68
Lateral half	49	29	57
Stage III:			
One side	24	11	46
Both sides	40	11	28

Table 22.6. Complications most likely from irradiation

Complication	No.	%	Dead
Gastric ulcer	7	4.6	6*
Intestinal obstruction or perforation	2	1.3	1
"Persistent" diarrhea	27	17.9	0
Other, not serious	20	13.2	0

* Only two died from irradiation complications, see text.

In Stage IIb we differentiated between tumors localized to the medial half and those which extended out to the lateral half of the parametrium. In Stage III we differentiated between those affecting only one side of the parametrium and those which affected both sides. This parametrial extension and prognosis in 71 Stage IIb cases and 64 Stage III cases is shown in Table 22.5. The results are quite clear: The larger the tumor, the poorer the prognosis. Stage IIb tumors affecting only the

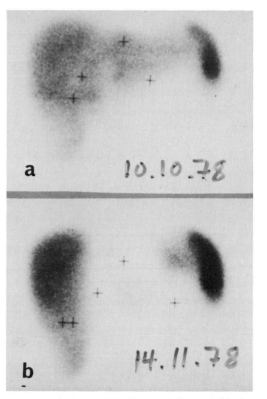

Fig. 22.4. Scintigram of the liver (a) before and (b) after 50 Gy periaortic irradiation.

medial half had a survival rate of 68% as compared to 57% for those which extended to the lateral half. In Stage III, patients with unilateral tumors fared better than those with bilateral tumors.

Of the total of 69 patients with Stage III lesions the crude survival rate during the observation period was 36%. Two patients died from intercurrent disease. Once again it was observed that patients having tumors that made it possible to combine radium with external irradiation, had a better prognosis than those receiving external irradiation alone. Increasing the pelvic dose to 60 Gy had no effect, all of these patients died.

Only 11 patients with Stage IV disease were evaluable. To date, two of the eleven remain alive. Both received radium and external radiation.

COMPLICATIONS

The most common complication was persistent diarrhoea which occurred in 18% of the cases (Table 22.6). By "persistent" we mean that during the follow-up the patients complained of diarrhoea more than two months after treatment. Sometimes the diarrhoea lasted up to six months. Other complications which were not considered serious were nausea, vomiting, and/or diarrhoea during therapy. In some cases, intravenous fluids had to be administered to compensate for electrolyte and water loss. In two patients, we observed intestinal obstruction and perforation, and one

patient died. Surprisingly, the most common major complication was gastric ulcer. Two of the seven patients listed in Table 22.6 had had gastric ulcer for some years before treatment. Of these seven patients, six are now dead. However, it should be emphasized that only two died from complications, the other four from recurrence of the cancer. That periaortic irradiation affects the organs in the upper abdomen is shown in Fig. 22.4.

We have compared data from the series of Stages IIb–IV cases treated during the years 1971–73 with the series from 1975–77. We used the actuarial method of calculating the survival curves. It is sad to discover that, in the latter series receiving periaortic radiotherapy, there is no significant increase in survival. However, before reaching a final conclusion, we must continue our series for several more years to gather more data. We have reduced the maximum dose to the periaortic region to 40 Gy. We do not recommend increasing the pelvic dose to 60 Gy in patients with large tumors, since none of the patients who received this dose in our series, have survived. It must be concluded that only in those cases in which it is possible to treat the primary tumor by external radiotherapy and by intracavitary sources, can the results be expected to improve by including the periaortic regions in the radiation field. External irradiation by itself cannot compete with combined intracavitary and external radiation.

23

Carcinoma of the cervix in the young patient

The concept that young women with cancer of the cervix have a poorer prognosis is widely held and supported by extensive studies e.g. Kottmeier and Lindell (1, 2). However, in our study on the combined treatment of Stage Ib carcinoma of the cervix published in 1973 (3) it was clearly shown that at this early stage of the disease there was no difference in the 5-year survival rate between the different age groups. The latest study on the problem of age and prognosis in patients with squamous cell carcinoma of the uterine cervix was published in 1977 (4).

In the Norwegian Radium Hospital 2,002 cases of cervical carcinoma were treated during the years 1963–68. The patients were divided into three age groups, with the specific aim of studying the prognosis of the young patients. The distribution of histologic tumor types was the same in all age groups. The young patients had a more favorable stage distribution and, as a group, a better prognosis than the older ones, but within each stage the same 5-year survival rate was found for all age groups. The period studied was relatively short (6 years), but modern therapy was available to all patients.

In Table 23.1 the distribution of clinical stages in relation to age is shown. A distinction was made between patients above 35 years of age and those below. In the total material of 2,002 cases only 139 patients were 35 years of age or younger. The vast majority of cases were squamous cell carcinomas (92.5%). Next in frequency were the adenocarcinomas (5%). The remainder, 2.5%, were adenoacanthomas, adenosquamous or undifferentiated tumors. The histologic distribution was the same in all age groups.

Treatment methods within the different stages

Table 23.1. The relationship between age and stage in a total of 2002 patients with carcinoma of the cervix treated in the Norwegian Radium Hospital during the years 1963–68

Stage	18–34 years No.	18–34 years %	Total series No.	Total series %
I	91	65.5	939	46.9
II	39	28.0	745	37.2
III	6	4.3	224	11.2
IV	3	2.2	94	4.7
Total	139	100.0	2002	100.0

Table 23.2. Relationship between age, stage and 5-year survival rate calculated after the life table method

Stage	Total No.	Age 18–34 Per cent survival	Age 35–54 Per cent survival	Age 55–89 Per cent survival	Total Per cent survival
Ia	147	100.0	99.0	100.0	99.0
Ib	892	80.0	87.0	84.0	85.0
Ia + Ib	939	83.5*	89.0*	84.0*	87.0*
IIa	371	82.0	63.0	75.0	69.0
IIb	374	45.0	62.0	53.0	55.0
IIa + IIb	745	72.0*	63.0*	63.0*	65.0*
III	224	33.0	26.0	27.0	27.0
IV	94	0.0	3.0	4.0	3.0
Total	2002	76.0	76.0	59.0	70.0

* Difference between survival rates not significant

were the same, although perhaps more patients in the younger age groups in the earlier stages were subjected to combined radiological-surgical treatment. Table 23.2 shows the 5-year survival rate according to the life table method among the three age groups and the total study population.

The material presented is unselected and large enough for statistical significance. The principles of therapy were not altered during the study period, and supervoltage therapy was available to all patients. If younger women have biologically more malignant tumors, the effect that this should have on mortality is neutralized by modern therapy.

The latest study from Scandinavia on age and prognosis in cervical cancer was published by Gynning et al. in 1983 (5). They found that in Stage Ib the prognosis was worse for patients under 35 years when radiotherapy alone was given. However, in a series of 274 cases treated by preoperative radiation and radical surgery, the prognosis for the young patients was slightly better than for the patients older than 35 years. The observations made in our own material may be due to the fact that in the early stages of the disease, combined treatment was always preferred.

24

Carcinoma of the cervix in pregnancy

Carcinoma of the cervix detected during pregnancy has always been a controversial problem. During the first 24 weeks the patients will usually be treated as non-pregnant women. The only exception is that during radiotherapy, either with intracavitary sources or external irradiation, abortion will occur. During the first 10–12 weeks some clinics prefer to induce abortion before therapy is started. During the second trimester from 12 to 24 weeks the argument is that the foetus is so big that tears can occur in the cancer infiltrated cervix, and thus there is risk of spread of the disease. But there are no observations in the literature that really support such a concept. There are also reports with induction of abortion during the second trimester without any significant decrease in survival rate as compared to those who prefer to give external radiotherapy until abortion occurs spontaneously.

During the third trimester it is usual that every effort is made to preserve both the life of the child and the mother. The most crucial time is between 25 and 30 weeks of pregnancy. During the first weeks of the third trimester many authors prefer to wait until the foetus is more mature, perform caesarian section, and subsequently treat the cervical lesion.

In earlier years, carcinoma of the cervix during pregnancy could be detected in all clinical stages. After the invent of cytology and the use of smears during the women's first consultation during pregnancy, most lesions are detected in Stage 0 or Stage Ia. This is clearly illustrated in two series from the Norwegian Radium Hospital, the first from the years 1956–70 and the second from 1971–80 (not published).

MATERIAL

In the first 15-year period, altogether 44 patients were diagnosed as having carcinoma of the cervix during pregnancy. Of these lesions, 6 were in Stage 0, 27 in Stage I, 9 in Stage II, 1 in Stage III and 1 in Stage IV.

Ten of the patients were in the age group 25–29 years, 31 in the age group 30–39 years, and 3 in the age group 40–45 years. The youngest patient was 26 years of age, the oldest 43 years of age.

Squamous cell carcinoma was diagnosed in 42 cases and undifferentiated lesion in 2 cases.

Of the total series 18 were in the first trimester, 11 in the second and 13 in the third; 2 cases were detected post partum.

During the first period of study, the Stage 0 lesions (CIN III) in the first trimester were all treated with legal abortion, followed in five cases by conization and in one case by simple hysterectomy. This policy changed during the 1970s. Use of the colposcope in particular, has made it possible to follow the patients during pregnancy and rather treat their intraepithelial lesion 6–8 weeks after delivery.

The number of cases seen each year varied between two and three. This should be related to the total number of invasive cervical carcinomas seen in the hospital, which during the same time period varied between approximately 200 and 350 each year. The total number of births in the country varied between 55,000 and 65,000 a year. This gives an incidence of cervical cancer in pregnancy of between approximately 3/100,000 and 5/100,000.

It is not surprising with the small number of cases seen that the approaches to the problem of treatment have varied a great deal. During the first trimester, 12 patients had a Stage Ib lesion. In three of these which were earlier than 10 weeks, legal abortion was performed followed by intracavitary radium and radical hysterectomy with lymphadenectomy. In one case hysterectomy had been performed before referral to the hospital because of a supposed diagnosis of a bleeding myoma protruding through the cervical canal. This patient received external radiotherapy. One patient was treated with primary Wertheim operation and lymphadenectomy. She had a very small tumor. The rest of the patients in the first trimester, seven cases, were all treated with primary radium which induced abortion. Intracavitary irradiation was followed six weeks later by Wertheim hysterectomy and lymphadenectomy. All of these 12 patients in Stage Ib treated in the first trimester are alive and well.

One patient in the first trimester had a Stage IV carcinoma of the cervix with metastases to the supraclavicular area on the left side. An explorative laparotomy was performed, and it was found that there were extensive metastases to the pelvic wall and alongside the periaortic region. She died less than one year after operation.

In the second trimester there were eight Stage I lesions and three Stage II lesions. In one case radical hysterectomy and lymphadenectomy had to be performed as an emergency because of heavy bleeding. Unfortunately, the tumor was transected and at the same time metastases were found in the pelvis. She died in the course of one year.

In two cases the foetus was removed by caesarian section followed by intracavitary radium and radical surgery in one case, and by radium only in another case with a very small tumor. Radium and radical surgery was performed in four cases. Radium and external irradiation was given in another four cases. Only the case mentioned above, where the tumor was transected, died from her disease.

Caesarian section was performed before treatment of the cervical lesion in all 12 cases in the third trimester, 6 of which were in Stage I and 6 in Stage II. In 9 of the 12 the woman was delivered of a living child. One child died nine weeks after ceasarian section because of prematurity. Caesarian section was followed in all cases by intracavitary radium. A Wertheim operation was performed in 5 cases, and in 7 cases it was decided that external high-voltage radiotherapy should be given. Of this total of 12 cases in the third trimester, 4 died from cancer. Two of these patients had already proven metastases to the pelvic wall during the Wertheim operation.

The two patients in whom the tumor was detected *post partum* were both treated with intracavitary radium and radical surgery. In one of the patients metastases were found on the pelvic wall, and she developed lung metastases and metastases to the supraclavicular region one year later.

CONCLUSION

The series comprised a total of 38 patients with invasive cervical carcinoma. Of these, 27 were in clinical Stage I; only one of these died from cancer, and she had metastases on the pelvic wall which were detected during operation. There were nine Stage II lesions, four of which died from cancer. During operation, spread to the pelvis was found in two of these four cases. There was one patient with an extensive Stage III tumor, and one with a Stage IV tumor, and both of these died within the first year after treatment.

Altogether it seems that carcinoma of the cervix during pregnancy has approximately the same prognosis, stage for stage, as for the patients who are not pregnant. In our series we have preferred combined radiological-surgical treatment in most cases. Therapeutic abortion in the first and second trimesters can be performed either immediately or be induced by intracavitary or external irradiation.

MICROCARCINOMA DURING PREGNANCY

During the years 1971–80 a total of 18 patients were admitted with a diagnosis of carcinoma of the cervix Stage Ia during pregnancy. Of these as many as ten were in the first trimester, three in the second, two in the third, and in three cases the tumor was detected *post partum*. The relatively large number of cases which were found early in pregnancy is undoubtedly related to the fact that many of these patients consulted their doctor with a request for legal abortion. Routine smear discovered the lesion, and they were referred to the Norwegian Radium Hospital for treatment.

All patients except one had a squamous cell carcinoma. An adenosquamous lesion was found in this single case.

Abortion was induced in all patients in the first

and second trimesters. In one patient conization was the only treatment. All the other patients in the first and second trimesters underwent hysterectomy, and in two cases also lymphadenectomy. The reason for performing lymphadenectomy was the finding of tumor cells in vessels.

The two patients in the third trimester underwent caesarian section. Both of them were eight months pregnant, and they were delivered of a living child. In one case the caesarian section was followed immediately by radical hysterectomy with lymphadenectomy. The other patient was treated by simple hysterectomy six weeks after the caesarian section.

Of the three patients who were treated for their microinvasive carcinoma *post partum,* two were operated with Wertheim hysterectomy and lymphadenectomy because of invasion of tumor cells in endothelial lined spaces. The remaining patient was treated by conization only.

The results for this small series of microcarcinoma during pregnancy must be characterized as excellent. There have been no recurrences, and all patients are today living and well.

25

Effect of irradiation on the foeto-placental unit

During our studies of malignant tumors during pregnancy it was found of interest to investigate the effect of irradiation on the foetus and the placenta. From earlier studies within this field it seemed as if foetal death was due to a direct effect of irradiation on the brain tissue. Altogether seven patients were studied during the years 1966–78 (1). They received external irradiation to a pelvic field or to an abdominal field not including the kidneys. The diagnosis, patient age and gestational age are shown in Table 25.1.

The calculated mid-pelvic dose in six patients was 30 Gy, in one patient 34 Gy. In five patients the placenta was completely within the irradiated volume. In the other two, approximately one half of the placenta was irradiated.

Before, during and after irradiation, pelvic angiography was performed to demonstrate the uteroplacental circulation and the placental size. During irradiation estriol, human chorionic gonadotrophin and pregnanediol excretion in the urine were examined. In two patients serum levels of progesterone and human chorionic somatomammotrophine were also measured, and in one case total estrogen, estradiol and estriol measurements were performed.

Spontaneous abortion occurred in five patients

after a dose of 30 Gy, and two were operated upon within two weeks of the cessation of irradiation, before abortion had occurred.

RESULTS

The uterus grew normally in all patients throughout the treatment period. The X-ray films exposed after 10 and 30 Gy did reveal a decrease in the size of the placenta and also a slight decrease in the maternal circulation. At the end of 30 Gy radiation therapy, radiography demonstrated deformation of the foetal scull in three of the patients, and an unnatural position of the head in a fourth. In the other patients the foetus still appeared normal when abortion occurred.

The values of HCG, progesterone and estriol showed no definite changes during the first two weeks of irradiation. In the third week all the hormone analyses showed a decrease except for human chorionic somatomammotrophine (Fig. 25.1). The value of this last hormone remained constant during the whole period of irradiation. Between the fourth and fifth weeks of irradiation, i.e. between 20 and 30 Gy of radiotherapy, a dramatic fall in the other hormones was observed

Table 25.1. Type of genital carcinoma, patient age and gestational age in 7 pregnant patients treated by high voltage irradiation.

Type of carcinoma	Age (years)	Gestation (weeks)
Adenocarcinoma of the ovary Stage I	20	11
Adenocarcinoma of the ovary Stage I	19	16
Squamous cell carcinoma of the cervix Stage I	37	16
Adenocarcinoma of the ovary Stage III	28	20
Squamous cell carcinoma of the cervix Stage I	31	20
Squamous cell carcinoma of the cervix Stage I	23	25
Squamous cell carcinoma of the cervix Stage I	36	27

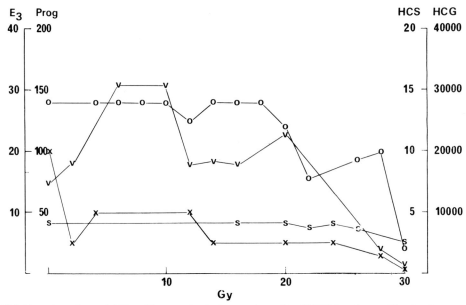

Fig. 25.1. Excretion of estriol (E₃) and human chorionic gonadotrophin (HCG) in urine, and levels of progesterone (Prog) and human chorionic somatomammotrophin (HCS) in serum during irradiation of a pregnant patient. E_3, μmol/l=v, HCG, IU/l=x, Prog, nmol/l=o, HCS, μg/ml=s. From (1) and by courtesy of Acta Radiol Oncol.

indicating a sharp decrease in the production of these hormones by the foeto-placental unit.

In all cases, microscopy of the uterus showed dilated vessels in the uterine wall without obliterative process, intimal fibrosis or thrombosis. The placenta was severely degenerated with obliteration of the villous vessels, particularly in the terminal villi, generalized fibrosis, focal calcification and syncytial degeneration. In one case microscopy of the foetal tissues was performed. Hyperemia in all organs was found, but no parenchymatous degeneration or specific abnormalities

in the large or small vessels. Due to a general autolysis the brain was not examined.

This study seems to indicate that damage to the foetal central nervous system but also placental insufficiency may be responsible for the intrauterine foetal death during external radiotherapy. It also shows that spontaneous abortion occurs relatively late in the course of external radiotherapy in foetuses during the first and second trimesters. Spontaneous abortion occurs much earlier when intracavitary radiotherapy with radium sources is applied.

26
Adenocarcinoma cervicis uteri

Adenocarcinoma of the uterine cervix generally constitutes about 5% of all cervical carcinomas. In 1963, Bergsjø (1) published a series of 169 patients with adenocarcinoma of the cervix uteri treated in the Norwegian Radium Hospital during the years 1945–60. This group comprised 4.1% of the total number of cervical carcinomas admitted during the same period. From 1963 to 1968, 2,002 cases of carcinoma of the cervix were treated in our institution. Of these, 102 (5.1%) were adenocarcinomas (2). In both series, the patients with adenocarcinomas had a higher mean age than patients with squamous cell carcinoma. It has been claimed that adenocarcinoma of the cervix has become more frequent during recent decades. This has not been experienced at the Norwegian Radium Hospital. An increase from 4.1% to 5% during the time period 1945–68 is not statistically significant.

If we compare the stage distribution during these two periods, there has been no significant difference. On the other hand, in the earlier stages of the disease there has been a significant increase in 5-year survival. This may be related to a more aggressive attitude in the treatment of adenocarcinomas. It seems as if surgery should be applied more frequently in this histological type of the disease. During the years 1945–56, 52% of the Stage I lesions survived for five years compared with 83% during the years 1963–68, when surgery was applied much more frequently.

Our experience indicates that these patients are at more risk than patients with squamous cell carcinomas. It seems that the introduction of supervoltage therapy has had no appreciable effect on mortality for those patients treated with radiotherapy alone. In contradistinction to squamous cell carcinoma, adenocarcinoma seems to take a more malignant course in elderly patients, and there is evidence that the development of adenocarcinoma of the cervix in postmenopausal women is a particularly malignant process biologically different from adenocarcinomas in younger women.

27

Carcinoembryonic antigen (CEA) determinations in carcinoma of the cervix

I 1965 Gold and Freedman (1) described a protein which was found in adenocarcinoma of the colon and in embryonic digestive tissue during the first two trimesters of pregnancy. It was given the name carcinoembryonic antigen (CEA), and it belongs to the so-called oncofetal antigens. CEA was first believed to be a specific antigen in cancer of the colon and rectum. However, further studies showed that it was an antigen common to several varieties of malignant tumors (2, 3). Hansen et al. (4) developed a radioimmunoassay ("CEA-ROCHE") for determining the antigen in the plasma of patients with different types of cancer; they also studied the plasma levels in healthy persons.

Khoo and Mackay (5, 6) were among the first to report the value of this tumor marker in gynecologic cancers. Van Nagell et al. in 1982 (7), and Kjørstad in 1984 (8), have reviewed the literature on the usefulness of CEA determinations in gynecologic oncology to date and presented their own investigations.

The first papers on CEA studies in carcinoma of the cervix and corpus uteri from the Norwegian Radium Hospital appeared in 1977 and 1978 (9, 10), further publications followed in 1982, 1983 and 1984 (11, 12, 13). An attempt to summarize the most important observations made in our unit throughout the last 7–8 years will be given here. Emphasis will be placed on the *clinical* use of CEA in carcinoma of the cervix.

SENSITIVITY AND SPECIFICITY

Carcinoembryonic antigen is not a cancer specific protein. It can be found in minute quantities in the plasma of healthy volunteers. Most authors using the radioimmunoassay method of Hansen

et al. (4) agree that CEA levels up to 2.5 µg/l should be considered "normal" and levels above 2.5 µg/l "abnormal". "Abnormal" values, however, are found not just in cancer patients but also in some cases of heavy smokers, in patients with liver disease, in those with an inflammatory bowel disease and obstructive lung disease. There are still many unsolved problems concerning the production, release and metabolism of CEA. Van Nagell et al. (7) compiled data from 11 publications and concluded that levels higher than 2.5 µg/l were observed in 11% of healthy volunteers, in 18% of patients with benign gynecologic disease, in 53% of patients with carcinoma of the cervix, in 37% of patients with endometrial cancer and in 46% of those with ovarian cancer. Their conclusion was that CEA determinations cannot be used as a screening method for any of the major groups of gynecologic cancer. The most important clinical role of CEA today is probably as a monitor of disease status in patients whose tumors produce and release CEA so that a high concentration of antigen can be found in plasma prior to therapy. But even in this clinical situation the usefulness of serial CEA determinations is equivocal (8).

SQUAMOUS CELL CARCINOMA OF THE CERVIX

Pretreatment CEA levels

The relationship between the stage of the disease and the pretreatment levels of CEA was studied in 205 patients with invasive cervical cancer and 30 patients with cervical intraepithelial neoplasia. The control material comprised 91 healthy blood donors. A modified CEA-ROCHE RIA test was used (10). An upper reference value of 3.5 µg/l was determined by analyzing test samples of the 91 blood donors and adding 2 SD to the mean value found.

Of the control material, 98% had CEA levels below 3.5 µg/l. The corresponding figure for those with CIN lesions was 87%. With the increasing stage of the disease, which usually means an increasing volume of the tumor, high abnormal CEA levels were found in growing numbers. For the 205 patients with invasive lesions, the pretreatment range was from 0.5 to 107 µg/l. Values of 20 µg/l were seen in only three patients, however, all with very large tumors. In the 30 patients with CIN lesions, the range was from 0.8 to 4.6 µg/l

It may be concluded that the pretreatment level of CEA is only a rough indicator of the extent of the disease in squamous cell carcinoma of the cervix. However, in cases of early disease, significant additional information may be gained from the levels of CEA. In 51 Stage Ib lesions radical hysterectomy with lymphadenectomy was performed. Only 2 out of 36 patients (6%) without metastases had values over 5 µg/l compared with 6 out of 15 (40%) with disease that had spread to the lymph nodes.

Posttreatment CEA levels

The above-mentioned study of pretreatment values of CEA was published in 1978 (10), and four years later the prognostic significance of such measurements and the value of serial determinations of CEA after treatment were discussed (11). Altogether 195 patients with squamous cell carcinoma of the cervix treated in the Norwegian Radium Hospital 1976–78 were screened for plasma CEA levels before treatment, and followed with CEA determinations at regular intervals of three months for the first year, twice yearly thereafter, or more often if recurrence was suspected clinically. All patients with suspected recurrence were admitted for evaluation. Patients who had been treated for other malignant diseases or who had conditions known to influence CEA levels such as liver, bowel, or obstructive lung diseases were excluded from the material.

A total of 178 patients were followed for a full three years, and in Table 27.1 the percentage of patients without evidence of disease after this observation period is presented in relation to the

Table 27.1. Results of follow-up at three years for patients with squamous cell carcinoma of the cervix in relation to initial plasma values of CEA

Stage	CEA ≤ 5.0 µg/l		CEA > 5.0 µg/l	
	No.	% NED	No.	% NED
Ib	47	85*	17	47*
Ib and IIa	90	80*	25	52*
IIa + IIb	37	73†	19	47†
IIb–IV	36	53†	27	30†

* P < 0.005. † P < 0.100. % NED: Percentage of patients within group without evidence of disease at the end of three years observation. No patients in Stage Ia had levels > 5.0 µg/l or recurrence.

pretreatment values of CEA. In this table the cutoff level for "normal" values of CEA has been set at 5 µg/l, because levels between 2.5 µg/l and 5 µg/l gave equivocal results. It is obvious that in the earlier stages of the disease, Stages Ib and IIa, initial plasma levels above 5 µg/l have a deleterious influence on prognosis. In Stages IIb–IV, the pretreatment values of CEA are of doubtful prognostic significance.

It is seldom, however, that CEA values increase after therapy without tumor recurrence. This is in agreement with a number of studies reported in the literature.

The crucial point is that such an increase usually occurs several months before the site of the recurrence is found, and that we still have no chemotherapeutic agent which has been shown to eradicate such early recurrences of squamous cell carcinoma of the cervix. Fortunately, false positive tests are extremely rare, although we have seen a few such cases which have brought both patients and ourselves into a difficult dilemma.

ADENOCARCINOMA CERVICIS UTERI

As early as 1977 Kjørstad and Ørjasæter (9) were able to demonstrate that endometrial carcinoma is a poor CEA producer, while endocervical adenocarcinoma is a very reliable producer. In adenocarcinoma of the endocervix 68% had values exceeding the "normal" 2.5 µg/l. The highest recorded value was 108 µg/l. No patient with disease confined to the cervix had a value over 4 µg/

l. Out of 25 cases operated with radical hysterectomy and lymphadenectomy, eight had lymph node metastases, and all of these showed CEA levels above 5 μg/l. Two had levels above 10 μg/l and four had levels above 20 μg/l.

In a later follow-up study (12) comprising 54 patients with endocervical adenocarcinoma (all stages), it was found that no patient, regardless of stage, with an initial value over 15 μg/l survived. In the range between 5 and 15 μg/l the recurrence rate was 67%. This should be compared with a 5-year survival of 90% in those with pretreatment CEA values below 5 μg/l. In a patient with Stage Ia cervical adenocarcinoma (microcarcinoma) the pretreatment value was 5.8 μg/l. Radical surgery revealed no lymph node metastases. However, CEA after operation was still as high as 5 μg/l. Six years later she was readmitted with massive lung metastases (14). CEA at that time was 15,000 μg/l.

THE FUTURE USE OF CEA DETERMINATIONS

In retrospect it seems as though, especially in the earlier stages of disease with squamous cell carcinoma of the cervix, both pretreatment values and follow-up with serial determinations may be of importance.

Kjørstad and Ørjasæter (13) have also studied the low values of CEA found in the advanced stages of the disease. Their findings are equivocal and are hardly of any importance for our decision upon therapy. It is striking, however, that patients with an advanced stage and a pretreatment value less than 2.5 μg/l seem to have a poor prognosis.

In adenocarcinoma of the cervix all patients should have CEA determinations both pretreatment and in the follow-up period.

In corpus carcinoma CEA determinations are scarcely of any importance.

28
Endometrial carcinoma

STAGING

Stage 0. – Atypical endometrial hyperplasia (carcinoma in situ). Histological findings suspicious of malignancy.

Stage I. – The carcinoma is confined to the corpus.

Stage Ia. – The length of the uterine cavity is 8 cm or less.

Stage Ib. – The length of the uterine cavity is > 8 cm.

Stage II. – The carcinoma has involved the corpus and the cervix, but has not extended outside the uterus.

Stage III. – The carcinoma has extended outside the uterus, but not outside the true pelvis.

Stage IV. – The carcinoma has extended outside the true pelvis or has obviously involved the mucosa of the bladder or rectum.

Stage IVa. – Spread of the growth to adjacent organs: urinary bladder, rectum, sigmoid, or small bowel.

Stage IVb. – Spread to distant organs.

Cases of carcinoma of the corpus should be grouped with regard to the degree of differentiation of the adenocarcinoma as follows:

G1 – Highly differentiated adenomatous carcinoma.

G2 – Moderately differentiated adenomatous carcinoma with partly solid areas.

G3 – Predominantly solid or entirely undifferentiated carcinoma.

(see Figs. 28.1 and 28.2)

Cases of uterine sarcomas, pure or mixed, and choriocarcinomas should be reported separately.

Notes on the staging

The extension of the carcinoma to the endocervix is confirmed by fractionated curettage. Scraping of the cervix should be the first step of the curettage, and the specimens from the cervix should be examined separately. Occasionally it may be difficult to decide whether the endocervix is involved by the cancer or not. In such cases, the simultaneous presence of normal cervical glands and cancer in the same fragment of tissue will give the final diagnosis.

The presence of metastases in the vagina or in the ovary is sufficient evidence in itself to allot a case to Stage III.

EPIDEMIOLOGY

In contrast to carcinoma of the cervix, endometrial carcinoma is a hormone-dependent tumor. There is substantial evidence that long-term unopposed estrogen stimulation is a factor that can influence the development of endometrial carcinoma. Many observations suggest that there is an abnormality in the hypothalamic-pituitary-ovarian hormonal axis. The patients are usually postmenopausal, obese, show impaired fertility and a relatively high percentage have prediabetes or diabetes. During their younger years, and especially before menopause, a history of irregular menstruation with anovulatory bleedings can be obtained. Hypertension is also more common among women with endometrial cancer compared to the normal population. Another factor that indicates the hormonal factor in endometrial cancer is that young women with Stein-Leventhal syndrome, which is associated with menstrual irregularities, infertility, obesity, and hirsutism, have a relatively high frequency of endometrial carcinoma. The same holds true for those patients with estrogen producing tumors, especially theco-

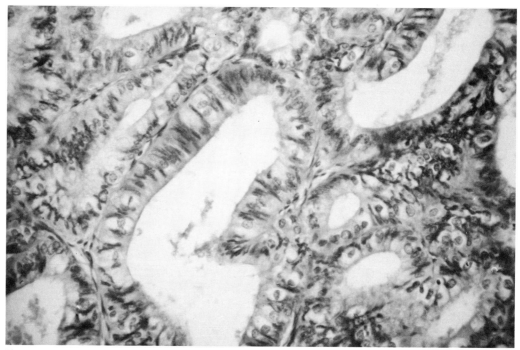

Fig. 28.1. Example of endometrial carcinoma Grade 1–2.

mas and granulosa-thecacell tumors of the ovaries. Pathogenetically, a prolonged and/or increased stimulation by estrogens seems to be the most important factor. It has been shown that androstendion can act as a precursor of estron. This conversion most probably takes place in fat tissue, and may explain the relatively high frequency of obesity among patients with endometrial carcinoma. Since 1975 several epidemiological reports have appeared indicating an association between exogenous estrogen use and endometrial cancer. The association appears to be strongest for local disease and the highly differentiated lesions, and weakest for the most invasive disease with poorly differentiated tumors.

INCIDENCE

In many Western countries carcinoma of the endometrium now ranks first as the most common malignancy arising from the female genital tract. This is due to an increase in the number of patients with endometrial cancer, but also to a significant decline in the incidence of invasive cervical cancer. The cause of this increase is obscure. It may be

due to the fact that a larger proportion of the population is now postmenopausal, and endometrial carcinoma is known to be more frequent after 50–60 years of age. In addition, there are many indications that the increased use of exogenous estrogens to combat menopausal symptoms may be a factor of importance.

Data from the Cancer Registry of Norway show that there has been an increase in the reported cases of carcinoma of the corpus in this country. In Fig. 28.3 the total number of endometrial carcinomas reported to the Registry during the years 1955–80 is shown. In 1978 endometrial carcinoma accounted for 5.5% of all female malignancies. The total age-adjusted incidence rate nearly doubled during the period 1955–78, and the annual percentage change for the age-adjusted incidence rate was greater than for any other female genital cancer. The age-specific rates showed a consistent increase above the age of 45, and there was a slight tendency to even greater increase in incidence in the last 10 years of the period. This increase has also influenced the clinical material at the Norwegian Radium Hospital. In 1950 a total of 86 patients with endometrial

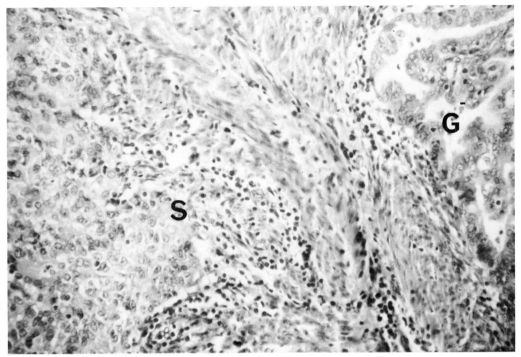

Fig. 28.2. Example of endometrial carcinoma Grade 3. S: solid area, G: glandular structures.

carcinoma were treated as compared to 304 in 1984 (Fig. 1.3, p. 13). This sharp increase in the numbers seen in our hospital has also been influenced by a higher referral rate.

DIAGNOSIS

As mentioned above, endometrial carcinoma is a disease of postmenopausal women. The highest

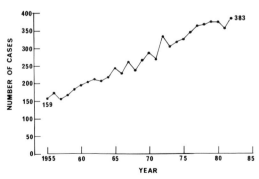

Fig. 28.3. Number of new cases of endometrial carcinoma reported to the Norwegian Cancer Registry in the period 1955–82.

incidence is seen between the sixth and seventh decades. Seventy-five percent of the patients are over 50 years of age, and only 4–5% younger than 40 years. Approximately 25% of the women are still menstruating.

Intermenstrual bleeding, sanguinary discharge or postmenopausal bleeding are the main clinical features of endometrial cancer. A bleeding anomaly occurs in about 90–95% of the cases. Purulent discharge or pyometra is also very suggestive of endometrial cancer, especially in postmenopausal women. Pain is a late symptom and occurs mainly when the disease infiltrates nerves or bony structures in the pelvis. Fortunately, the later stages of the disease are very uncommon. The stage distri-

Table 28.1. Stage distribution of 580 cases of endometrial carcinoma treated in the years 1973–75.

Stage	No.	Per cent
Stage I	342	59.0
Stage II	199	34.3
Stage III	21	3.6
Stage IV	18	3.1

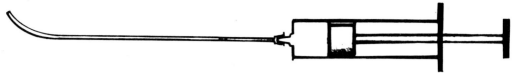

Fig. 28.4. Cannula and disposable syringe for obtaining cytologic smear material from the endometrial cavity.

Endoscann

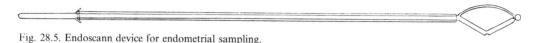

Fig. 28.5. Endoscann device for endometrial sampling.

bution of 580 cases treated during the years 1973–75 is shown in Table 28.1.

It is wise to remember the following three sentences when diagnosis of corpus carcinoma is being made:

1. Irregular bleeding before the climacteric years *may be* due to endometrial carcinoma.
2. Irregular bleeding during the climacteric years *is often* due to carcinoma of the endometrium.
3. Postmenopausal bleeding *is* endometrial carcinoma until this has been disproved by adequate diagnostic methods.

Clinical examination of the patient with bimanual palpation of the uterus will sometimes reveal an enlargement and a softening of the body of the uterus. It is, however, frequently very difficult to palpate these women because of their obesity. The best results of clinical examination are obtained when both the bladder and the rectum have been thoroughly emptied, and the palpation is performed under anesthesia. In Stage III disease, parametrial infiltration, vaginal extension or an enlarged ovary may be found.

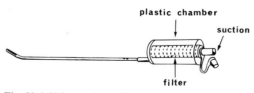

plastic chamber

suction

filter

Fig. 28.6. Vabra aspirator for suction curettage.

CYTOLOGY

There is unanimous agreement that cytologic smears taken from the cervix or the vagina will seldom reveal an early adenocarcinoma of the corpus. In larger materials, about 50–60% of the cases of endometrial carcinoma, early or late, may be detected by such smears. It should be remembered, however, that if endometrial cells, normal or atypical, are found in smears from the vagina in postmenopausal women, this is very suggestive of an endometrial carcinoma.

Much better results regarding both sensitivity and specificity of a cytologic smear are obtained when the smear is taken from the endometrial cavity. Several devices have been constructed for obtaining a representative smear from the endometrium. The simplest device is a cannula which can be inserted into the cavity and connected to a disposable syringe. If the cannula is moved around in the cavity and aspiration is performed, endometrial cells may be aspirated and afterwards spread out on an ordinary slide for cytologic examination (Fig. 28.4). The so-called endoscann is a more dependable device (Fig. 28.5). On an outpatient basis we have found this very useful. Endoscann smears are obtained by turning the device around when inserted into the endometrial cavity. Controlled studies have shown that the endoscann method of obtaining cellular material is almost as reliable as an ordinary fractionated curettage. There is very slight discomfort connected with this method.

CURETTAGE

Before the endoscann method became available, for several years, on an outpatient basis, we used the so-called suction curettage or Vabra aspiration (Fig. 28.6). The Vabra cannula is so small that it can be inserted through the cervical canal without any dilatation. When the tip of the cannula is inside the uterus, suction is applied and the cannula is moved back and forth and rotated so that an almost ordinary curettage can be performed. On an outpatient basis without anesthesia, some patients experience discomfort, and some may even faint during manipulation of the cannula. The percentage of such complications, however, is relatively low, less than 5%. The material obtained is much more abundant than cytological material obtained by an endoscann device.

If there are suspicious symptoms, such as postmenopausal bleeding, which cannot be explained by gynecological examination, colposcopy, endoscann cytology or Vabra aspiration, it will be necessary to perform a fractionated curettage under anesthesia. Fractionated curettage must, of course, also be performed when a patient is admitted to hospital after a positive smear. Scraping of the endocervix should be performed before dilatation of the cervical canal and curettage of the endometrium. The specimen obtained from the endocervix should be kept separated from the curettings from the endometrial cavity. For some years the Stockholm school of gynecologic oncology distinguished between lesions completely located to the endometrial cavity, those which involved the isthmus, and those which also involved the endocervical canal. It is, however, very difficult to make such a distinction so that most gynecologic oncology departments today only distinguish between a Stage I carcinoma of the endometrium localized to the endometrial cavity, and those with involvement of the isthmus and/or the endocervical canal (Stage II).

RECEPTOR STUDIES

Today it seems as if determination of estrogen and progesteron receptors may in the future influence our management of endometrial cancer, and possibly be included in our staging. Receptor negative tumors have a poorer prognosis than receptor positive tumors.

29
Endometrial carcinoma Stage 0

There has been considerable debate about the existence of an endometrial lesion which can be compared to cervical intraepithelial neoplasia. Nevertheless, both retrospective and prospective studies have shown that about 10–15% of what in earlier years was called atypical endometrial hyperplasia may in the course of time, develop into endometrial adenocarcinoma. In the author's opinion it would be of great help for the clinician if the histopathologist were to grade the precursors to invasive adenocarcinoma of the endometrium, and, for example, use the term "Endometrial Intraepithelial Neoplasia, Grades I, II and III" (EIN, I–III). Such a histopathological system may give the clinician a much more concise picture of what is going on in the endometrium during e.g. unopposed continuous estrogen stimulation.

EIN grades I–III should probably always be treated. This would be in concordance with the concept of cervical, vaginal and vulvar intraepithelial neoplasia. It must be admitted that it is difficult to make such a distinction when only examining curettings. However, Fox (1) is of the opinion that there are a number of findings which stand out as being of real significance, e.g. the presence of true intraglandular epithelial bridges, devoid of stromal support, the presence of polymorphs and nuclear debris within glandular lumens, and cellular anarchy. When Fox introduces the term "cellular anarchy", he describes this as the piling up of cells with rounded, irregular nuclei and scanty cytoplasm into sheets and masses, which is sometimes seen focally within a gland that appears otherwise to have a fairly regular epithelium. A further valid differentiating point is the presence of abnormal mitotic figures. Such a lesion would have a great potentiality for developing into an adenocarcinoma or can be seen adjacent to an adenocarcinoma already invading into the myometrium. If any degree of atypical endometrial hyperplasia is found in a postmenopausal woman where most of the endometrial cavity shows an atrophic epithelium, then this is highly suggestive of the beginning of an invasive cancer. Cases that evolve into an invasive adenocarcinoma often show very superficial myometrial invasion, and such cases can be compared to a microinvasive carcinoma of the cervix. It is quite clear that also this nomenclature will meet with many opponents. Perhaps some prospective and also retrospective studies in the future can clarify whether this new nomenclature is worthwhile in clinical practice.

DIAGNOSIS

The symptoms of EIN are the same as for a fully developed adenocarcinoma. In particular, irregular bleeding and/or postmenopausal bleeding are the leading symptoms in the diagnosis. It is extremely seldom that these patients develop pyometra, and they never have any pain. The ultimate diagnosis will be made on fractionated curettage, but a general practitioner will often be able to obtain a satisfactory specimen by the endocyte method, so that the diagnosis of endometrial adenocarcinoma is suspected before the patient is admitted to hospital.

TREATMENT

Since these women are usually climacteric or postmenopausal, the rational treatment is hysterectomy with bilateral oophorectomy. In the younger age groups it should not be necessary to remove the ovaries, because an intraepithelial lesion, and even a highly differentiated adenocarcinoma with superficial invasion in the myometrium, never spreads to the ovaries.

An alternative method in the older patients with contraindications against operation could be to use the Heyman method of radium packing. The only disadvantage in such cases is that one will never be able to determine whether it really was a Stage 0 lesion, or if there was invasion into the myometrium.

Hormonal treatment of recurrences of carcinoma of the endometrium became popular at the beginning of the 1960s. The first publication from the Norwegian Radium Hospital about this method was published in 1965 by Bergsjø (2). In 1967 we started to treat carcinoma of the corpus Stage 0 with progestagens only. Progestagens were given to all cases with a diagnosis of atypical adenomatous hyperplasia. The histopathologist used the criteria of Novak and Woodruff (3) for this lesion: Crowding of glands, increased pseudo-stratification of gland epithelium or actual stratifi-cation including intraluminal budding and varying degrees of cellular atypia. Progression, persistence or regression of these changes as well as presence or absence of desidual stromal reaction after hormone treatment was registered. The gestagen preparation used during these years was hydroxyprogesteroncaproate. After an initial injection of 1,000 mg, weekly doses of 500 mg were given i.m. for 12 weeks to a total dose of 7,000 mg. Control curettage was performed after administration of total doses of 4,000 and 7,000 mg. If invasive lesion occurred during treatment or if persistent atypical adenomatous hyperplasia was present after termination of hormone therapy, hysterectomy was performed (4). Today, only relatively young, premenopausal women with atypical adenomatous hyperplasia are treated with progestagens. The majority of the Stage 0 cases undergo immediate hysterectomy.

30
Endometrial carcinoma Stage I

If fractionated curettage, clinical examination and X-ray of the lungs, skeleton and urography indicate that the tumor is only located to the endometrial cavity, the case is classified as endometrial carcinoma Stage I. In all series published this is fortunately the most frequent stage of this disease. In the eighteenth volume of the *Annual Report* (1) 11,501 cases of carcinoma of the corpus were reported in the years 1973–75 inclusive. Of these, 74.3% belonged to Stage I. Stage distribution for the whole material is shown in Table 30.1. Survival studies performed by the Cancer Registry of Norway for the years 1968–75 showed that 2,327 cases were reported from the whole country, constituting 5.1% of all female malignances. Of these 2,327 cases, 1,587 were treated in the Norwegian Radium Hospital, which means that 68.2% of all endometrial carcinomas in the country were treated in our institution. The stage distribution for 580 cases treated in 1973–75 is shown in Table 28.1, p. 155. More cases in our material were allotted to Stage II than in the total series published in volume 18 of the *Annual Report*. The reason for this is most probably related to the interpretation of cervical curettings. It should be mentioned that in the *Annual Report* there are great discrepancies between the reported frequency of Stage II lesions from institution to institution. The figures vary from 3.1% to 51.6%.

Survival studies performed by the Cancer Registry of Norway from 1953 to 1975 show that the survival rates increased significantly during the study period (Fig. 30.1).

The results of treatment of endometrial carcinoma Stage I at the Norwegian Radium Hospital have been published in 1966 (2), 1969 (3), 1976 (4), and 1980 (5). The 1976 and 1980 publications dealt with a controlled clinical trial which started in 1968. Data from the latter paper will be summarized here.

THE VALUE OF EXTERNAL IRRADIATION IN STAGE I ENDOMETRIAL CARCINOMA

Review of the literature discloses that great differences of opinion exist about how to treat endometrial carcinoma. Surgery, consisting of total hysterectomy and bilateral salpingo-oophorectomy is generally accepted as the cornerstone of treatment. However, there are few institutions which do not add some form of radiotherapy, either preoperatively or postoperatively. If radium packing is used, there are also differences of opinion about when hysterectomy should be performed. The time period between the packing and surgery varies from one to six weeks. External radiotherapy may also be given preoperatively. Another regime is primary surgery followed by vaginal radium and external irradiation to a pelvic field. For many years this regime was the method used in the Norwegian Radium Hospital. However, external radiotherapy was not given to all patients, only to those with deep myometrial infiltration. The philosophy was that deep myometrial infiltration usually gives rise to a considerable frequency of metastases to the pelvic lymph nodes. In a study of 140 patients with Stage I lesions,

Table 30.1. Carcinoma of the corpus uteri. Distribution by stage and 5-year survival rate in the different stages (1).

Stage	Patients treated		5-year survival	
	No.	%	No.	%
I	8550	74.3	6340	74.2
II	1690	14.7	970	57.4
III	822	7.2	240	29.2
IV	314	2.7	30	9.6
No stage	125	1.1	76	60.8
Total	11501	100.0	7656	66.6

Creasman et al. found an overall incidence of 11.4% pelvic lymph node metastases. With deep myometrial infiltration the frequency was 43% (6).

When the controlled clinical trial started in 1968, we found that there was considerable evidence in the literature that recurrences in the vagina might be significantly reduced by giving postoperative vaginal radium irradiation. It was therefore decided that all patients should have this form of radiotherapy. The main aim of the study was to see if it was possible to define the group of patients which really benefited from external radiotherapy after primary surgery. Our experience with pelvic lymph node dissection in the younger age groups in carcinoma of the cervix indicated that lymphadenectomy in the older, and frequently obese patients with endometrial carcinoma should not be performed. Another question which was discussed before the trial was set up was whether the hysterectomy should be simple or radical. We did not believe that radical hysterectomy was a procedure that should be performed in old, obese patients with Stage I endometrial carcinomas. Some years later, in 1974, Rutledge (7) discussed the role of radical hysterectomy in adenocarcinoma of the endometrium. He concluded that the high cure rate being obtained by conservative hysterectomy indicated that most patients did not need the more hazardous radical hysterectomy. Furthermore, the older patients with associated diseases limit the applicability of radical hysterectomy. Our decision to make simple hysterectomy the only surgical treatment of preference has later been confirmed by a study by

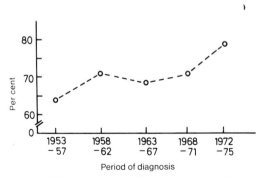

Fig. 30.1. Five-year survival for patients with endometrial carcinoma in Norway in the period 1953–75.

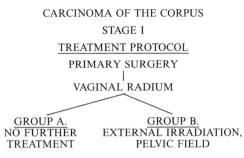

Fig. 30.2. Treatment protocol for 540 patients with endometrial carcinoma Stage I treated in the years 1968–74.

Iversen and Holter (8). In a series of 34 patients with Stage I adenocarcinoma of the corpus selected for radical hysterectomy combined with pelvic lymphadenectomy, the 5-year survival rate was not more than 80%, but, more important, there were 15% with urinary tract complications.

TREATMENT PROTOCOL AND MATERIAL

From 1968 to 1974, 540 patients referred to the Norwegian Radium Hospital for primary and/or secondary treatment of Stage I carcinoma of the corpus uteri were included in the trial. Altogether 18 cases that belonged to the FIGO clinical Stage I, but with proved metastases at surgery, were excluded. The treatment protocol is shown in Fig. 30.2.

Primary treatment consisted of abdominal hysterectomy and bilateral salpingo-oophorectomy. About one week postoperatively all patients received intravaginal radium irradiation with an applicator which delivered approximately 60 Gy to the surface of the vaginal wall. Randomization was performed at the start of radium application. The control Group A received no further treatment, Group B received external irradiation to a pelvic field, 40 Gy.

The histological material from surgery specimens was graded according to the FIGO rules. In 518 cases it was possible to divide the series into two groups according to the depth of tumor infiltration into the myometrium: (1) Infiltration of up to half of the myometrial thickness, and (2) infiltration of more than half of the myometrial thickness.

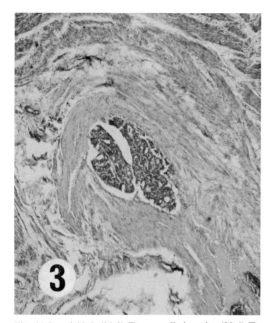
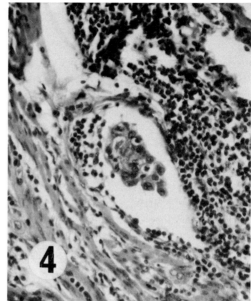

Fig. 30.3 and 30.4. (30.3) Tumor cells in vein. (30.4) Tumor cells in lymph vessel.

During the last part of the study interest was focused on tumor cell invasion of blood and/or lymph vessels. In 151 consecutive cases the presence of such invasion was carefully investigated (Fig. 30.3 and 30.4).

RESULTS

Follow-up examinations were performed four times the first year, twice the second year, and once yearly afterwards. No patients were lost to follow-up. The majority of the patients with recurrences were examined in the Norwegian Radium Hospital before death, and additional therapy was instituted. To allow inclusion in the analysis of those patients successfully treated for recurrence during the observation period, the concept of a "Death and Recurrence Rate" (DRR) was introduced. All recurrences detected between three and nine years of follow-up were included in the DRR. This may make interpretation of the results more reliable than the survival rate alone. Survival was calculated by the life table method (Fig. 30.5).

Of the 540 patients, 277 were allocated to Group A and 263 to Group B. Factors influencing the prognosis was similar in the two groups and included age distribution, weight distribution,

uterine cavity length, myometrial infiltration, and histologic grade. This verified a proper randomization.

During the 2–10 year follow-up no significant difference in survival was found between treatment groups A and B. After five years the survival rates were 91 and 89% respectively, and after nine years 90 and 87%. The DRR was 12.3% in Group A and 11.8% in Group B.

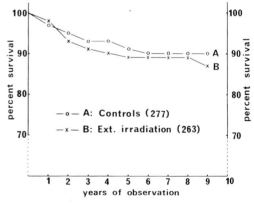

Fig. 30.5. Actuarial survival curves for patients treated by hysterectomy and vaginal irradiation (A), and for group of patients which in addition received external irradiation to a pelvic field (B). From (5) and reproduced by courtesy of Academic Press Inc.

Table 30.2. Death and recurrence rate, death rate, vaginal and pelvic recurrence, and distant metastasis for patients with histologic grade 1 and 2 tumors infiltrating less or more than half the myometrium

Treatment group	Myometrial infiltration ≤ 0.5					Myometrial infiltration > 0.5				
	No. of patients	DRR (%)	Deaths of cancer (%)	Vaginal and pelvic recurrence (%)	Distant metastasis (%)	No. of patients	DRR (%)	Deaths of cancer (%)	Vaginal and pelvic recurrence (%)	Distant metastasis (%)
A	126	5.6	2.3	4.0	1.6	51	13.7	7.8	9.8	3.9
B	131	7.6	6.9	2.3	6.9	32	15.6	9.4	9.4	9.4

DRR = death and recurrence rate (see text).

A thorough analysis of the material showed that the two most important prognostic factors are histologic grade and depth of myometrial infiltration. It was found of interest to combine these two factors. These analyses are shown in Tables 30.2 and 30.3. The prognoses for patients with Grade 1 and Grade 2 lesions were found almost identical, and, therefore, these two groups were considered as a single entity. Table 30.2 shows that patients with histologic Grade 1 and Grade 2 tumors do not benefit by additional external irradiation irrespective of depth of myometrial infiltration. More patients died of corpus cancer in Group B than in Group A because a significantly higher number of patients in Group B developed distant metastases. This was in accordance with the preliminary results presented in 1976 (4).

Furthermore, no positive effect was produced by pelvic irradiation in patients with histologic Grade 3 tumors infiltrating less than half the myometrial wall (Table 30.3). Only patients with poorly differentiated tumors infiltrating more

than half the myometrial wall showed a higher survival rate in Group B (where pelvic irradiation was given) than in Group A. The figures in Table 30.2 and 30.3 show that additional external irradiation provides significantly better pelvic control of the disease. This advantage, however, is outweighed by a higher number of distant metastases in Group B, resulting in the same survival rate in the two treatment groups.

TUMOR CELLS IN ENDOTHELIAL LINED SPACES

In the last 151 consecutive patients of this clinical trial, the surgical specimens were carefully studied for tumor cells in blood or lymph vessels. Vessel invasion was found in 30 patients (19.9%). The DRR for these 30 patients was 26.7% (8 patients), which is significantly higher at the 5% level compared to the 9.1% (11 patients) DRR for the remaining 121 patients.

Table 30.3. Death and recurrence rate, death rate, vaginal and pelvic recurrence, and distant metastasis for patients with histologic grade 3 tumors infiltrating less or more than half the myometrium

Treatment group	Myometrial infiltration ≤ 0.5					Myometrial infiltration > 0.5				
	No. of patients	DRR (%)	Deaths of cancer (%)	Vaginal and pelvic recurrence (%)	Distant metastasis (%)	No. of patients	DRR (%)	Deaths of cancer (%)	Vaginal and pelvic recurrence (%)	Distant metastasis (%)
A	36	11.1	8.3	5.6	5.6	51	31.4	27.5	19.6	15.7
B	47	19.1	17.0	2.1	17.0	44	18.2	18.2	4.5	13.6

DRR = death and recurrence rate.

CONCLUSION

The observations made in this controlled clinical trial confirm data that have been published in earlier studies. It was found that older patients have a poorer prognosis than those in the younger age groups. Furthermore, significantly more patients over 60 years of age had tumors infiltrating deeper than half the myometrial thickness. This observation might explain their poorer prognosis, which was not influenced by external pelvic irradiation.

The size of the uterine cavity was found to be of less prognostic importance than traditionally believed, although there were slightly more recurrences observed in patients with a uterine cavity length of more than 8 cm. The observed difference, however, was not significant.

The most important prognostic factors were the histologic grade and the depth of myometrial infiltration. The Grade 3 lesions were found to be more apt to penetrate deep into the myometrium.

A new observation is that the occurrence of tumor cells in blood or lymph vessels in the myometrial wall was, as in other gynecologic tumors, related to a significantly higher number of recurrences and deaths.

A highly significant improvement in pelvic control was obtained in patients receiving additional external irradiation. On the other hand, patients receiving external irradiation developed a higher number of distant metastases. The reason for this is obscure. It may be that external irradiation influences the immunologic defense mechanism of the patient. Another explanation, as shown by Engeset in animal studies (9), may be a progressive reduction of the barrier function of the lymph nodes after irradiation. This phenomenon might also contribute to the shorter interval for recurrent disease in the group of patients receiving external irradiation.

On the basis of the data presented here, the following treatment protocol is recommended:

1. Patients with Stage I endometrial carcinoma should undergo primary hysterectomy and salpingo-oophorectomy followed by vaginal radiation.
2. Patients with Grade 3 lesions infiltrating more than half of the myometrial thickness should receive external irradiation to the pelvic lymph nodes with a tumoricidal dose of 40 Gy.
3. The therapeutic consequence of the finding of tumor cells in vascular spaces is not quite clear. The prognosis of the patients in whom vascular invasion was found was poor and therefore pelvic irradiation is also recommended in these cases. It is highly probable that they have more metastases to the lymph nodes than patients with no vascular invasion.
4. Patients with tumors infiltrating more or less through the myometrium, irrespective of histologic grade, probably should also receive external irradiation. All other patients should only by treated with vaginal intracavitary radiotherapy and no external irradiation.

By following this treatment protocol a large number of patients will avoid having to have external radiotherapy and nevertheless have a good prognosis. When recurrences in the pelvis occur, one may give radiotherapy, progestagens, antiestrogens and/or cytostatics. It seems quite clear from the present study that giving external radiotherapy to all patients with endometrial carcinoma Stage I does not influence the survival rate.

Since the study referred to above was published, vaginal irradiation has been given by the Cathetron afterloading machine, using cobolt sources. More than 500 patients have been treated, and the local vaginal recurrence rate has been only about 1%. Complications have been rare, and both for the patients and the personnel this method is most acceptable.

Adjuvant therapy in Stage I endometrial carcinoma with progestagens has been found of no value in a large controlled clinical study comprising more than 1100 patients (not published). Recent receptor studies, however, indicate that lack of estrogen and/or progesteron receptors carries a bad prognosis. Receptor determinations should therefore be carried out on a larger scale in future.

31
Peritoneal cytology

In a study from the Norwegian Radium Hospital in 1956, Dahle (1) pointed to the fact that, theoretically, fragments of endometrial carcinoma may pass through the lumina of the Fallopian tubes and cause implantations in the peritoneal cavity. This type of spread had been discussed in the literature for many years when he performed his study of peritoneal cytology. The method he used was described as follows:

> Just after opening the abdomen, the intestines were packed away from the pelvic cavity with gauze pads, clamps were vertically applied at each side of the fundus of the uterus to the broad ligament, and the uterus pulled forward towards the symphysis. Then the Douglas cul de sac was washed with 20 ml of physiologic saline solution. Before performing the hysterectomy, the tubes were removed, and the washings and the tubes were immediately sent for cytologic examination.

This procedure was applied in 21 patients with endometrial carcinoma Stage I. He found that in 7 cases there were tumor cells in the pouch of Douglas, and in 11 cases there were tumor cells in one or both tubes, 6 unilateral and 5 bilateral cases. He suggested that such tumor cells might give rise to recurrences in the peritoneal cavity and recommended that one should use radioactive colloidal gold to prevent this. However, soon after his article was published, he left the hospital, and his idea was not followed up by his successor. His work has been taken up later by the Gynecologic Oncology Group (GOG), which in 1981 published a similar study of 167 patients with clinical Stage I carcinoma of the endometrium. Twenty-six (15.5%) of these had malignant cells identified on cytologic examinations of peritoneal washings. Recurrence developed in 10 of these 26 (34%) compared to 14 of 141 (9.9%) patients with negative cytologic testing (2). The GOG recommended that patients with positive peritoneal cytology possibly should be treated with intraperitoneal radioactive chromic phosphate suspension. But, in this connection, it should be mentioned that in our controlled clinical trial of 540 patients, only 9 (1.7%) had a recurrence in the upper abdomen. Furthermore, in 1983 Yazigi, Piver and Blumenson (3) reported a peritoneal cytology study performed on 93 patients with Stage I endometrial cancer seen at Roswell Park Memorial Institute. Ten patients (11%) had positive cytology for neoplastic cells. All patients were followed for a minimum of 10 years or until death from cancer or intercurrent disease. No patient received treatment for positive cytology. There was one recurrence in the patients with positive cytology (10%), and six recurrences in the negative group (7.2%). They concluded that malignant peritoneal cytology does not seem to be a prognostic indicator in Stage I endometrial cancer. It should be realized that the cytopathologic diagnosis of malignant cells in peritoneal washings is often controversial.

32
Endometrial carcinoma Stage II

In 1941 Heyman, Reuterwall and Benner for the first time recommended that fractional curettage should be performed in all cases of endometrial carcinoma so that involvement of the cervix could be determined. They found a subgroup which they called "cancer corporis et colli uteri", subsequently termed Stage II endometrial carcinoma. The interpretation of the endocervical curettings may frequently be a problem for the histopathologist. There are at least three possible findings in the endocervical specimen: (1) Endocervical tissue with no associated endometrial cancer, (2) endocervical gland-bearing tissue with free-floating tumor cells, and (3) endocervical gland-bearing tissue contiguous with endometrial cancer demonstrating a true Stage II disease. For the clinician the problem arises when he receives a report of free-floating tumor cells, whether this is only contamination of the endocervix by the shedding of a Stage I cancer located in the corpus above, or conversely such free-floating tumor cells might have been detached from the endocervix in the presence of a true Stage II cancer.

The only paper on this problem from our institution was published in 1982 (1). Not only the histopathological evaluation of endocervical curettings, but also other prognostic factors and the value of combined radiological surgical treatment were evaluated in a prospective randomized clinical trial.

It is well known that, in endometrial adenocarcinoma, extension to the cervix seems to adversely affect the survival rate. In the latest report from the Norwegian Radium Hospital (2) a total of 580 cases of endometrial carcinoma were studied. The 5-year crude survival rate for Stage I lesions was 84.2% compared to 66.3% for the Stage II lesions. The poorer prognosis for Stage II disease can be explained partly by the higher incidence of pelvic lymph node metastases than in Stage I disease.

It has also been shown that a tumor which has extended into the cervix is usually relatively large with deep infiltration of the myometrium.

MATERIAL AND METHODS

During the years 1968–76, 185 patients with Stage II carcinoma of the corpus were referred to the Norwegian Radium Hospital. Eleven patients were excluded from the analysis. Five patients were found during operation to have extension of the disease beyond the uterus, and six were unable to complete the treatment program. Thus, 174 patients were left for analysis and follow-up. Altogether 135 patients received all their treatment in our hospital. Treatment consisted of a modified Heyman packing with 10 mg radium capsules, followed six weeks later by total abdominal hysterectomy and bilateral salpingo-oophorectomy. During the second week after surgery, vaginal irradiation with a radium applicator was employed delivering a homogenous dose of 60 Gy to the surface of the inner two thirds of the vaginal wall. After the end of vaginal radium treatment the patients were randomized to one of the following groups:

Group A: No further treatment.
Group B: External whole pelvic irradiation with a total midpelvic dose of 40 Gy with shielding of the bladder and rectum after 20 Gy. Five fractions a week were given in the course of four weeks.

The endocervical curettings and the operative specimens were classified according to the WHO International Histologic Classification of tumors. Of the 174 cases, 78 showed only free-floating tumor cells in the cervical curettings. Of these 78 cases, 75 were ordinary adenocarcinomas, 1 adenosquamous carcinoma, and 2 clear cell carcinomas.

The remaining 96 cases showed endocervical gland-bearing tissue contiguous with endometrial cancer and/or infiltration into the stroma of the surgical specimen. Of these 96 cases 84 were classified as ordinary adenocarcinomas, 5 as adenosquamous carcinomas, and in 7 cases clear cell carcinomas were found. An analysis of the factors influencing prognosis, treatment complications and survival was performed separately for the 84 invasive adenocarcinomas and the 75 cases with only free-floating tumor cells in the cervical curettings.

It was found that the DRR was significantly higher in patients with a uterine cavity > 8 cm (35.0% vs. 17.5%).

Surprisingly it did not seem that whole pelvic irradiation did improve prognosis. It should be emphasized, however, that the series studied is too small for an adequate statistical analysis. The 5-year survival rates were identical among treated and non-treated (Fig. 32.1). The group with only free-floating tumor cells in the cervix had a 5-year survival rate identical with Stage I endometrial carcinoma from the same time period (Group C. Fig. 32.1).

In 10 cases the cervix was grossly invaded by the tumor. Four of these patients died of cancer (40%). This should be compared with a DRR in the rest of the series of 17.5%. In Table 32.1 and

Table 32.1. Adenocarcinoma of the corpus uteri with extension to the cervix*

Histologic grade	No. of patients	DRR (%)	Vessel invasion (%)
G1	6	16.7	16.7
G2	58	19.0	19.0
G3	20	25.0	50.0
Total	84	20.2	26.2

* Relationship between histologic grade, death and recurrence rate (DRR) and frequency of vessel invasion.

Table 32.2. Adenocarcinoma of the corpus with infiltration into the cervix*

Myometrial infiltration**	No. of patients	DRR (%)	G3 tumors (%)	Vessel invasion (%)
)$\frac{1}{2}$	31	12.9	9.7	12.9
>$\frac{1}{2}$	22	31.8	27.3	68.2
?	31	19.4	35.5	9.7
Total	84	20.2	23.8	26.2

* Relationship between myometrial infiltration, death and recurrence rate (DRR) and frequency of G3 tumors and vessel invasion.
**)$\frac{1}{2}$ = less or equal to half the myometrial thickness, >$\frac{1}{2}$ = more than half the myometrial thickness, ? = no tumor left after preoperative radium packing.

32.2 the relationship between histologic grade, vessel invasion and DRR is shown. As can be seen, there were more G3 lesions in this series than in the endometrial carcinoma Stage I series. The DRR increased with the increasing grade of the disease and with the occurrence of vessel invasion.

The depth of infiltration into the myometrium could be assessed in 53 patients. In the rest of the series there was no residual tumor six weeks after radium packing. The DRR was adversely affected by deep myometrial infiltration. Furthermore, both G3 tumors and vessel invasion were much more frequent in those with myometrial infiltration of more than half the myometrial thickness.

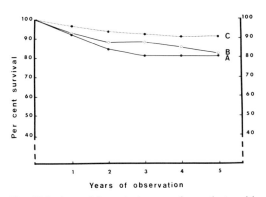

Fig. 32.1. Actuarial survival curves for patients with carcinoma of the corpus Stage II. A: Treated by radium packing and hysterectomy. B: Additional pelvic irradiation. C: Group of patients with free floating tumor cells in cervical curettings, see text. From (1) and reproduced by courtesy of Academic Press Inc.

CARCINOMA OF OTHER HISTOLOGICAL TYPES

Five patients with confirmed cervical involvement were found to have adenosquamous carcinoma.

Their mean age was 63 years. In only one patient was vessel invasion found. This patient suffered lateral pelvic wall recurrence and died after 11 months.

Clear cell carcinoma was found in seven patients. Their mean age was 65 years. Two of the patients had deeply infiltrating tumors, and two showed vessel invasion. Significantly more patients (4/7) died in this group than in the group of patients with ordinary adenocarcinoma (16/84). The DRR was 57.1% as compared to 18.8% for the ordinary adenocarcinomas.

In recent years we have in accordance with other studies found that the so-called serous papillary carcinoma of the endometrium can be separated as a specially poor prognostic group.

CONCLUSION

If only free-floating tumor cells are found in the endocervical scraping, the patient may be treated as for an endometrial carcinoma Stage I, i.e. with primary surgery. Also, if there is only microscopic evidence of infiltration into the gland-bearing tissue and no grossly visible tumor, primary surgery can be performed. In these cases, however, it might be wise to do a modified extended hysterectomy with removal of at least part of the parametria on both sides. A true radical Wertheim hysterectomy should not be necessary.

In 10 of our 174 patients we found that the cervix was grossly involved, either by inspection or by the findings of endocervical scraping. In some cases the tumor could be seen protruding through the external os, and in other cases abundant material was obtained from a cavity in the endocervix. Such cases could be treated in several ways. If one prefers primary surgery, this should certainly be performed as a radical hysterectomy and with pelvic lymphadenectomy. If lymphadenectomy is difficult, external irradiation should be given. Those who do not adhere to primary radical surgery, may either give radium packing or external radiotherapy preoperatively. Pelvic and periaortic node sampling is also recommended. Unfortunately, we have no experience with this procedure, but several series from the United States seem to indicate that such sampling may give the clinician additional information of importance for the decision on further therapy after surgery (3).

Endometrial carcinoma Stage III

According to the definition of the International Federation of Gynecology and Obstetrics (FIGO), classification and staging should always be based on careful clinical examination and should be performed before any definite treatment is started. Carcinoma of the corpus uteri Stage III is defined as a lesion that has extended outside the uterus, but not outside the true pelvis. There should be no involvement of the mucosa of the bladder or the rectum. In carcinoma of the corpus, however, the patients are usually obese, and it is frequently difficult to decide by ordinary bimanual palpation if the lesion has extended outside the uterus. The presence of metastases in for example the ovary or the Fallopian tube are frequently only diagnosed at operation or by histologic examination of the operation specimen. In some reports these cases are included in the total Stage III group, although these patients might carry a significantly better prognosis. This certainly is one of the reasons why the results of treatment in Stage III carcinoma, as presented in the eighteenth *Annual Report* (1), vary between 16 and 45%. The Norwegian Radium Hospital reported 21 cases, and 6 of these (28.6%) survived for five years.

During the years 1960–77 a total of 3,393 cases of carcinoma of the corpus were treated in the Norwegian Radium Hospital. One hundred and seventy-five patients had tumor extension outside the uterus, but not outside the true pelvis. One hundred and eight of these patients had clinical Stage III disease, and in 67 patients, originally classified as Stages I or II, the intrapelvic extrauterine tumor spread was first detected at surgery or histopathological examination of the operation specimen (surgical-pathological Stage III). This means that there were 3.2% of *clinical* Stage III disease in this large series of 3,393 patients. In the eighteenth *Annual Report,* Stage III lesions comprise between 0 and 33% of cases treated in the different institutions. Most institutions report a frequency of between 5 and 10%. It was found of interest to compare the results in patients with *clinical Stage III* and those with *surgical-pathological Stage III* disease (2).

MATERIAL AND METHODS

From 1960 to 1977, a total of 108 patients had clinical Stage III, and 67 patients had surgical-pathological Stage III disease. The distribution by site of extrauterine tumor extension in these two groups is shown in Table 33.1. The majority of patients who presented with clinical Stage III disease, had vaginal and/or parametrial involvement. In patients with surgical-pathological Stage III the adnexa were the most frequent sites of spread.

The mode of treatment for the two groups of patients varied and is summarized in Table 33.2. In the choice of primary treatment the site and the extent of the extrauterine tumor extension and the general condition of the patient were of major importance. If possible, surgery was performed, and consisted of total abdominal hysterectomy and bilateral salpingo-oophorectomy (106 cases). After surgery, 99 of the 106 patients underwent radiotherapy consisting of megavoltage irradiation to a pelvic field with a total dose of 40–50 Gy in 4–5 weeks. In patients with vaginal extension of the tumor, external irradiation was combined with intravaginal radium irradiation. Of the clinical Stage III patients, 64% were inoperable because of the tumor extension, and radiotherapy was the treatment of choice. The majority of these patients were treated with radium packing, and this was followed by megavoltage external irradiation to a total dose of 40–50 Gy in 4–5 weeks with central shielding after 20 Gy.

In the later part of the study period, the use of progestagens was introduced. Seventy-six of the

Table 33.1. Distribution by site of extra-uterine tumor extension

Site of extra-uterine tumor extension	Clinical stage III		Surgical-pathological stage III	
	No.	%	No.	%
Vagina	42	39	1	1
Parametrium	31	29	2	3
Ovary and/or tube	4	4	46	69
Pelveo-peritoneal surface	–	–	8	12
Multiple sites	31	29	10	15
Total	108	100	67	100

Table 33.2 Treatment modalities

Mode of treatment	Clinical stage III		Surgical-pathological stage III	
	No.	%	No.	%
Surgery + irradiation	35 (16)*	32 (15)	64 (25)	96 (37)
Irradiation	66 (32)	61 (30)	–	–
Surgery	4 (1)	4 (1)	3 (2)	4 (3)
Progestagens	3	3	–	–
Total	108 (49)	100 (46)	67 (27)	100 (40)

* in brackets, numbers and percentages of patients who received progestagional agents.

175 patients received hydroxyprogesteroncaproate as part of their initial treatment. The drug was administered by injection, 1000 mg daily during the first week, followed by 1000 mg every week for three months, and thereafter every second week for at least one year.

The histologic classification of the tumors was based mainly on the first fractional curettage specimen, because preoperative irradiation had either destroyed or altered the appearance of the tumor, and because in many patients no operation was performed. The tumors were graded according to the FIGO system. There were 12 cases of adenosquamous carcinoma, and 8 cases of clear cell carcinoma.

When possible, the maximum depth of tumor infiltration in the myometrium was assessed and recorded as less, equal, or deeper than half the myometrial thickness. In all cases, vessel invasion was recorded as present or not.

RESULTS

The 5-year actuarial survival rates were 16% for clinical Stage III and 40% for surgical-pathologi-

cal Stage III (Fig. 33.1). Most of the patients who died from their disease, did so in the course of the first two years after treatment.

In both series, the deaths from cancer were related to the well known prognostic factors, age, histologic grade, myometrial infiltration, cervical involvement and tumor cells in vessels. Patients

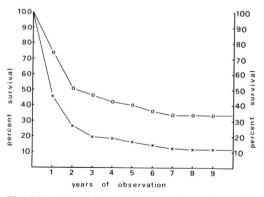

Fig. 33.1. Actuarial survival curves for patients with carcinoma of the corpus Stage III. o – o: Surgical-pathological Stage III (N=67). x – x: Clinical Stage III (N=108). From (2) and reproduced by courtesy of Academic Press Inc.

older than 60 years of age did less well than those below 60 years of age in both series. It was striking that there were no cases with histologic Grade 1 in the clinical Stage III series. The death rate was the same for patients with Grade 2 lesions as for those with Grade 3 lesions. In the surgical-pathological Stage III, however, the same difference as in Stages I and II disease was found. More patients died from cancer when they had Grade 3 lesions as compared to Grades I and II lesions (81% vs. 50%). The prognosis for patients with adenosquamous or clear cell carcinomas was poor in both series.

Adjuvant progestagen therapy was given in 52 of the 108 clinical Stage III, and in 27 of the 67 surgical-pathological Stage III patients. It is difficult to evaluate the results. However, it seems that if the tumor has extended so much outside the uterus that surgery cannot be performed, adjuvant progestagen therapy does not increase the survival rate. In patients treated with combined surgery and irradiation, addition of progestagens seemed to be of some benefit.

In conclusion, it may be claimed that surgical-pathological Stage III carcinoma of the endometrium should always be considered as a separate group when reporting endometrial cancer, because the prognosis differs significantly from that of clinical Stage III. Complete surgical eradication of the tumor is of great prognostic importance in both clinical and surgical-pathological Stage III endometrial cancer. Surgery combined with radiotherapy is currently the best available treatment. In both groups a staging periaortic lymphadenectomy or lymph node biopsy should be considered to decide on periaortic irradiation, for example.

Adjuvant progestational therapy seems to be of some benefit, especially when all macroscopic tumor tissue has been removed. There is, however, an obvious need for systematic clinical studies on the value of different adjuvant chemotherapeutic regimes and/or antiestrogens.

34
Endometrial carcinoma Stage IV

In Stage IV endometrial cancer the tumor has extended outside the true pelvis or has obviously involved the mucosa of the bladder and/or rectum. In the eighteenth *Annual Report* a total of 11,501 patients with carcinoma of the corpus were reported as being treated. Out of these, 314 (2.7%) belonged to Stage IV. The 5-year survival rate for the Stage IV cases was 9.6%.

The low incidence of Stage IV cancer contributes to the poor experience of many gynecologists with these patients. From 1960 to 1977 altogether 3,393 cases of corpus cancer were seen in the Norwegian Radium Hospital out of which 83 (2.4%) belonged to Stage IV (1).

Postmenopausal bleeding was the first symptom in 87% of the patients, and in 37% the only symptom. Other symptoms include low abdominal pain, vaginal discharge, increasing abdominal size, enlarged lymph glands and deteriorating con-

dition of the patient. In 52% there was a patient delay of more than three months, and in 25% the symptoms had lasted for more than one year before a physician was consulted.

Great variations in the sites of extrauterine tumor extension and in the medical condition of the patient led to greatly individualized treatment regimes. Broadly outlined, radiotherapy, surgery combined with radiotherapy and progestagens were used.

SURVIVAL

Seventy-seven percent of all patients died within the first year of diagnosis. The actuarial 5-year survival rate was 10%.

Most of the patients were unsuitable for surgery (73%). Radiotherapy therefore played an impor-

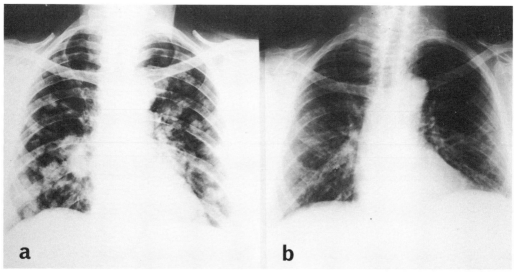

Fig. 34.1. Stage IV carcinoma of the corpus with lung metastases (a). Disappearance of metastases after three months treatment with hydroxyprogesteronecaproate.

tant role in the treatment. It was the main method for 50 patients, and combined with progestagens in 30 of these. Control of pelvic disease was achieved in 13 of these 50 patients (25%), and 4 of them were alive without evidence of disease at the end of the observation period ranging from 3 to 19 years.

Radiotherapy can also play an important role in the control of extrapelvic tumor. In five patients with supraclavicular and two patients with axillary lymph node metastases, complete clinical remission was achieved by radiotherapy.

The value of progestagen treatment is clearly demonstrated in our series. In 20 of the 83 patients such treatment was considered successful for more than three months. Five of eight cases had lung metastases which completely disappeared after treatment with hydroxyprogesteroncaproate (Fig. 34.1). Another patient, also with lung metastases and involvement of the bladder mucosa, received intracavitary radium, pelvic irradiation and progestagens. She had recurrence of her lung metastases, and progestagen treatment was continued.

She died of her cancer nine years after primary treatment.

Although we achieved only 10% 5-year survival, there is no doubt that the treatment protocol with surgery, if possible, and radiotherapy combined with progestagens, in most cases gives good palliation. There was a definite improvement in the quality of life also for those who died from their disease.

Nevertheless, there is no doubt that there is a great need for systemic therapy in these patients, not only with progestagens, but also with cytostatics. In recurrent disease we have seen complete response of for example lung metastases in approximately 30% of the cases with 5-fluorouracil. Other drugs which have been used with some success in advanced or recurrent endometrial carcinoma are cyclophosphamide, melphalan, adriamycin and cis-platinum. In particular, adriamycin in combination with other drugs has become popular in many places in the United States (2). To date, we have no personal experience with antiestrogens such as tamoxifen (3).

35
Recurrent endometrial adenocarcinoma

For many years little attention was paid to recurrent adenocarcinoma of the endometrium. This has certainly been due to the fact that more than 80% with endometrial cancer have localized disease with an overall 5-year survival rate of about 75%. During the last decade, however, growing interest in the treatment of recurrences of corpus cancer has been reflected in an increasing number of papers dealing with this problem. There are several reasons for this. Firstly, endometrial carcinoma has become more and more common in Western countries. Furthermore, the introduction of hormone and, in later years, also chemotherapy for recurrences has shown that even with distant metastases some patients can be cured. This is especially so with lung metastases.

To evaluate our own experience with recurrent disease a study based on 379 patients admitted to our hospital from 1960 to 1977 was reviewed (1). Recurrence was defined as re-growth of endometrial cancer after an apparently complete remission following primary treatment, and lasting for at least three months. Patients with residual disease after the initial treatment were excluded.

TREATMENT

In 117 of the 379 patients no treatment was given for the following reasons: too extensive disease, the deteriorating medical condition of the patient, or previous radiotherapy of the site of recurrence.

In the course of one year, 90% of the untreated patients were dead, as compared to 50% of those who received some form of treatment for their recurrence. Twenty-nine of the 262 treated patients (11.1%) were alive at the end of the observation period, which ranged from 3 to 19 years. Radiotherapy was the most common method of treatment (64%). Six percent of these patients also had surgery. Surgery plays a minor, but significant part when used in cases with localized operable recurrent disease. In these patients prognosis is relatively good. Of 29 patients treated with surgery 10 are alive without evidence of disease at the end of the observation period.

The best treatment results were obtained in patients with vaginal vault recurrences, uterine recurrences, or recurrences in the outer part of the vagina resulting in 24, 21 and 14% survivors, respectively, without evidence of disease at the end of the observation period.

All in all, the prognosis for the patients with recurrent endometrial cancer treated by the current surgical, radiotherapeutic and hormonal methods, is poor. Only 11.1% of the 262 treated patients survived during the observation period of from 3 to 19 years. If the current management of advanced and recurrent endometrial cancer is to be improved, adjuvant chemotherapy with cytotoxic drugs would seem to be a reasonable choice. There are not many publications available on this topic. It seems, however, that alkylating agents such as cyclophosphamide and melphalan, and 5-fluorouracil appear to have some activity. More recently adriamycin has proved to have a significant activity. Also cis-platinum has been found to be active in advanced and recurrent endometrial cancer. Recently, combination chemotherapy has come into use. Antiestrogens also have a place in the recurrent endometrial carcinomas.

At present, receptor studies are being carried out in our hospital to evaluate whether it is possible to select cases for hormone treatment when recurrences occur. To date, the results are inconclusive. It is the author's opinion that adjuvant hormone therapy should not only be based on receptor values. Nor should it be forgotten that the anabolic progestagens frequently induce a state of physical well-being even if survival is not significantly increased.

36
Sarcoma of the uterus

EPIDEMIOLOGY

Sarcomas of the uterus are rare. In Norway there are approximately ten cases a year, or 0.5/100,000, which is comparable to rates found in other parts of the Western world. Between 2 and 4% of all malignant tumors of the uterus are sarcomas. Almost all cases detected in Norway are referred to the Norwegian Radium Hospital, either for primary treatment or for secondary treatment after surgery has been performed elsewhere. However, since uterine sarcomas are so rare, the experience gained even in a large cancer-referral institution is still quite limited.

STAGING

We have used the same staging procedure for sarcomas of the uterus as for carcinoma of the uterine corpus.

Stage I. – Tumor is limited to the corpus.
Stage II. – Tumor has grown down into the cervical canal.
Stage III. – Tumor has extended beyond the uterus, but is still confined within the true pelvis.
Stage IV. – Tumor has invaded either the bladder or the rectum or has spread outside the pelvis.
Stage IVa. – Spread to bladder and/or rectum.
Stage IVb. – Distant metastases.

HISTOLOGY

The most commonly used classification for uterine sarcomas today is that first proposed by Ober in 1959 (1), and later modified by Kempson (2). Ober suggested that uterine sarcomas should be categorized according to their cell type and site of origin. The tumors can be either pure or mixed, the latter being composed of more than one cell type. Homologous tumors contain tissue elements entirely indigenous to the uterus, whereas heterologous tumors contain tissue elements that are foreign to the uterus. Because many of the sarcomas included in Ober's classification are extremely rare, and since there are many subgroups, we have followed the Gynecologic Oncology Group in the United States by simplifying the classification as shown in Table 36.1. The leiomyosarcomas as well as the endometrial stromal sarcomas and mixed homologous Müllerian sarcomas all contain tissue found in the normal uterus, while the mixed heterologous Müllerian sarcomas, also called mixed mesodermal tumors, contain tissue that is alien to the uterus.

Rhabdomyosarcoma (sarcoma botryoides) is the most common pure heterologous sarcoma. It is a very rare tumor, and can occur at all ages, primarily in young girls. We have no experience with this type of sarcoma, because the girls are treated by pediatric surgeons.

The incidence of malignant mixed Müllerian tumors is thought to be increasing, and at our hospital these tumors are encountered as often as leiomyosarcomas at present. In earlier series, leiomyosarcoma was the most frequent type of sarcoma. This is in accordance with most series presented in the world literature, where, in general, leiomyosarcoma is the most common, followed by malignant mixed Müllerian tumor and endometrial stromal sarcoma.

Leiomyosarcomas typically are solitary masses, and about 60% are intramural, some are submucosal and some subserosal. Very occasionally we have found leiomyosarcomas developing in pre-existing leiomyomas. If this is the case, the patients have a good prognosis.

In later years we have counted the mitotic rate in all leiomyosarcomas, and we agree that tumors with a mitotic rate of 5 or more per 10 high power

Table 36.1. Classification of uterine sarcomas

Leiomyosarcomas
Endometrial stromal sarcomas
Mixed homologous Müllerian sarcomas
  (carcinosarcoma)
Mixed heterologous Müllerian sarcomas
  (mixed mesodermal sarcoma)
Other uterine sarcomas

Table 36.3. Uterine sarcomas, 1968–74 series, treated by surgery, radiation and actinomycin D.

Tumor extension	Total No.	No. alive
Localized tumor	40	21
Non-localized tumor	33	3
Total	73	23

fields (HPF) have a potential for recurrence or metastasis and should be designated leiomyosarcomas. In contrast, those tumors with 4 or fewer mitotic figures per 10 HPF are almost invariably benign.

The origin of mixed Müllerian tumors has still not been clarified. One theory claims that such tumors arise from embryonal rests, while another theory, which is more commonly accepted, claims that such tumors are derived from the mesenchymal cells lying just below the endometrial epithelium. The mixed homologous Müllerian sarcomas are also called carcinosarcomas, and over the years we have tried to differentiate between these and so-called mixed heterologous Müllerian sarcomas, which may contain elements of rhabdomyosarcoma, chondrosarcoma or other elements that are foreign to the uterus. Also in the mixed Müllerian sarcomas the most commonly used histopathological criteria for determination of malignancy are hypercellularity, nuclear atypism and prominent mitotic activity.

Endometrial stromal sarcomas are composed exclusively of neoplastic endometrial stromal cells. They are subclassified in accordance with the appearance of their margins (circumscribed or infiltrating) and also on their mitotic rate. Often those tumors with an infiltrating border, but a low mitotic rate, have been termed endolymphatic stromal myosis or endometrial stromatosis. These tumors have a better prognosis than the true endometrial stromal sarcomas, which always have a high mitotic rate.

It is well known that all the sarcomas found in the uterus may spread by contiguous growth, hematological spread or lymphogenous spread. The leiomyosarcomas usually invade vessels and spread to the liver, lungs, bone or brain. The mixed Müllerian sarcomas, especially the homologous type (carcinosarcoma), also spread via the blood route, but frequently lymphatic spread to the pelvic lymph nodes will also be found. This makes us believe that perhaps these tumors may benefit from additional radiotherapy. The same holds true for the endometrial stromal sarcomas.

Over the years we have also seen a few cases of so-called benign metastasizing leiomyomas. These tumors usually stop growing when the uterus and both ovaries are removed, so that they are no longer influenced by estrogen. In a few cases we have also tried progestagen treatment with some effect.

Table 36.2. Data on the two series. In 1947–1962 the patients received radiotherapy after surgery, in the 1968–1974 period they in addition received treatment with actinomycin D.

Type of sarcoma	1947–1962		1968–1974	
	Total no. cases	No. alive	Total no. cases	No. alive
Leiomyosarcoma	58	14	39	6
Endometrial stromal sarcoma	0	0	7	6
Mixed Müllerian sarcoma	33	11	26	4
Unclassified	9	0	1	0
Total	100	25	73	16

We have no experience with pure heterologous sarcomas in the uterus, such a rhabdomyosarcomas, chondrosarcomas or osteosarcomas. We have, however, seen cases of mixed heterologous Müllerian sarcomas, which have contained areas of rhabdomyosarcoma. These tumors have a very poor prognosis.

TREATMENT METHODS

In 1983 the results were published of three studies on the treatment of sarcoma of the uterus at the Norwegian Radium Hospital. The periods studied were 1947–62, 1968–74 and 1975–81 (3).

During the first study period, 1947–62, treatment was based on surgery combined with external irradiation to a pelvic field. During most of these years, conventional radiotherapy with a four field technique was used. High-voltage machines were introduced in 1957–58. The 5-year survival rate was only 7% for the group in which the surgical borders were not free of malignancy or the sarcoma had already spread to other organs.

In the second study period, 1968–74, actinomycin D was added to external irradiation. It was thought that actinomycin D could possibly cure microscopic metastases and also act as a radiosensitizer. At the time this study started, actinomycin

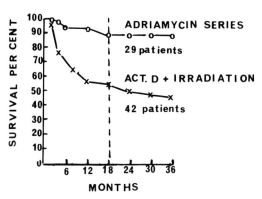

Fig. 36.2. Results of adjuvant chemotherapy with adriamycin in sarcoma of the uterus Stage I compared with earlier series treated with actinomycin D and pelvic irradiation. From (3) and reproduced by courtesy of Raven Press.

D was one of the few drugs which was considered effective in the therapy of sarcomas.

The exact data from these two series are shown in Table 36.2. We found that the addition of actinomycin D did not produce better treatment results. When metastases were found during surgery, or if radical surgery was impossible, several combined treatment schemes were used with little or no success. This is clearly shown in Table 36.3. While 50% of those with localized tumor survived for five years, only 2 out of 33 with non-localized tumor did so.

We divided the material from the actinomycin D series, 1968–74, into those classified as mixed Müllerian sarcoma and leiomyosarcoma. Fig. 36.1 shows that only approximately 30% in both groups survived for five years. Those with non-localized tumors are also included in these curves.

The most recent series, 1976–80, showed that today women with sarcoma are slightly younger than women in previous years. Among the leiomyosarcoma patients seven were premenopausal and the average age of this group, comprising 20 cases, was 51 years. The average age of women with endometrial stromal sarcoma was 53, and five were premenopausal, while the average age of those with mixed mesodermal tumors was 59, and three were premenopausal. In all three series the vast majority of the patients initially consulted a physician because of bleeding or bleeding with discharge. Other symptoms were pain, increasing girth and in a few cases urinary symptoms with

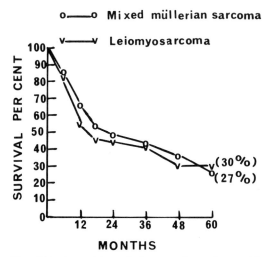

Fig. 36.1. Actuarial survival curves for patients with mixed Müllerian sarcoma and leiomyosarcoma treated with hysterectomy, irradiation and actinomycin D. From (3) and reproduced by courtesy of Raven Press, New York.

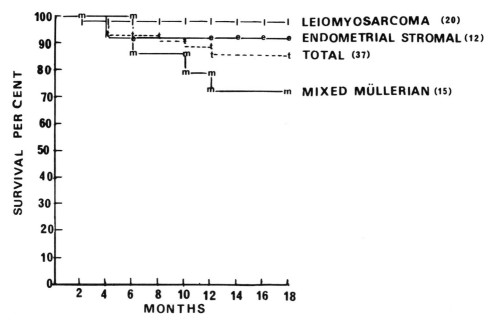

Fig. 36.3. Actuarial survival curves for different histological types of sarcoma of the uterus Stage I treated with adjuvant chemotherapy with adriamycin. From (3) and reproduced by courtesy of Raven Press.

frequent micturition. The diagnosis in most patients with mixed mesodermal tumors was established as a result of curettage, which was not the case in patients with leiomyosarcoma, in which case the operative specimen was often needed to make the final diagnosis.

Since the first two series did not show any significant effect either of surgery followed by radiotherapy or radiotherapy combined with actinomycin D, we began searching for other drugs. In 1975 adriamycin had become available in our country, and we decided that all patients with localized sarcomas should receive adjuvant chemotherapy with this drug. The schedule was 60 mg/m² adriamycin administered through a running intravenous flow every third week, and the maximum dose to be received by any patient was approximately 500 mg/m². This required that the patient be admitted to hospital every third week for approximately 7–9 months until the maximum dose was reached. We did not set up a controlled clinical trial because of the small number of patients admitted each year. We used the historical series, which received actinomycin D and irradiation, as a control group. In 1978, Omura and Blessing (5) showed that adriamycin alone can

provide a 27% response rate in recurrent disease. During our study period from 1975 to 1980 several other studies with adjuvant chemotherapy, either with adriamycin alone or in combination with dimethyltriazenoimidasol carboxamid (DTIC) or other drugs, were under way.

In Fig. 36.2 a comparison between the series receiving adriamycin as adjuvant chemotherapy and the series of localized tumors treated with actinomycin D and irradiation is shown. There was a remarkable difference in the survival rates between these two series.

In Fig. 36.3 the patients in the 1976–80 series are divided into the different histopathological groups. With adjuvant chemotherapy with adriamycin in localized tumors, leiomyosarcomas seem to have the best prognosis, while mixed Müllerian tumors have the poorest with a 70% survival rate after 18 months.

DISCUSSION

The results presented here must be somewhat sceptically evaluated. Several publications which have come out since our study cannot confirm that adriamycin alone or combined with e.g.

DTIC has a beneficial effect as adjuvant chemotherapy.

As regards the non-localized tumors, we are at present studying different drug combinations with or without radiotherapy. No results can be presented to date. Among the drugs we have used are cyclophosphamide, actinomycin D, adriamycin and vincristine. Thus far we have observed the disappearance of metastatic leiomyosarcomas in some patients receiving such combined treatment. It must be admitted, however, that sarcoma of the uterus must still be considered one of the most malignant tumors within gynecological oncology, and that we cannot present any treatment plan that really means a breakthrough in the treatment of these tumors.

37
Carcinoma of the ovary

STAGING

The staging of carcinoma of the ovary should be based on findings at clinical examination and surgical exploration. Histologic examination of possible spread outside the ovaries should be considered in the staging, as should cytology as far as effusions are concerned. It is desirable that biopsies should be taken from suspicious areas outside the pelvis. The finding of tumor cells in peritoneal effusions should not be considered sufficient to allocate a case to Stage III. Only positive biopsies outside the true pelvis should be taken into account when Stage III is being decided upon. However, the finding of tumor cells in effusions or in cytologic samples from the peritoneum above the pelvic brim, or e.g. at the dome of the diaphragm will influence the type of treatment.

At the meeting of the Cancer Committee of FIGO in Berlin September 1985, there was an unanimous agreement that in Stage I, only three subgroups should be recognized, not six, as has been the case for many years. On the other hand, the Committee also decided that in Stage III a division into three sub-groups should be introduced.

Stage I. – Growth limited to the ovaries

Stage Ia. – Growth limited to one ovary, capsule intact, no ascites, negative peritoneal washings.

Stage Ib. – Growth limited to both ovaries, capsules intact, no ascites, negative peritoneal washings.

Stage Ic. – Tumor in one or both ovaries with either tumor on the external surface, and/or rupture, spontaneous or during surgery, and/or ascites present, and/or positive peritoneal washings.

Ascites is peritoneal effusion, which in the opinion of the surgeon is pathological, exceeding the normal amount. Tumor cells should be demonstrated in the ascitic fluid.

If Stage Ic is based on positive peritoneal washings only, this should be reported.

Stage II. – Growth involving one or both ovaries with pelvic extension.

Stage IIa. – Extension and/or metastases to the uterus and/or tubes.

Stage IIb. – Extension to other pelvic tissues.

Stage IIc. – Tumor either Stage IIa or IIb, but with obvious ascites present which contains tumor cells.

Stage III. – Growth involving one or both ovaries with intraperitoneal metastases outside the pelvis and/or positive retroperitoneal nodes.

Tumor limited to the true pelvis with histologically proven metastases to small bowel or omentum.

Stage IIIa. – *Microscopic* spread to structures above the pelvic brim.

Stage IIIb. – Metastases above the pelvic brim less than 2 cm in diameter.

Stage IIIc. – All other cases of Stage III with metastases in the upper abdomen more than 2 cm in diameter.

Stage IV. – Growth involving one or both ovaries with distant metastases.

Parenchymal liver metastases equals Stage IV. If pleural effusion is present, there must be positive cytology to allot a case to Stage IV.

HISTOLOGICAL CLASSIFICATION OF THE COMMON PRIMARY EPITHELIAL TUMORS OF THE OVARY

Ovarian carcinoma is a common malignant tumor. It cannot be regarded as an entity. Therapeutic statistics on ovarian cancer are of limited value if attention is not paid to the histological type of the growth.

The cancer unit of the WHO has published a "histological typing of ovarian tumors" (1), which will help towards our understanding the pathology and behavior of ovarian neoplasms. The histopathological classification of epithelial tumors adopted by the WHO corresponds in principle with that proposed by FIGO.

It should be noted that cases of germ cell tumors, hormonal producing neoplasms such as granulosa-theca cell tumors, and metastatic carcinomas should be excluded from therapeutic statistics on ovarian carcinomas.

1. *Serous tumors*
(a) Serous benign cystadenomas.
(b) Serous cystadenomas with proliferating activity of the epithelial cells and nuclear abnormalities, but no infiltrative destructive growth (borderline cases, low potential malignancy).
(c) Serous cystadenocarcinomas.

2. *Mucinous tumors*
(a) Mucinous benign cystadenomas.
(b) Mucinous cystadenomas with proliferating activity of the epithelial cells and nuclear abnormalities, but with no infiltrative destructive growth (borderline cases, low potential malignancy).
(c) Mucinous cystadenocarcinomas.

3. *Endometrioid tumors*
(a) Endometrioid benign cysts.
(b) Endometrioid tumors with proliferating activity of the epithelial cells and nuclear abnormalities, but with no infiltrative destructive growth (borderline cases, low potential malignancy).
(c) Endometrioid adenocarcinomas.

4. *Clear cell tumors (mesonephroid tumors)*
(a) Benign clear cell tumors.
(b) Clear cell tumors with proliferating activity of the epithelial cells and nuclear abnormalities, but with no infiltrative destructive growth (borderline cases, low potential malignancy).
(c) Clear cell cystadenocarcinomas.

5. *Mixed epithelial tumors*
Tumors composed of a mixture of two or more of the malignant groups 1c, 2c, 3c or 4c described above and where none of them is predominant. Thus, a case should be listed as "mixed epithelial tumor" only if it is not possible to decide which is the predominant structure. The pathologist should always try to find out which is the leading structure and classify the case according to that element.

6. *Undifferentiated carcinoma*
Malignant structure that is too poorly differentiated to be placed in any of groups 1–5.

7. *No histology or unclassifiable*
Cases where explorative surgery has shown that obvious ovarian epithelial malignant tumor is present, but where no biopsy has been taken, or where the specimen is unclassifiable, e.g. because of necrosis.

Note: In some cases of anaplastic inoperable widespread malignant tumor it may be difficult for a gynecologist to decide the origin of the growth. Such cases should not be included in therapeutic statistics on carcinoma of the ovary. They should be classified as carcinoma abdominis.

EPIDEMIOLOGY

In many countries in Europe and in the United States ovarian cancer today is the leading cause of death among genital cancers. The incidence of ovarian cancer has also approached, or even surpassed, the incidence of cervical cancer in many countries.

Data from cancer registries around the world clearly show that ovarian cancer occurs with a considerably different frequency from country to country. Fig. 37.1 shows selected data from cancer registries in four different countries (2). It may be asked why the three Scandinavian countries, Denmark, Sweden and Norway, rank highest, while Japan has the lowest incidence of carcinoma of the ovary reported. There is no doubt that there must be ethnic differences. For example, in the United States the white population has a much higher incidence than the black, Spanish, Japanese or Chinese population. Of great interest is the fact that the Japanese in the United States have a higher incidence of ovarian carcinoma than the Japanese in their own country. A similar discrepancy between different ethnic groups is found in Singapore, where the Malaysians have a higher incidence than the Indian and the Chinese population. In India the incidence is very low in those areas where they have cancer registries, while in Israel a relatively high incidence rate is found among the Jews, but a very low incidence among the Muslims.

In 1974 (3) an epidemiologic study was performed in the Norwegian Radium Hospital concerning the incidence of ovarian neoplasia. A total of 1,141 cases were analyzed. We could not find any difference between the study population and the control population as to the age at menarche or menopause.

The most important observation was that the frequency of nulliparity among the patients with epithelial tumors of the ovary was much higher than in the total population in Norway, namely on an average 30% compared to 10%. Furthermore, there was a history of family cancer of the genital tract, breast or other sites, which was very high, on average, 32%. On the whole, it could not be proved that there are hereditary factors involved in the development of ovarian carcinoma. However, throughout the years we have found some

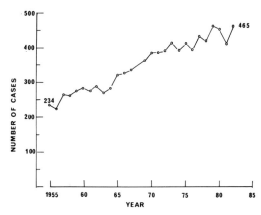

Fig. 37.2. Number of new cases of ovarian cancer reported to the Norwegian Cancer Registry in the period 1955–82.

families with epithelial carcinoma of the ovary, especially serous carcinomas, which have appeared in two or three generations, and/or in several sisters in the same generation. The same observation has been made in other countries (4).

It was concluded that the wide variation in the incidence of ovarian cancer reported by cancer registries throughout the world might in part be explained by differences in age distribution in the population studies. However, other factors, notably genetic, racial, dietary, cultural and ecologic variables may play a role. If, for example, in the future, American-born Japanese women are shown to develop ovarian cancer as frequently as white women, such epidemiological findings would tend to implicate environmental and dietary influences. However, emigrants cannot be regarded as a random sample of the country of origin.

The variation in incidence rates between specific histological types may be explained partly by differences in histopathological classification from country to country.

The observation that nulliparity was more frequent than expected in the group of patients with epithelial tumors of the ovary is of importance. Similar studies from other countries have shown that ovarian carcinoma is more common among infertile women, nulliparous women and women with only one or two children. In 1972, Fathalla (5) suggested that epithelial tumors might be due to incessant ovulation. It seems as if many preg-

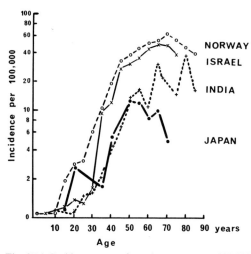

Fig. 37.1. Incidence rates of ovarian cancer per 100,000 in four different countries.

nancies in some way protect against the development of ovarian carcinoma of epithelial origin. The increasing incidence of ovarian cancer in many Western countries may have resulted from the decreasing average number of children born to successive generations of women.

We have no hard data which support the theory that "incessant ovulation" is a factor in promoting epithelial carcinoma of the ovary. The only factor which can support such a theory is that, in the Scandinavian countries of Denmark, Sweden and Norway, contraceptive practice has resulted in small families with between one and three children. This means that most of the females have only had a suppresion of ovulation throughout one to three pregnancies. Contraceptive practice in the Scandinavian countries was well developed before the advent of the pill. Thus, most females ovulated 400–500 times throughout their fertile years. Every time an ovum bursts through the surface epithelium of the ovary, a proliferative activity in the surface epithelial cells may be induced followed by the development of inclusion cysts. These inclusion cysts may possibly later develop into an epithelial tumor.

Carefully conducted epidemiological studies especially concerning those using oral contraceptives, which inhibit ovulation, will show if this is of value for the protection of developing ovarian carcinoma.

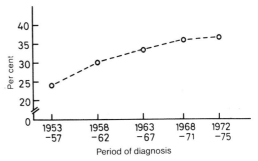

Fig. 37.4. Five-year survival rates for patients with ovarian cancer in Norway in the period 1953–75 (6).

INCIDENCE PATTERNS IN NORWAY

Today the population of Norway is a little more than 4 million people. The population increase has been relatively slow throughout the last 20 years. There has been a shift in the age distribution of the population, however, more and more people belonging to the older age groups. This may in part explain the fact that since the start of registration of carcinomas in Norway in 1952, there has been a steady increase in the total number of ovarian carcinomas being reported. In Fig. 37.2 it can be seen that the total number of ovarian carcinomas has increased from 234 in 1955 to 465 in 1984. The age-specific incidence rates of ovarian cancer in the years 1953–58 and 1972–76 is shown in Fig. 37.3. All cases of ovarian cancer are included in the two curves. Thus, both germ cell tumors, hormonal producing tumors and other rare tumors are included in the figures. However, about 90% of all cases belong to the epithelial ovarian carcinomas.

SURVIVAL STUDIES

During the years 1968–75 a total of 3,136 cases of ovarian carcinoma were analyzed for survival by the Cancer Registry of Norway (6).

There was an increase in incidence over time. It is possible that this increase is partly due to changes in the criteria of diagnosis and classification.

The death rates were fairly high during the first two years after diagnosis. After two years the relative survival rate was down to 46%. From

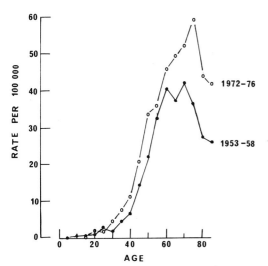

Fig. 37.3. Age-specific incidence rates of ovarian cancer in Norway in the periods 1953–58 and 1972–76.

then on the relative survival rate levelled off, being 41% at three years and 37% at five years. There was a moderate improvement in prognosis for this disease, particularly during the first year following diagnosis. The increase in survival was marked in cases under 45 years of age, whereas the survival rates for the older age groups showed only slight changes. There has been a continuous, although slight, improvement in prognosis during the last 20 years (Fig. 37.4). The 5-year relative survival rates decrease with increasing age, falling from 63% for the youngest to 20% for the older age group. This association of age with survival was consistent with stage of disease.

38
Malignant epithelial tumors of the ovary

The majority of ovarian carcinomas develop from the surface epithelium. Our own experience is that about 90% of malignant tumors of the ovary belong to this group. In a series of 1,137 cases seen in the Norwegian Radium Hospital during the years 1968–73, 86% were classified as epithelial carcinomas, 7.9% were undifferentiated carcinomas, most probably of epithelial origin, and only 6.1% belonged to the more specialized tumors developing from the germinal cells or from the granulosa-theca cells (1). The distribution by histology and stage of this large series is shown in Table 38.1. The majority of the tumors were classified as belonging to the serous group of carcinomas, either potentially malignant tumors or true carcinomas. Altogether 49.7% were classified as serous tumors, 18.2% as mucinous tumors, 12.4% as endometrioid tumors, and 5.8% as mesonephroid tumors (clear cell carcinomas). So-called potentially malignant tumors were found most frequently in the serous and mucinous lesions, about 6% in each group. Only three endometrioid tumors were classified as potentially malignant tumors. In the eighteenth volume of the *Annual Report* (2) the distribution by histology was as shown in Table 38.2.

CLINICAL FEATURES

Ovarian carcinoma rarely produces early characteristic symptoms or signs, with the result that at the time of diagnosis approximately 70% show spread to the peritoneal cavity either in the pelvic region or to the upper abdomen. Stage distribution in a series of 3,005 cases seen in the Norwegian Radium Hospital during the years 1970–80 is shown in Table 38.3. About 10% were in Stage IV, which means there were metastases outside the peritoneal cavity or to the parenchyma of the liver, and as many as 35% showed spread to the

upper abdomen, omentum, around the kidneys and/or to the dome of the diaphragm. This last place for spread is important to remember. Obviously, tumor cells from an ovarian carcinoma in the pelvic region may easily be detached and then follow the stream of fluid within the peritoneal cavity which passes upwards on both sides, lateral to the columna and the big vessels, and then the cells end up under the dome of the diaphragm. This may in some patients be the only place for implantation metastases.

There are at least two reasons for the poor stage distribution of the epithelial ovarian tumors. First, the patients have no distinct symptoms for a long time, and, secondly, we have no means of screening the female population for ovarian cancer. For several years at the Norwegian Radium Hospital we had a screening procedure for healthy women in the age groups from approximately 25 years up to 70 years. Almost 5,000 women took part in this screening. They all underwent:

1. The taking of a medical history followed by ordinary gynecological examination.
2. Taking of smears from the cervix and vagina and from the endometrial cavity.
3. Colposcopy.
4. The aspiration of fluid from the pouch of Douglas.

The aspiration smears from the pouch of Douglas aimed at detecting ovarian carcinoma. We did not find a single case with ovarian cancer by this method.

The most common symptoms in ovarian carcinoma are in our experience uncharacteristic lower abdominal pain, abdominal distension, increasing girth, and uncharacteristic symptoms from the bladder with frequent voiding, sometimes fol-

Table 38.1. Distribution by histology and stage in 1137 cases of ovarian cancer treated in the Norwegian Radium Hospital in 1968–73

Histology	Ia	Ib	Ic	IIa	Stage IIb	III	IV	Total	Per cent
Granulosacell tumor	30	1				3		34	3.0
Dysgerminoma	10	1				1		12	1.1
Malignant teratoma	6			2	4	10	1	23	2.0
Serous b.	44	12			4	5		65	5.7
Serous c.	57	30	11	15	65	283	38	499	44.0
Mucinous b.	66	4		1	2	4		77	6.8
Mucinous c.	52	6	8	3	18	37	5	129	11.4
Endometrioid b.	2			1				3	0.2
Endometrioid c.	40	9	5	14	31	29	10	138	12.1
Mesonephroid	29	3	2	1	16	12	4	67	5.8
Undifferentiated	5	5		1	10	44	25	90	7.9
Total	341	71	26	38	150	428	83	1137	
Per cent	30.0	6.3	2.3	3.4	13.2	37.5	7.3		100

lowed by dysuria. The most important factor which could possibly help in a better stage distribution and an earlier diagnosis of ovarian cancer would be that every doctor, whether a general practitioner, a gynecologist, a surgeon or an internist, always remember that uncharacteristic lower abdominal pain may be the first symptom of an ovarian cancer. If one always keeps this in mind and the fact that bladder symptoms may be due to ovarian cancer, then the next step is to perform a thorough gynecological examination under the best conditions. This means that both the bladder and the rectum should be emptied and the patient examined on a comfortable gyne-

cological examination table. Increasing abdominal girth and abdominal distension usually means either a very large tumor, or, more frequently, that there is already spread to the peritoneal cavity with production of ascites.

Strictly gynecological symptoms are rare. In epithelial ovarian tumors only approximately 10% may complain of bleeding symptoms with metrorrhagia or irregular menstrual periods. The most common epithelial tumors do not produce estrogens or other sexual hormones in an amount that would make it helpful to screen the women with hormonal tests. It is usually the granulosa-theca cell tumors or the pure thecomas that may induce either irregular bleeding in the premenopausal patient or postmenopausal metrorrhagia. Peculiarly enough, tumors metastasizing to the

Table 38.2. Distribution by histologic type in 7095 cases of epithelial carcinomas reported from the years 1976–1978 (2)

Histologic type	Total no.	Per cent
Serous carcinomas	3138	44.2
Mucinous carcinomas	838	11.8
Endometrioid carcinomas	1026	14.5
Clear cell carcinomas	303	4.3
Undifferentiated and unspecified carcinomas	1419	20.0
Serous borderline tumors	206	2.9
Mucinous borderline tumors	158	2.2
Other borderline tumors	7	0.1
Total	7095	100.0

Table 38.3. Stage distribution in a series of 3005 cases of carcinoma of the ovary, borderline lesions included, treated in the Norwegian Radium Hospital during the years 1970–1980.

Stage	No.	Per cent
Stage I	1200	39.9
Stage II	438	14.6
Stage III	974	32.4
Stage IV	258	8.6
Unknown	135	4.5
Total	3005	100.0

ovary from the gastrointestinal tract, especially those from the stomach, frequently induce a hyperproduction of estrogens in the ovarian stroma.

Sometimes torsion of a cystic tumor may cause intense pain. This is unfortunately rarely the case in epithelial ovarian carcinoma, but is more frequently seen with benign tumors of smaller size.

In some cases the first symptom may be enlargement of the inguinal lymph nodes or the lymph nodes in the supraclavicular region. It must be remembered that ovarian carcinoma spreads not only throughout the peritoneal cavity by seeding, but also through the lymphatic system. It is striking, however, how infrequent blood-born metastases are seen. The tumor remains in the peritoneal cavity for a very long period of time before distant metastases occur. In the late stages of the disease the woman becomes cachectic and often presents with a huge abdomen filled with ascitic fluid.

Ultrasound has been used very much in recent years, and may give valuable information about the site and type of an early tumor, especially if it is cystic. The more solid tumors with widespread disease in the peritoneal cavity are difficult to evaluate by ultrasound or by computer tomography. Nuclear magnetic resonance may prove to be the method of preference in the future, but today it is both expensive and time-consuming. I do not believe that these new methods should be used routinely in all patients. If there is clear-cut indication for laparotomy, it is better to evaluate the type and spread of disease during a surgical exploration of the abdominal cavity.

Fine-needle aspiration has been used in many clinics, and we have also used it for many years in the evaluation of ovarian tumors, spread from cervical cancer to the pelvic wall, spread to the lymph nodes in the inguinal or supraclavicular region, or spread to the liver. In ovarian tumors Kjellgren et al. (3) found that it was relatively easy by fine-needle aspiration cytology to decide if a tumor was benign or malignant, and also to give an indication of what type of histologic pattern the tumor had. We have performed a similar study (4). There is no doubt that fine-needle aspiration may give some information before an operation, but I would be reluctant to say that this should be performed routinely.

When the laparotomy is performed, it is important that the abdominal cavity should be systematically explored. The first step is to take peritoneal washings if there are no signs of tumor in the upper abdomen or spread in the pelvis. Thereafter a hand should be passed into the abdomen to carry out a systematic exploration to exclude obvious pathology. The method described by Asmussen and Miller (5) seems to be excellent. The drawings and description in their book on clinical gynecological urology are extremely good. They begin on the right side by pulling the great omentum to the patient's left side to allow exploration of the coecum and appendix. The principles are shown in Fig. 38.1. The ascending colon is followed upwards with a hand on its lateral side until the liver is felt. The lower aspect of the liver is then felt with the back of the fingers and the gall bladder palpated with a finger and thumb. The fingers then feel for the liver's anterior edge and pass between it and the costal margin so that the diaphragmatic surface can be felt with the fingers and the palm of the hand. As the hand passes medially, the fingers must be withdrawn a little to negotiate the ligamentum teres and then passed on to the upper surface of the left liver lobe. It is easy to come down again under the liver edge to

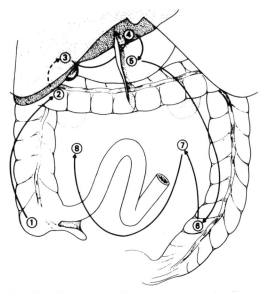

Fig. 38.1. Exploration of the abdominal cavity. From (5) and reproduced by courtesy of Blackwell Scientific Publications.

feel its lower aspect, the prepyloric and pyloric regions of the stomach and the beginning of the duodenum. The transverse and descending colon is then palpated until one reaches the sigmoid colon. The next step is to withdraw the hand and pass it behind the great omentum, first on the left and then on the right of the root of the mesentery. Then finally the two kidneys are explored.

If the situation is such that there seems to be no spread outside the ovaries, not only peritoneal washings should be taken, but also biopsies from the peritoneum of both colonic gutters and from the dome of the diaphragm. Biopsies should be taken from all suspicious parts where there are small whitish nodules.

If there is widespread disease, one must of course decide upon which type of operation should be performed. This will be discussed under "Management".

It is an advantage if one or a few biopsies from the primary tumor and its spread can be taken for frozen sections. This is not absolutely necessary, however, because the decision upon what to do in each case will depend much more upon the clinical judgement of the surgeon performing the operation, and of course also on the treatment protocol of the institution. In some clinics there is a tendency to be very reluctant to remove large tumor masses. It is recommended that the abdomen be closed and irradiation or chemotherapy given to reduce the tumor mass and then a second operation performed to see if there is a possibility of reductive surgery. Other surgeons are very radical and try to remove as much as possible during the first operation.

STUDIES ON OVARIAN EPITHELIAL CARCINOMAS IN THE NORWEGIAN RADIUM HOSPITAL

Our interest in this group of patients started in the mid-1950s when a high-voltage betatron machine was installed in the hospital. A few years later, at the beginning of the 1960s, chemotherapy with alkylating agents was introduced. Before this time, relatively few cases were referred to our hospital, but as shown in Fig. 38.2 there has been a rapid increase in referrals. In 1975–80 we treated approximately 300 new cases a year, which means

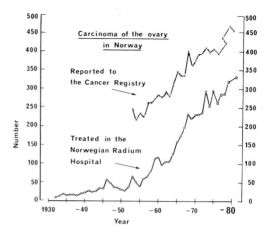

Fig. 38.2. Yearly number of patients with ovarian cancer reported to the Norwegian Cancer Registry and number of cases treated in the Norwegian Radium Hospital.

more than 2/3 of all the cases being detected in Norway.

In the 1950s radioactive colloidal gold was introduced into the treatment of ovarian cancer. To begin with, it was used for reducing the production of ascites in advanced cases, but also as an adjuvant treatment in the earlier stages. Several publications about the application of radioactive gold in ovarian cancer have emanated from the clinic over the years (6, 7).

The real background for our interest and experience in ovarian carcinoma started in the late 1960s, however, when the new histologic classification of ovarian epithelial tumors had been introduced. We made a retrospective survey of 990 cases which had been treated in the hospital up to 1965 (8). In this classification system it was emphasized that it is of great importance to keep separate the so-called borderline tumors.

Tumors of borderline malignancy are characterized by: (a) Stratification of the neoplastic epithelial cells, often accompanied by their detachment as cellular clusters, as well as nuclear abnormalities greater than those encountered in clearly benign tumors, and (b) a lack of destructive "invasion of the adjacent stroma". Borderline tumors could in many respects be compared to Stage 0 lesions of the cervix and the endometrium (Figs. 38.3 and 38.4).

As a rule there is no great difficulty in differen-

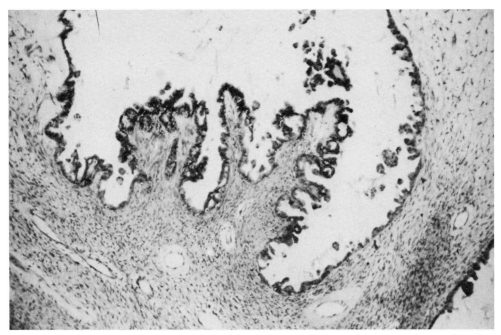

Fig. 38.3. Borderline serous carcinoma of the ovary with proliferating activity and nuclear abnormalities, but no signs of destructive invasion of the stroma.

tiating between serous and mucinous tumors. (Figs. 38.4 and 38.5). The essential difference is that if serous tumors secrete mucin, this is almost entirely extracellular, while only small quantities are visible in the apical portion of the cytoplasm of the neoplastic cells. In contrast, the great majority of mucinous tumors are characterized by the presence of considerable amounts of mucin within significant numbers of the neoplastic cells.

Endometrioid carcinomas are characterized in differentiated areas by the presence of regular tubular glands lined by stratified non-mucin containing epithelium. Occasionally strips of cells resembling the endocervical epithelium are encountered in small foci. Histologically benign or malignant squamous differentiation is often present and may provide an important diagnostic clue (Fig. 38.6). The squamous element may appear in the form of solid nests or masses of cells with small spindle-shaped nuclei. Occasionally an endometrioid carcinoma is highly papillar, creating a problem in differentiating from a serous papillary adenocarcinoma. The papillarity, however, is broader and more regular in the former, and other diagnostic features are typically present.

Clear cell carcinomas (mesonephroid tumors) are usually easily recognized forms of common epithelial carcinomas. The cells are large, fully hydral or rounded, containing glycogen and resembling the clear cells of a renal carcinoma. Distinctive hobnail cells lining cysts and tubules may also be found; these contain multiple papillae (Fig. 38.7).

The endodermal sinus tumor (yolk sack tumor), was considered for a long time to be a variation of clear cell carcinoma. They are rarely confused nowadays due to the important contributions of Teilum, who was the first to clearly distinguish them (9).

Today, Brenner tumors are also considered epithelial tumors. They have a low grade of malignancy. They are characterized by epithelial elements scattered throughout the stromal component. In rare cases the atypicality of the neoplastic cells and presence of invasion makes it necessary to include Brenner tumors in the group of malignant epithelial tumors. However, the vast majority of Brenner tumors have an extremely good prognosis although metastatic lesions have been described.

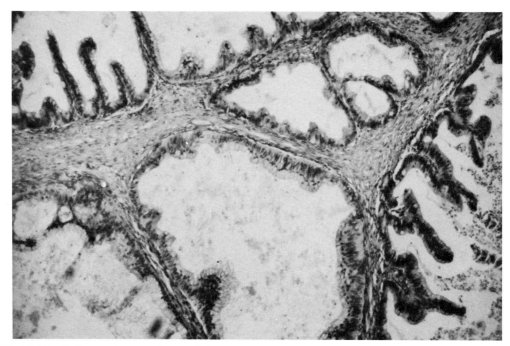

Fig. 38.4. Borderline mucinous carcinoma of the ovary with proliferating activity and nuclear abnormalities. Both cells and glands contain mucin.

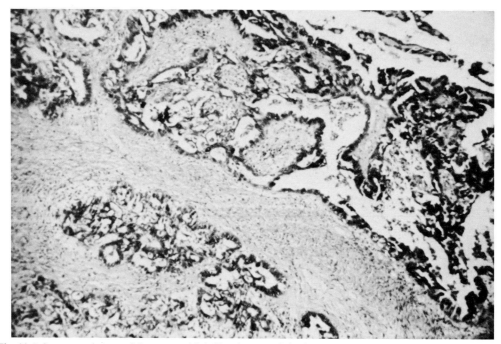

Fig. 38.5. Serous carcinoma of the ovary with infiltrative growth in the stroma.

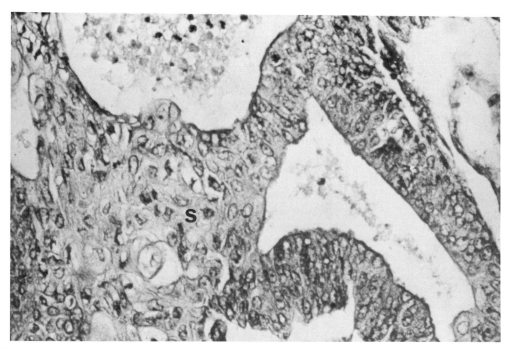

Fig. 38.6. Endometrioid carcinoma of the ovary resembling endometrial carcinoma of the uterus. Note area with squamous differentiation (s).

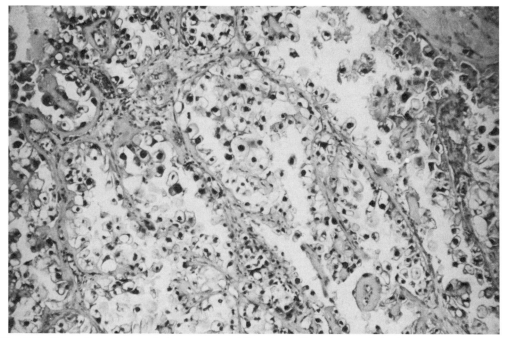

Fig. 38.7. Clear cell carcinoma of the ovary resembling clear cell carcinoma of the kidney. Large, clear cells containing glycogen with small, chromatin-rich nuclei. Typical hobnail cells dominate the picture.

The last group of epithelial tumors is the undifferentiated carcinomas. They have minimal differentiation (Fig. 38.8). Mucin, psammoma bodies and rare glands may be present, but not in a sufficient amount to categorize the tumor to one of the types described above. The undifferentiated carcinomas are sometimes confused with the diffuse granulosa-cell tumor. The best criterion for distinguishing them is the appearance of their nuclei. Those of the granulosa-cell tumor are typically round or angular, pale and often grooved, whereas those of the undifferentiated carcinomas are usually hyperchromatic with coarser, irregular chromatine and rarely contain grooves.

PROGNOSTIC FACTORS

Prognostic factors in ovarian cancer can be listed under the following headings: *Age, histology, stage, site and extent of metastases, radicality of the surgical intervention, response to additional radiotherapy or chemotherapy, immunologic factors.*

Age
In epithelial tumors of the ovary it has been shown that the 5-year survival rate is significantly better in the younger age groups stage by stage. One explanation for this is that the so-called borderline lesions are more common in young women than in older women (Fig. 38.9). This cannot be the only explanation, however. It is remarkable that even in Stage III carcinoma of the ovary young patients survived for a longer time than the older ones. As shown in Table 38.4, in a series of 252 Stage III epithelial carcinomas, 38% out of 71 women below 50 years of age survived for more than two years as compared to only 16.5% of 181 patients older than 50 years of age. Some immunologic factors are possibly the explanation for this difference.

Histology and prognosis
In a series of 990 epithelial carcinomas followed for 5–20 years, the potentially malignant tumors showed the best prognosis. The survival curves, however, show a small but steady decline during the entire observation period up to 20 years after primary treatment. The 5-year survival rate for the serous borderline tumors was 95%, while the 20-year actuarial survival rate was 78%. The corresponding figures for the borderline tumors of the mucinous type were 92% and 86% respectively. Among the truly invasive carcinomas, en-

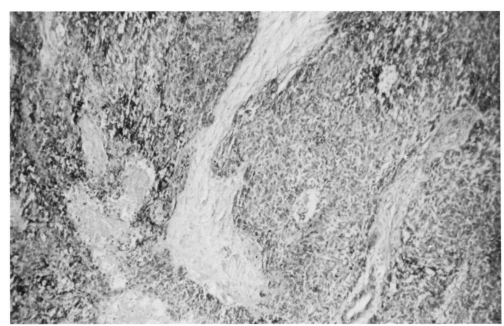

Fig. 38.8. Completely undifferentiated carcinoma of the ovary.

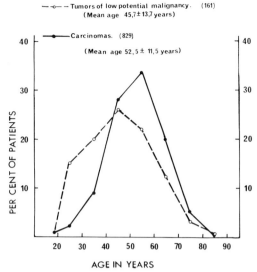

Fig. 38.9. Age distribution of tumors of low potential malignancy (borderline lesions) and of invasive carcinoma of the ovary. From (8) and reproduced by courtesy of Harper & Row, Publishers.

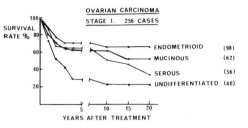

Fig. 38.10. Actuarial survival rates for four different histologic types of ovarian carcinoma Stage I.

dometrioid carcinomas had the best prognosis as long as there were no signs of spread, followed by the mucinous, serous and undifferentiated tumors in that order (Fig. 38.10). Serous carcinomas had a great tendency to a protracted clinical course with late recurrences up to 20 years after primary treatment. In Stage I the 5-year survival rate for the endometrioid tumors was 70%, for the serous 67%, and for the mucinous 64%. After 20 years of follow-up the actuarial survival rate for the endometrioid carcinomas was 67%, the mucinous carcinomas 55% and the serous carcinomas 36%. The worst prognosis was for the undifferentiated carcinomas, which even after three years of follow-up showed a survival rate of only 30%.

The degree of differentiation of the tumor is also an important prognostic indicator. This has been shown in many studies. In our own series of 252 Stage III epithelial carcinomas, 53.6% of 69 patients with a tumor classified as highly differentiated survived for more than two years, while only 19.1% of 89 cases with a tumor of medium differentiation, and 13.8% of 94 patients with a low degree of differentiation survived for more than two years (Table 38.5). Also in Stage I disease we have found a definite relationship between tumor differentiation and prognosis.

Stage
Stage of the disease has a great influence on survival rate. In our series of 990 cases we found a 5-year survival rate for all histological types as shown in Fig. 38.11. In Stage I about 60% of the patients were alive after five years, while in Stage II the corresponding figure was 45%, in Stage III 13% and in Stage IV 4%. The radicality of the primary operation was also of great importance. The observation that residual tumor after surgery of less than 2 cm in diameter carries a much better prognosis is in accordance with our experience.

Table 38.4. The relationship between age and prognosis as seen in a series of 252 Stage III epithelial carcinomas

| | Survival >2 years | | |
Age	No.	Per cent	Total No.
< 50 years	27	38.0	71
> 50 years	40	16.5	181
Total	67	26.6	252

Table 38.5. Differentiation and prognosis 252 Stage III epithelial carcinomas

| | Total | Survival >2 years | |
Differentiation	no.	No.	Per cent
High	69	37	53.6
Medium	89	17	19.1
Low	94	13	13.8
Total	252	67	26.6

In Stage I unilateral tumors had a significantly better prognosis than bilateral tumors or tumors with ascites present (Fig. 38.12).

Site and extent of metastases

There is no doubt that there are great differences in prognosis according to the site and extent of the spread. In Stage II, spread to the uterus only (Stage IIa) has a much better prognosis than if there is spread to the pouch of Douglas, to the rectum and/or sigmoid colon, to the pelvic wall and/or to the bladder peritoneum (Stage IIb). In a series from the Norwegian Radium Hospital treated in the years 1973–75, 21 out of 30 Stage IIa cases (70%) survived for five years compared to 32 out of 81 (39.5%) Stage IIb cases. During the same years 273 Stage III lesions were treated, and 42 (15.4%) survived for five years. In Stage III, however, there is a great variation of the spread. Those cases which show microscopic or macroscopic spread to the omentum only, have a survival rate which can be compared to the Stage IIb cases.

PSAMMOMA BODIES IN SEROUS CARCINOMA OF THE OVARY

The occurrence of areas of microscopic calcification (psammoma bodies) in serous carcinoma of the ovary is well known (Fig. 38.13). When we reviewed our series of 990 patients with ovarian cancer (8), we were puzzled by the fact that in many of the cases with long-term survival, psammoma bodies were found by microscopic examination. We did not find any reports in the literature, which clearly showed that these calcified bodies are a criterion of a low degree of malignancy. To study this problem in detail, blind histological subgrouping according to the presence or absence of psammoma bodies was performed.

In only 1 out of 205 endometrioid tumors and in none of 59 clear cell tumors or 155 undifferentiated carcinomas, were calcified granules found.

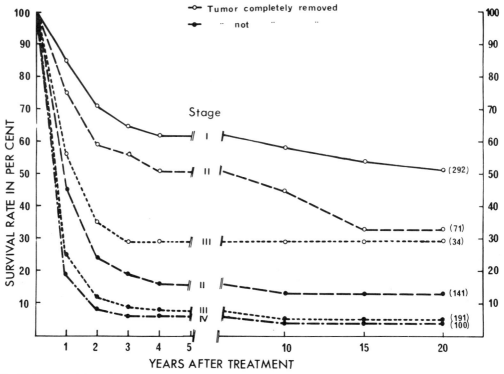

Fig. 38.11. Actuarial survival rate in relation to stage and operability. Numbers of patients in parentheses. From (8). and reproduced by courtesy of Harper & Row, Publishers.

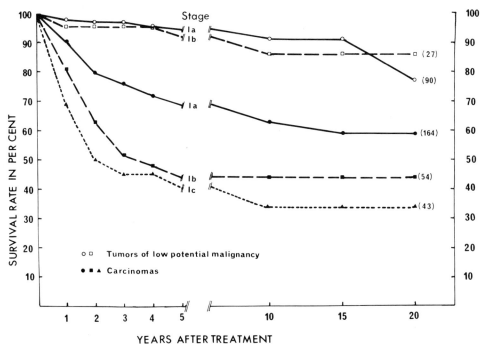

Fig. 38.12. Actuarial survival rates for borderline lesions Stages Ia and Ib, and for invasive ovarian carcinomas Stage Ia, Ib and Ic. Numbers of patient in parentheses. From (8) and reproduced by courtesy of Harper & Row, Publishers.

However, the frequency of psammoma bodies in serous carcinomas was 92 out of 283 (32.5%) and in serous tumors of low potential malignancy 17 out of 74 (23%).

Cumulative survival curves for the series of true invasive carcinomas with or without psammoma bodies are shown in Fig. 38.14. There was a remarkable and significant difference of about 20%, which was already demonstrable 2–3 years after primary treatment, and which persisted for 15 years of follow-up.

In future studies on the value of different treatment methods in cancer of the ovary, the occurrence of psammoma bodies in serous carcinomas should possibly be taken into account. The development of such calcifications may reflect a specific tumor host reaction.

CARCINOMA OF THE OVARY AND ENDOMETRIOSIS

Sampson described endometrioid carcinomas of the ovary for the first time in 1925 (10). At a conference in Stockholm in 1961 Santesson proposed that these tumors should be classified as an entity separate from the serous carcinomas. The microscopic similarity between endometrioid ovarian carcinoma and endometrial carcinoma is striking, but this does not necessarily indicate a common histogenesis. On the other hand, while there is a general agreement that serous and mucinous carcinomas may develop from benign or semimalignant ovarian adenomas of a corresponding histological pattern, the theory that endometrioid carcinoma has its benign counterpart in ovarian endometriosis is not generally accepted. According to some investigators this may be true in the majority of cases, but others claim that endometrioid carcinoma represents a special category of serous carcinoma. It is difficult to prove that an endometrioid carcinoma has developed directly from endometriosis. The ultimate proof is a tumor area in which there is clear microscopic evidence of this kind of malignant transformation.

As shown in Table 38.6, endometriosis was almost without exception found only in connection

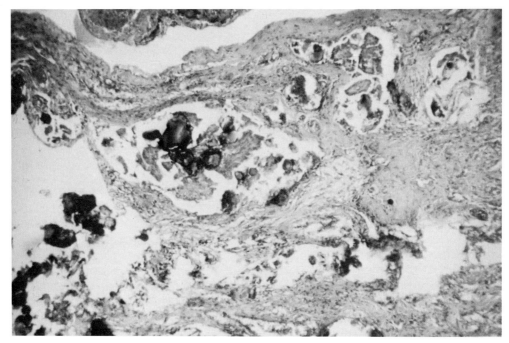

Fig. 38.13. Psammoma bodies in serous carcinoma of the ovary.

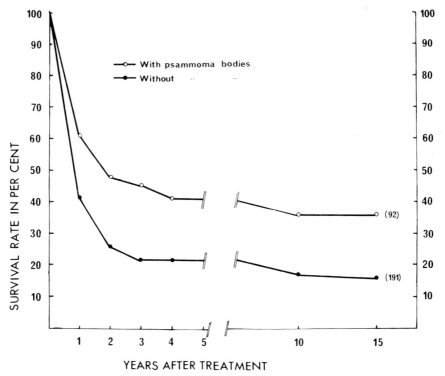

Fig. 38.14. Actuarial survival rate for 92 patients with serous carcinoma with psammoma bodies and 191 cases without psammoma bodies, all stages.

Table 38.6. Distribution by tumor type and the occurrence of endometriosis

Histologic diagnosis	Total No.	With endometriosis No.	With endometriosis Per cent
Serous borderline lesions	74	0	0.0
Serous carcinomas	283	0	0.0
Mucinous borderline lesions	80	0	0.0
Mucinous carcinomas	123	1	0.8
Endometrioid borderline lesions	7	1	14.3
Endometrioid carcinomas	205	19	9.3
Clear cell carcinomas	59	14	23.7
Undifferentiated carcinomas	155	0	0.0
Sinus endodermal tumors	4	0	0.0
Total	990	35	3.5

with endometrioid and clear cell (mesonephroid) carcinomas. One single case of endometriosis was revealed amongst a total of 203 mucinous tumors, and none in the groups of serous and undifferentiated lesions. Seven endometrioid tumors were classified as potentially malignant lesions, six of which belonged to the clinical Stage I. In one of these, concomitant ovarian endometriosis was found. In the series of 205 cases of endometrioid carcinoma, the incidence of endometriosis was 9.3% (Table 38.7). Endometriosis was most frequently found in the clinical Stage Ib, and the difference between the incidence rate of 29.4% in this stage and that of the other clinical stages was statistically significant.

The occurrence of endometriosis did not seem to influence the prognosis. Of great importance, however, was the radical nature of the primary operation.

Table 38.7. Endometrioid carcinoma. Relation between stage and the occurrence of histologically proven endometriosis.

Stage	Total No.	Per cent	With endometriosis No.	With endometriosis Per cent
I	98	47.8	12	12.2
II	51	24.8	6	11.8
III	42	20.5	0	0.0
IV	14	6.8	1	7.1
Total	205	100.0	19	9.3

CLEAR CELL TUMORS OF THE OVARY

In earlier years, clear cell tumors were frequently called mesonephroid tumors of the ovary. The term "mesonephroma ovarii" was introduced by Schiller in 1939 (11) to designate a tumor considered to be of mesonephric origin, because it had tufts and a tubular structure similar to developing glomeruli and tubules. This theory of histogenesis has been challenged by many authors, some of whom are of the opinion that mesonephromas represent variants of serous tumors of the ovary or, in other words, that these lesions are of Müllerian origin.

In our own series of 990 patients with epithelial ovarian carcinomas, 59 cases (6%) were classified as clear cell adenocarcinoma of the ovary. All patients were treated surgically. In addition they received some form of irradiation therapy.

Survival curves for the different clinical stages are depicted in Fig. 38.15. The most important indication of prognosis was the extent of the tumor. The results for Stage I tumors were as good as those in other epithelial carcinomas of the ovary in Stage I. With tumor spread beyond the ovaries, however, prognosis was worse than that for other differentiated malignant epithelial tumors.

Several investigators have pointed out that ovarian endometriosis occurs with remarkable frequency in clear cell carcinoma. In our series of 59 patients the frequency of endometriosis was 23.7%.

The high frequency of concomitant ovarian endometriosis supports, to a certain degree, the theory that clear cell carcinomas of the ovary are related to endometrioid tumors, and that the origin of such tumors may be the Müllerian epithelium.

MANAGEMENT

Surgery

The cornerstone in the treatment of epithelial tumors of the ovary is still surgery. This seems to be generally accepted. Morrow (12), in an extensive review of malignant and borderline epithelial tumors of the ovary, clearly demonstrated the influence resectability has on survival.

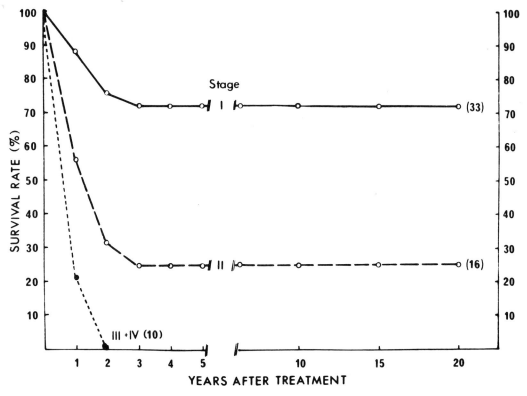

Fig. 38.15. Actuarial survival rate related to stage in 59 cases of clear cell carcinoma of the ovary.

Throughout the years we have experienced that even in Stage Ia both ovaries should be removed if the lesion is a true carcinoma of more than Grade I. The other ovary, which macroscopically may look normal, will in about 5–10% of the cases harbor a microscopically malignant lesion. This percentage is even higher if it is a serous carcinoma.

Furthermore, we also recommend the removal of the uterus. True carcinoma of the ovary not infrequently metastasizes to the uterus and vice versa. In an unpublished study we discovered that pure endometrial metastases are very seldom found. In Stages II and III, serosal metastases are common, and also metastases to the endometrium may be found so frequently that hysterectomy should be performed routinely. Another reason for removing the uterus is that there is always a possibility of endometrial carcinoma developing often many years later. The risk of this event is definitely higher in patients who have been suc-

cessfully treated for ovarian cancer. It should also be taken into account that if the ovaries have been removed, then hormone therapy should often be instituted in the younger patients, and if estrogens are included in such therapy, bleeding episodes from the uterus may be a problem.

There can be no dispute that the greater omentum is a common site of metastases from ovarian carcinoma. Therefore we recommend greater omentectomy as a routine procedure. Another reason for this recommendation is the fact that the omentum plays an important role in the production of ascites, especially when macroscopic metastases are found to this site during the primary operation or when recurrences occur. A third reason which has been important in our Unit throughout the years, is that this will facilitate an even distribution of radioactive colloids in the peritoneal cavity. The omentum is an expendable organ, and the theory that omentectomy may increase the risk of postoperative bowel obstruction has never been proven. We have had no problems which would support this theory. Greater omentectomy has now been used routinely in the Norwegian Radium Hospital during surgery for ovarian cancer in more than 3,000 cases.

Thus, the routine operation for true epithelial carcinoma of the ovary which we recommend is: *total hysterectomy, bilateral oophorectomy and greater omentectomy.*

Conservative surgery, which means removal of only one ovary and the ipsilateral tube, should be restricted to young women of childbearing age who want to preserve the possibility of pregnancy. Before deciding upon conservative surgery, certain prerequisites must be fulfilled. The epithelial tumor must either be a borderline lesion or a Grade 1 true carcinoma. The tumor must be unilateral with no excrescences on the surface and no signs of ascites (Stage Ia). Peritoneal washings must be negative. In many articles and textbooks, borderline lesions are described as non-malignant. This is not correct. If women treated for serous or mucinous borderline lesions are followed for 15–20 years, even in Stage I, between 10 and 15% die from their disease (8). Furthermore, in supposedly Stage Ia serous borderline tumors, a microscopic lesion may sometimes be found in the contralateral macroscopically normal ovary.

In unilateral borderline lesions and Grade 1 true carcinomas where unilateral oophorectomy has been performed with the aim of preserving fertility, it would possibly be wise to follow-up these cases with yearly laparoscopic examinations and peritoneal washings until the patient has given birth to one or two children, and then remove the remaining ovary. There is no doubt that these women are at a relatively high risk of developing a true carcinoma in the remaining ovary. There are no data available which really can prove this hypothesis. Our experience is that a biopsy of the ovary which looks macroscopically normal is not reliable.

Tumor reductive surgery. As mentioned previously, the standard treatment of carcinoma of the ovary is bilateral salpingo-oophorectomy, total hysterectomy and omentectomy. Unfortunately in Stages IIb and III this is not sufficient to remove all tumor tissue. The chance of cure is minimal if tumor tissue is left behind, even if modern radio-

therapy or chemotherapy is added. In 1968 Munnell (13) introduced the term "maximal surgical effort". In the 1970s the value of so-called "debulking" or "tumor reductive surgery" has been extensively discussed. In a comprehensive statistical analysis Griffiths in 1975 (14) found that the histologic grade and the actual size of the residual tumor (metastases) were the most important factors for survival. Today it is generally accepted that if the diameter of the remaining metastases is larger than approximately 2 cm, the response to radiotherapy or chemotherapy is poor. Our attitude for many years has been that the most aggressive surgery should be restricted to those cases in which all or nearly all of the gross tumor can be excised. In these cases an improved response to radiotherapy or chemotherapy can be expected.

Another indication for tumor debulking is the possible prevention of ascites reproduction and also the relief of discomfort associated with tumor. The most important factor for ascites reproduction is the tumor bulk in the omentum. Usually a simple excision of the greater omentum is sufficient. If the infiltration of the omentum is extensive, however, it may be wise to also remove the lesser omentum from the greater curvature of the stomach.

Resection of intestines should usually be avoided. Sometimes intestinal obstruction may force the surgeon to do a resection and anastomosis. The incidence of subsequent fistula in such cases is unfortunately relatively high.

It should be emphasized that adequate surgery for advanced ovarian cancer cannot be performed without adequate exposure, which means a midline excision which extends frequently far proximal to the umbilicus, even up to the xiphoid. Sometimes the spread is so extensive that the standard removal of both ovaries, the uterus and omentum cannot be performed. A biopsy should then be taken, and a second laparotomy may be tried either after radiotherapy or chemotherapy over a specific time (see later). In some cases spread to the pouch of Douglas and around the cervix is so extensive that it is wise not to try to perform total hysterectomy, but rather a supravaginal amputation.

Candidates for tumor reductive surgery are frequently in a poor general condition with anemia, hypoproteinemia and dehydration. It is therefore necessary to bring the patient into a better physiologic status before anesthesia and surgery. This has become much easier since the development of total parenteral nutrition.

Furthermore, it is also necessary, in addition to an evaluation of the blood status, to have at least a chest film, intravenous pyelogram and barium enema. Upper gastrointestinal series and specialized tests such as bone scan, ultrasound, computer tomography, nuclear magnetic resonance, etc., should be performed as indicated and not routinely when indication for laparotomy exists.

Radiation therapy
The place of radiotherapy in the treatment of ovarian carcinoma has still not been established. Since the advent of chemotherapy, many authors report that they have completely abandoned all types of radiation therapy. Others, however, recommend total abdominal radiation in both the early and late stages of the disease. Some prefer to use radiocolloids in the early Stages I and II. Since way back in the 1930s, patients have been referred to our Hospital for either primary or postoperative radiotherapy, mostly the latter. During the earlier years irradiation was not standardized and was given by conventional 250 kV machines. In 1957 a high-voltage machine was installed. A few years earlier instillation of radio-

active colloidal gold was introduced. In 1971 an analysis of the results of treatment by these three modalities was published (6). The study was retrospective and the choice of radiotherapy was not at random. The observations made, however, were striking and are shown in Tables 38.8 and 38.9. The influence of rupture of the tumor was also investigated (Table 38.10). The results seem to indicate that intraperitoneal instillation of radioactive gold improved the chances of cure in cases where no macroscopic tumor tissue was left behind, and also had a positive effect in cases with rupture of the tumor.

Radiocolloids. The results of the above-mentioned study seemed convincing. However, to ascertain the value of treatment with radiocolloids, a prospective randomized trial was started in 1968 comparing pelvic irradiation, 50 Gy, with a reduced pelvic dose, 30 Gy, combined with intraperitoneal instillation of Au[198], 100 mCi (7). Only Stage I and Stage II lesions were included. During the years 1968–74 altogether 418 patients entered this trial. Distribution by Stage (Stage Ia,b,c, IIa,b), histological type and age were similar in the two treatment groups. The Stage I series comprised 175 invasive carcinomas and 83 tumors of low potential malignancy. The Stage II series comprised 160 invasive carcinomas and 5 tumors of low potential malignancy.

No significant difference in 5-year survival rate was found for the patients with Stage I lesions

Table 38.8. Carcinoma of the ovary. Five-year survival in relation to type of radiotherapy. Tumor completely removed

| | Roentgen 250 kV | | | Betatron 31 MeV | | | Radioactive Au[198] | | |
	No.	Alive	%	No.	Alive	%	No.	Alive	%
Stage I	55	28	51	98	62	63	51	43	84
Stage II	17	7	41	23	7	30	15	8	53
Stage III	–	–		9	2	22	15	6	38

Table 38.9. Carcinoma of the ovary. Five-year survival in relation to type of radiotherapy. Non-radical surgery

| | Roentgen 250 kV | | | Betatron 31 MeV | | | Radioactive Au[198] | | |
	No.	Alive	%	No.	Alive	%	No.	Alive	%
Stage II	25	7	28	57	11	19	14	1	7
Stage III	20	1	5	75	5	7	42	4	10
Stage IV	10	1	10	49	4	8	20	1	5

Table 38.10. Comparison of 5-year survival rates according to the life table technique for cases of Stage I carcinoma with and without rupture of tumor

Therapy	Rupture of tumor				No rupture of tumor			
	No. of cases	Dead	Too short observation	Survival rate	No. of cases	Dead	Too short observation	Survival rate
Roentgen 250 kV	6	4	0	33.3%	49	25	1	48.6%
Betatron 31 MeV	25	11	0	55.9%	73	24	3	66.7%
Betatron 31 MeV and radioactive gold	21	3	1	85.0%	30	4	1	86.3%
Total	52	18	1	64.8%	152	53	5	64.6%

(Fig. 38.16). However, this was due to more patients dying from complications in the radiocolloid group. If only cancer deaths were counted, radiocolloid treatment was definitely better than pelvic irradiation. It was also observed that Stage Ia serous tumors, Stage Ib and Stage Ic tumors, all histological types, and ruptured tumors, did significantly better when treated with Au[198] (Table 38.11). Furthermore, the 5-year survival for patients with Stage II lesions treated with gold was 54.1% compared to 40% for those receiving external irradiation only (Fig. 38.17).

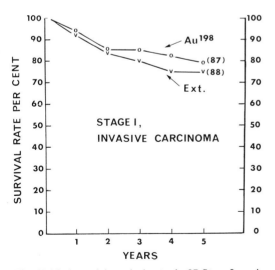

Fig. 38.16. Actuarial survival rates in 87 Stage I carcinoma of the ovary receiving postoperative treatment with radioactive gold and in 88 patients receiving postoperative pelvic irradiation. Randomized clinical trial, see text. From (7) and reproduced by courtesy of C. V. Mosby, Company.

After a closer scrutiny of this prospective trial, it was obvious that the irradiation dose in the gold series should be reduced. This was first carried out by omitting the additional external irradiation, 30 Gy. Later on, we have replaced the gammaemitter Au[198], with the pure betaemitter, P[32]. This was also of benefit to the personnel because of the reduced radiation hazard.

The 5-year survival rate for the latest two series treated with radiocolloids was 88% for Stages Ia and Ib. This compares well with other series reported from different institutions both in Europe and the United States. Dembo and Busch (16) have published a number of articles from the Princess Margaret Hospital, Toronto, recommending total abdominal irradiation in so-called intermediate and high-risk cases of ovarian carcinoma. They take not only the stage of the disease into account, but also age, pathology and grade. This certainly is a sophisticated and much more rational way of selecting patients for additional radiotherapy after surgery. For the purpose of comparison, our results in Stages Ib, Ic, IIa and IIb have been compared with those of the Toronto group. The disease-free interval and survival were similar in the two series. At the Norwegian Radium Hospital selected cases have been given total abdominal irradiation after the Princess Margaret Hospital schedule. It is our impression that the patients suffer more from nausea and gastrointestinal complications during this type of extensive external irradiation than those patients receiving radioactive phosphorus. Furthermore, the treatment with external irradiation takes much longer time and is more expensive than treatment with radiocolloids. Our conclusion is that in those cases which are

Table 38.11. The relationship between histologic type, rupture of tumor and deaths in Stage I ovarian carcinoma

Histology invasive ca.	Gold			External radiation		
	Total No.	Deaths No.	%	Total No.	Deaths No.	%
Serous	18	1	5.6	24	7	29.1
Mucinous	22	1	4.6	26	3	11.5
Endometrioid	28	6	21.5	23	4	17.4
Mesonephroid	18	5	27.6	14	6	42.8
Undifferentiated	1	0	0	1	1	(100)
Ruptured tumor	19	1	5.3	16	6	37.5

macroscopically disease-free and where there are no adhesions which may cause loculation of the isotope, radioactive phosphorus can safely be given. Furthermore, in tumors which have ruptured, the isotope may well have more to offer than external irradiation. Borderline lesions and low grade carcinomas Stage Ia and Ib should not be given any type of additional irradiation.

There has been considerable dispute about the distribution of radioactivity after intraperitoneal administration of radiocolloids. In 1984 an investigation of this problem was published (17). The whole-body distribution of radioactivity after intraperitoneal instillation of P^{32} labelled with chromic hydroxide particles was determined in 21 patients. Gamma-camera imaging of the abdominal distribution revealed that the administration procedure was critical for obtaining a homogeneous plating of the radiocolloids on the serosal surface of the peritoneum. When liquid is introduced into the peritoneum, because of gravity most of it will be confined to the lower part of the cavity. By moving the patient during or shortly after the instillation, this may be overcome, but is not always easy to do. To achieve an even distribution, the suspension of particles should be diluted before administration, and the colloid should be instilled through multiple outlets also sprinkling the suspension over the upper part of the abdominal cavity. In addition, it was found that the amount of P^{32} in peripheral blood increased for seven days after instillations followed by a continuous decrease. The bone marrow concentration was from two to five times as high as that in blood, but the total amounts were too small to give significant radiation doses. Radioac-

tive phosphorus should not be applied when there are intraperitoneal adhesions. Our practice is to apply the solution in one liter of saline immediately after laparotomy. The catheter is introduced through a separate stab wound and placed across the upper abdominal cavity.

Preoperative external irradiation

It is the opinion of the author that the value of radiocolloid treatment or treatment with external irradiation after the Princess Margaret Hospital schedule is well established today in patients with no macroscopic signs of residual tumor. Also pa-

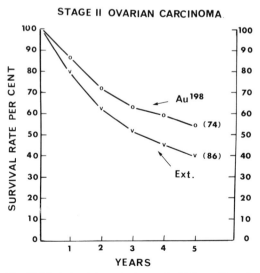

Fig. 38.17. Actuarial survival rates in 74 Stage II carcinoma of the ovary receiving postoperative treatment with radioactive gold and in 86 cases receiving postoperative pelvic irradiation. Randomized clinical trial, see text. From (7) and reproduced by courtesy of C. V. Mosby, Company.

tients with ascites, positive peritoneal washings, rupture of tumor or positive peritoneal biopsies from the upper abdomen should be considered candidates for such additional radiotherapy. Borderline or low grade lesions Stages Ia and Ib should be excluded, as well as young women with Stage Ia true carcinomas of higher grade.

A much more controversial problem is the role of radiation therapy in the advanced stages of the disease where large tumor masses are left behind after surgery. The question often arises whether it may be possible to do an adequate debulking operation after having given a specific dose of external irradiation. In our Hospital this question has been studied in a series of 456 patients with Stage III epithelial tumors treated during the years 1968–73 (18). Status at admission for these patients is shown in Table 38.12. The term "complete pelvic surgery" means that at primary surgery it was possible to remove both ovaries, the uterus and the greater omentum. In these cases, however, more or less extensive metastases (usually much larger than 2 cm in diameter) were left behind in the abdomen, in the renal hiluses or over the dome of the diaphragm. Those cases found inoperable either at surgery or by clinical examination, and those where only partial tumor resection could be performed, received 30 Gy external radiation over four weeks to a so-called large abdominal field. The liver and the dome of the diaphragm were not included in the field, and the kidneys were shielded after 20 Gy. Two weeks after the conclusion of radiotherapy, another attempt at surgery was made. In approximately one third of the cases deemed completely inoperable at the first

operation, complete pelvic surgery could be performed. For those with a clinical diagnosis of inoperability, the ovaries, uterus and omentum could be removed in nearly 50%. There seems to be no doubt that the type of radiotherapy given enhanced operability, but not to an extent that only minimal residual disease was left behind. It must also be emphasized that spread to the liver surface or the diaphragm did not receive any irradiation.

Even if the response rate to preoperative irradiation seemed promising, during the follow-up only a small increase in salvage rate was found (Table 38.13). In those patients who had "successful" surgery at the second attempt, there was a shift towards prolonged survival during the first two years compared to those who were still inoperable. The best 5-year survival rate was found in the group where "complete pelvic surgery" could be performed at the first laparotomy. It was concluded that operability is undoubtedly influenced by external irradiation preoperatively, but increased long-term survival in advanced ovarian cancer is very small.

Of the 456 patients described in Table 38.12, 299 were selected for a prospective, randomized study. The aim of the trial was to compare the results of maximum external irradiation to a large abdominal field, 50 Gy, with a reduced dose of external irradiation, 30 Gy, followed immediately after surgery by chemotherapy with an alkylating agent (thio-tepa) (19). The results of this study showed that maximum radiotherapy is not superior to a reduced dose of irradiation combined with an alkylating agent (Fig. 38.18). This combination therapy saves time and eliminates many of the risks and inconveniences of radiotherapy. In many centers radiotherapy in advanced ovarian cancer has been abandoned, and treatment is based on single drug or in later years, mostly multiple drug therapy. The combined radiological and cytostatic therapy in our own study from 1978 compares well with such treatment protocols as regards survival rates. The degree of palliation is harder to assess as both multiple drug chemotherapy and maximum radiotherapy have different side effects. Our patients tolerated external radiation up to 30 Gy well. In many cases ascites was reduced and the general condition of the pa-

Table 38.12. Status at admission for 456 patients with ovarian carcinoma Stage III treated with abdominal external irradiation

Treatment group	Number	Per cent
Complete pelvic surgery*	154	33.7
Partial tumour resection	157	34.5
Inoperable, biopsy only	96	21.0
inoperable disease	49	10.7
Total	456	100.0

* Total abdominal hysterectomy, bilateral salpingo-oophorectomy, and omentectomy.

Table 38.13. Survival rate correlated with the outcome of type of surgery at primary operation and after 3000 rads external irradiation to a large abdominal field

Treatment group	No.	Survival		
		1 year (%)	2 years (%)	5 years (%)
"Complete pelvic surgery" at first laparotomy. No preoperative irradiation.	154	51	32	24
Inoperable at first laparotomy. "Complete pelvic surgery" after 3,000 rads	36	42	27	13
Inoperable at first and second laparotomy. 3,000 rads between laparotomies	34	28	17	5
Clinical diagnosis of inoperability. 3,000 rads before laparotomy	49	45	32	15

tients improved. In the group receiving 50 Gy, however, the frequency of side effects was high with loss of weight, electrolyte disturbances due to vomiting and diarrhea, and lowering of the serum proteins.

After concluding this study, therefore, we have for some years used only chemotherapy for preoperative and for postoperative treatment of advanced ovarian cancer. We have tried both single drug and multiple drug therapy with different chemotherapeutic agents. Still, there is no doubt that in selected cases with advanced disease, radiotherapy may give palliation, especially in cases where the response to chemotherapy is poor. Thus, radiotherapy is not completely abandoned, but it is difficult to clearly define those cases which should be candidates for palliative radiotherapy.

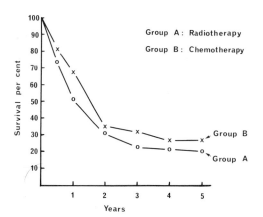

Fig. 38.18. Actuarial survival rates for Stage III carcinoma of the ovary treated with 30 Gy abdominal irradiation followed by chemotherapy with thiotepa (Group B), and for patients treated postoperatively with 50 Gy abdominal irradiation.

Chemotherapy

A bewildering number of drugs which have been shown to be effective in the treatment of epithelial tumors of the ovary are today available for the gynecologic oncologist. Likewise there is a bewildering number of reports on different multiple drug schedules. This is clearly shown, for example, in the reviews by Morrow (12) and by Lewis, Blessing and Kellner (20).

During the 1970s the concept of Phase I, Phase II and Phase III studies developed. The objective of Phase I studies is to establish a safe and tolerable dosage schedule. In Phase II studies the tumor response rates are measured. The intent of Phase III studies is mainly to compare the efficacy of the new therapy with that of existing treatment methods. Phase III studies are also used to compare two or three different new treatment schedules with multiple drugs. Most studies published to date have utilized response rates as end-points. A complete response (CR) is defined as disappearance of all evidence of disease for at least one month. Partial response (PR) means more than 50% reduction in the product of the largest diameters of each tumor mass for more than one month. Stable disease (SD) means no change or a reduction of less than 50%, and progressive disease (PD) is defined as more than 50% increase in the product of the two larger diameters of any tumor mass, or the appearance of a new lesion.

There is no doubt that the response rates have their greatest utility as end-points in Phase II studies, providing a rapid and simple answer to whether the treatment is active, and also indicating the frequency and grade of a short-term effect. For Phase III studies, however, the author agrees completely with Dembo and Busch (16) that greater precision should be required to assess treatment activity than in Phase II studies. The stakes are higher, because the "best arm" of a Phase III study usually becomes the new standard therapy. The comparison of actuarial survival curves is the best method of evaluating treatment efficacy in any Phase III study of ovarian cancer, preferably with a 5-year follow-up. The next best end-point is the survival time, i.e. the time from diagnosis to death. The relapse-free interval, which measures the time to new evidence of active disease, is a useful end-point for interim reporting. Almost all patients who develop recurrent ovarian cancer die of their disease, and the majority of the relapses occur within five years of initial treatment.

The majority of patients with advanced disease where metastases larger than approximately 2–3 cm in diameter are left behind after initial surgery will die in the course of 1–3 years irrespective of type of additional treatment, whether this consists of radiotherapy, single or multiple drug chemotherapy. Such non-curative therapy must be evaluated with regard to palliation and prolongation of life. In this situation a conflict often results. In particular a multiple drug regime which prolongs life for a couple of months may be so toxic that the reduced quality of life outweighs the increased survival time. This should always be taken into account in ovarian cancer patients with large residual disease when the relative merits of single and multiple drug chemotherapy are being weighed. This philosophy has undoubtedly influenced the development of chemotherapy in epithelial ovarian cancer at the Norwegian Radium Hospital. We have been slow to accept enthusi-

Table 38.14. Randomized series of 301 patients with ovarian carcinoma Stage I and II where all macroscopic tumor tissue were removed at operation.

Treatment group	Postoperative radiotherapy		Total No.
	External irradiation	Isotope instillation	
Thiotepa	42	109	151
No chemotherapy	46	104	150
Total	88	213	301

Table 38.15. Site of recurrence in patients treated with adjuvant chemotherapy and controls

Treatment group	Recurrence			
	Pelvis	Abdomen	Distant	Total
Thiotepa	20	5	13	38
No chemotherapy	18	8	11	37
Total	38	13	24	75

astic reports on new drugs or on different multiple drug regimes.

Adjuvant chemotherapy. In the following, this term is only used about chemotherapy given after supposedly radical removal of all tumor tissue. The purpose is to eradicate possible microscopic metastases which we know are present in a certain percentage of apparently successfully operated Stage I and Stage II cases. Treatment with radiocolloids must also be regarded as adjuvant therapy, as described previously.

During the years 1975–81, 301 patients with ovarian cancer Stages I and II were randomly allocated to one of two groups after radical surgery and postoperative irradition (21). The treatment group received two courses of an alkylating agent, thio-tepa, two weeks apart, followed by 15 mg biweekly for six months. The control group received no chemotherapy. The material is shown in Table 38.14. All patients were scheduled for radiocolloid treatment, but in 88 cases referred from other hospitals, postoperative adhesions made it preferable to use external irradiation.

The average duration of follow-up was five years, with a minimum of two years. A total of 75 recurrences were observed (25%). These were evenly distributed with 38 in the treatment group and 37 in the control group (Table 38.15). Sixty-eight patients with recurrences died, 35 in the treatment group and 33 in the control group. Neither time till recurrence nor survival were different in the two groups.

Taking into account all the well-known prognostic factors, randomization was found balanced. It seems therefore safe to conclude that the alkylating agent thio-tepa, administered as described, had no added protective effect against recurrence. In more advanced disease it is our experience that the drug gives a response rate (CR + PR) of about 30% if it is given after the same schedule as in this controlled clinical trial.

The adjuvant trial with thio-tepa was closed in 1981. A new prospective randomized trial was started in 1982, comparing radioactive phosphorus instillation with cis-platinum chemotherapy as adjuvant therapy in radically treated Stage I and Stage II ovarian cancer. No results are available as yet.

Chemotherapy of advanced disease. In the early 1960s few cytostatic drugs were available in Norway. At that time alkylating drugs were recommended in the treatment of advanced ovarian cancer. In our country only cyclophosphamide and thio-tepa were on the market. Since cyclophosphamide was known to give extensive hair-loss in a large number of the patients, it was decided that thio-tepa should be the drug of choice. In these early years thio-tepa was given mostly for palliation, and there were no strict treatment protocols. Because remarkable effect was sometimes seen with the complete disappearance of even large metastases, it was decided, in 1968, to compare treatment with thio-tepa with maximum radiotherapy in cases where tumor reductive surgery had been performed, but where metastases were still left behind in the upper abdomen. The results of this study have already been described (p. 202). Since it was realized that chemotherapy in such advanced cases gave the same 5-year survival and had fewer side effects than maximum radiotherapy, it was decided to start a new treatment protocol. All patients in which so-called "complete pelvic surgery" had been performed were scheduled for treatment with thio-tepa. When recurrence was detected, the patients were randomized to either adriamycin or hexamethylmelamine. Inoperable cases received thio-tepa over a period of 10 weeks. A second-look surgery was then performed, and the patients were divided into responders and non-responders. Responders were randomized to either continued single drug chemotherapy with thio-tepa, or to combination chemotherapy with thio-tepa and adriamycin. Non-responders were randomized to treatment with either adriamycin or hexamethylmelamine. When one regime failed, the patients were changed over to the alternative regime. The results of this study have not been published. It was soon found, however, that neither adriamycin nor hexamethylmelamine were useful as second-line chemotherapeutic agents. Only a few responders were observed. Furthermore, both adriamycin and hexamethylmelamine had relatively high numbers of toxic effects. A drawback with adriamycin is also that treatment with this agent can only be carried out over a limited time period because of heart toxicity. Altogether the results were disappointing, even in the series receiving a combination of thio-tepa and adriamycin. This trial has therefore also been concluded.

Our philosophy of treatment in advanced epithelial tumors of the ovary has always been "nil nocere". We have tried several new drugs both in Phase I and Phase II studies, and have found that some of them have similar response rates in single drug studies as alkylating agents. In our unit today, cis-platinum is compared with thio-tepa in advanced disease. There seems to be no doubt that cis-platinum has one of the highest response rates in Phase II studies. However, it remains to be proven that cis-platinum really gives a higher *long-term* survival than the much less toxic and more easily administered alkylating agents. Even if a large number of publications on different multiple drug schemes show high response rates and a prolonged short-term survival, the quality of life with such intensive chemotherapeutic regimes has never been adequately assessed. It should be remembered for example that sequential treatment with an alkylating agent and cis-platinum give the same long-term survival as when combined treatment with an alkylating agent and cis-platinum is carried out immediately after surgery.

We have been reluctant to treat advanced ovarian cancer with multiple drug regimes because of the philosophy expressed above.

39
Granulosa-theca cell tumors of the ovary

EPIDEMIOLOGY

Granulosa-theca cell tumors represent the largest group of functioning ovarian tumors. With rare exceptions, pure theca cell tumors are benign. The majority of these lesions are of mixed granulosa and theca cells, and the prognosis is dependent on the malignant granulosa cell. Many have failed to separate the benign theca cell tumors from the granulosa cell group. In comparing incidence figures from Norway (1) and Sweden one finds an incidence of 0.6/100,000 and 1.7/100,000 respectively. This must reflect different histologic criteria.

Granulosa-theca cell tumors comprise from 3 to 10% of all malignant ovarian tumors. It must be emphasized that if there is a granulosa cell element in the tumor, it must be considered a malignant ovarian tumor. It has been stated that a diffuse growth pattern of the granulosa cells indicates a poor prognosis, but this is not generally accepted. The place of radiotherapy in the treatment of granulosa cell tumors is also a controversial question.

In 1979 a series of 118 cases of granulosa-theca cell tumors of the ovary with long-term follow-up were presented from the Norwegian Radium Hospital (2).

MATERIAL AND METHODS

The 118 cases of granulosa cell tumors of the ovary were followed-up for from 5 to more than 30 years.

A review was made of 85 cases treated in the Norwegian Radium Hospital, and 92 cases treated in other hospitals. Pure thecomas were excluded, but not mixed granulosa-theca cell tumors, where the histology of the granulosa cell component was evaluated. The degree of cellular atypia was evaluated according to nuclear and cellular pleomorphism and arbitrarily graded as absent, (0), slight (+), moderate (+ +), and severe (+ + +). Mitoses per 10 high-power fields (HPF) were counted in areas where they were most abundant.

The original surgical records were reviewed and the patient staged according to the FIGO system.

SYMPTOMS

The mean age at diagnosis was 53.7 years. The ages ranged from 18 to 79 years. Sixty-two women (52.5%) were postmenopausal at the time of diagnosis, while seven additional patients above 50 years had had a hysterectomy several years before the menopause. Only 12 patients (10.2%) were less than 40 years.

The most common presenting symptom was abnormal uterine bleeding, in 41% of all patients as postmenopausal bleeding. In 10 of the premenopausal patients oligo- or amenorrhoea preceded the diagnosis. One third of the patients noted abdominal distension or pain, and nearly 8% had acute pain because of torsion or rupture of a cyst.

HISTOLOGY

The tumors were mostly unilateral with no side predominance. Bilateral tumors were seen in only six cases (5%). Many of the tumors within Stage I were rather large. About $\frac{1}{4}$ were greater than 15 cm in diameter. The tumors often showed both solid and cystic areas with hemorrhage or necrosis.

Usually several of the common histological patterns were seen in the same tumor. The characteristic Call-Exner bodies formed by granulosa cells surrounding small cystic areas containing cell debris occurred in about two thirds of the cases

(Fig. 39.1). The diffuse or so-called "sarcomatoid" growth pattern was found in 50% of the tumors. The diffuse areas showed slightly more atypia and a higher number of mitoses than those with Call-Exner bodies.

Endometrial tissue was obtained shortly before or at the initial laparotomy from 64 patients. Cystic glandular hyperplasia occurred in 41 endometria (64% of those examined), while another 13 postmenopausal cases had slightly estrogen stimulated endometria. One case of atypical adenomatous hyperplasia and two endometrial adenocarcinomas were found (1.6% and 3.1% respectively). Two other patients had been treated with hysterectomy because of endometrial adenocarcinoma several years before the diagnosis of granulosa cell tumor.

Table 39.1. Type of treatment in 118 cases of granulosa cell tumors

Treatment	No. of cases		
	NRH*	Others	Total
Unilat.[a]	1	26	27
Unilat. + Rad.	13	3	16
Bilat.	3	21	24
Bilat. + Rad.	44	3	47
Bilat. + Gold	1		1
Rad. only	3		3
Total	65	53	118

[a] Unilat., unilateral salpingo-oophorectomy; Bilat., bilateral salpingo-oophorectomy; Rad., radiotherapy; Gold, radioactive gold.
* NRH: Norwegian Radium Hospital.

TREATMENT

All patients underwent an exploratory laparotomy. The treatment varied considerably (Table 39.1). In the earlier period of this series surgery was often conservative, and the patients treated outside the Norwegian Radium Hospital more often had only one ovary removed. In the last 40 years radiation techniques have changed considerably, explaining the lack of uniformity in the radiotherapy. Most patients had a tumor dose of approximately 40 Gy delivered to the midpelvis. Those treated outside the Norwegian Radium Hospital rarely received irradiation.

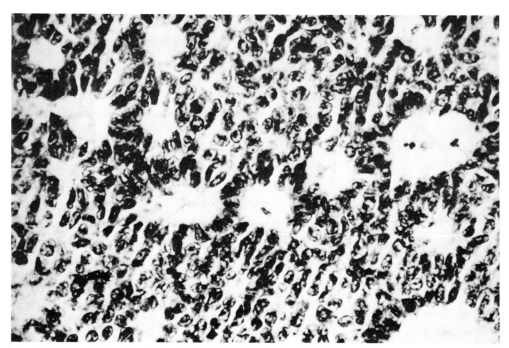

Fig. 39.1. Granulosa cell tumor of the ovary with typical Call Exner bodies. From (2) and reproduced by courtesy of Academic Press Inc.

RESULTS

Fifty patients died, 31 from their granulosa cell tumor, 15 of these within five years. For the whole series the observed 5-year survival was 80.5%, while the relative survival was 82.3%.

Recurrence in the pelvis or spread outside the pelvis was seen in 25 cases. Four of these patients are alive with no evidence of disease, one of them 14 years after the recurrence. Three patients had recurrences 19, 20, and 22 years after primary operation. One patient died from ruptured liver metastasis 23 years after the primary diagnosis, and 10 years after surgical removal of a recurrence in the other ovary. The only extra abdominal metastasis in this series was to the pleura. The time between the primary diagnosis and recurrence varied from 1 to 22 years with a mean of 8.9 years, while the interval between recurrence and death was from 0 to 10 years with a mean of 2.6 years.

In an evaluation of how clinical and histopathological findings relate to prognosis, the following observations were made. The difference between stage of disease and survival was statistically significant, when death from all causes is

Table 39.2. Tumor size and prognosis

| Size (cm) | No. of cases | Deaths | |
		From tumor	From other causes
< 5	15	2	2
5–10	44	8	9
10–15	25	6	2
> 15	32	15	6
Unknown	2	0	0
Total	118	31	19

included and also when death from granulosa cell tumor only are taken into consideration (Fig. 39.2). There seemed to be a relation between large tumor size and risk of death from tumor (Table 39.2).

The mortality increased with increasing mitotic rates and with increased cellular atypia (Fig. 39.3 and 39.4). Areas with the diffuse growth pattern indicated a poor prognosis when deaths from all causes were included.

The difference in observed and relative survival rates respectively for Stage I patients treated by surgery alone and by surgery combined with radiotherapy, were not statistically significant.

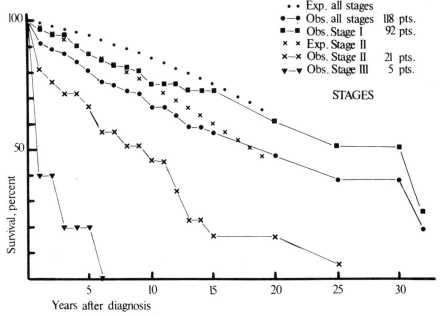

Fig. 39.2. Actuarial survival rate in the different stages of the disease. From (2) and reproduced by courtesy of Academic Press Inc.

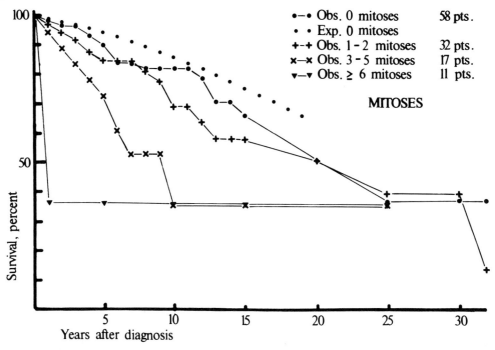

Fig. 39.3. Survival rate related to mitotic activity. From (2) and reproduced by courtesy of Academic Press Inc.

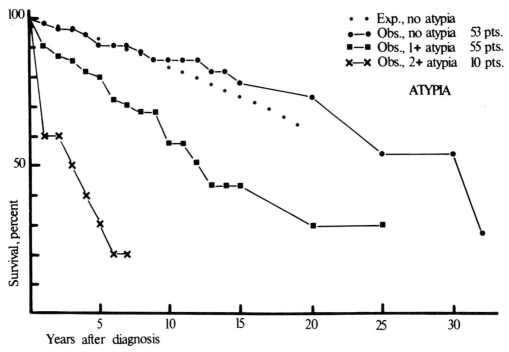

Fig. 39.4. Survival rate related to atypia. From (2) and reproduced by courtesy of Academic Press Inc.

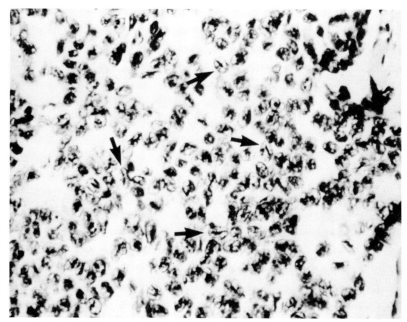

Fig. 39.5. Granulosa cells with typical nuclear grooves (arrows). From (2) and reproduced by courtesy of Academic Press Inc.

DISCUSSION

In conclusion, the histological diagnosis of a granulosa cell tumor is usually easy. Call-Exner bodies are pathognomonic, but are only present in about one half of the cases. There are many other characteristic growth patterns. Nuclei of well-differentiated granulosa cell tumors often show a longitudinal nuclear groove (Fig. 39.5). The diffuse growth pattern may be difficult to separate from thecomas. Reticulum stain may be of considerable help as fibres tend to surround single thecoma cells and groups of granulosa cells.

The clinical stage is of great prognostic significance; so also is tumor size. The size of the tumor may vary considerably within each stage. Patients below 40 years of age at diagnosis are reported to have a better prognosis than the older ones, and the present series confirms this. A positive relationship between atypia and mitotic index and recurrence rate has been reported (3). In our study we found that three or more mitoses per 10 HPF indicated a higher risk, and the mortality increased with the mitotic index. The finding of atypia also influenced the prognosis. The patients with diffuse growth pattern in their tumors had a

slightly lower survival rate than those without. Our relative survival rates resemble those of Sjöstedt and Wallén (4), but differ from the findings of Norris and Taylor (5), who excluded postoperative deaths and deaths from causes other than granulosa cell tumors before calculating life table survival rates. Evidence of estrogen stimulation of the endometrium is commonly found in these patients. In this series of 118 patients, severe atypia or adenocarcinoma of the endometrium was found in 4.7%. Fox et al. (6) reported 1.7%. Gusberg and Kardon (7), however, found a much higher frequency of 27.5%.

There are no absolute prognostic factors to direct treatment policy. Our series gives no evidence that radiotherapy helps any patients in Stage I. Previous studies have shown a beneficial effect of irradiation in patients with advanced stages, residual tumor tissue or recurrent disease, or when more than 50% "anaplastic cells" are found in the specimen. Our observations are in agreement with this. Routine postoperative irradiation has been proposed in postmenopausal patients. We do not agree with this if the patient has a Stage I tumor except if there is a high degree of atypia and/or a large number of mitoses.

40
Dysgerminoma

For many years confusion existed among pathologists as to the classification of the germ cell tumors of the ovary. This was first and foremost due to their rarity. The reported series were small, heterogeneous mixtures of different tumors. The diagnosis was uncertain and treatment met with little success. In 1973 the WHO introduced a new classification of germ cell tumors of the ovary. This classification is shown in Table 40.1. The largest group of malignant germ cell tumors treated in our hospital throughout the years is the dysgerminomas followed by the malignant teratomas, the endodermal sinus tumors and embryonal carcinomas. All of these tumors usually afflict girls and young women.

In 1951 four cases of dysgerminoma were reported from our hospital (1), three of these were cured with a combination of surgery and radiotherapy. The second series was reported in 1964 (2), and it was concluded that in girls or young women unilateral oophorectomy followed by radiotherapy to the ipsilateral side and the periaortic lymph nodes should be the treatment of choice. In 1983 a series of 45 pure dysgerminomas were collected, all of which were followed for from 2 to 25 years (3). This series will be described in detail.

CLINICAL FEATURES

Age distribution. The youngest patient was 11 years and the oldest 40 years. The average age was 22 years. At the time of diagnosis 39 patients were menstruating regularly, three were prepubertal and two aged 21 and 22 had primary amenorrhoea. One 20-year-old patient had a previously diagnosed XXY intersex. Of 25 married patients 21 were parous. Eight were pregnant at the time of diagnosis.

Symptoms. As in other reported series, increasing abdominal size and/or pain were the main symptoms. Five tumors were found on routine medical examination. Of the pregnant patients, two presented with obstructed labor, whilst five experienced abdominal pain during pregnancy; one tumor was detected on examination after the patient had requested legal abortion.

Stage distribution. Throughout the years we have used the FIGO staging also for dysgerminomas. Table 40.2 shows the stage distribution for the 45 patients in this series. Of the 39 patients in Stage I, four had bilateral tumors. This compares well with other series, where bilateral tumors are found in between 10 and 20% of cases. Ascites was found in only one patient in Stage I.

Tumor size. Both in the present series and in the other two series reported from our hospital it was found that the tumor was relatively large when first detected (Table 40.3). Only one patient had a tumor less than 5 cm in diameter. The majority

---

Table 40.1. WHO classification of germ cell tumors of the ovary

1. Dysgerminoma
2. Endodermal sinus tumor (yolk sac tumor)
3. Embryonal carcinoma
4. Polyembryoma
5. Choriocarcinoma
6. Teratomas
   a. Immature (solid, cystic or both)
   b. Mature
      i Solid
      ii Cystic
         Mature cystic teratoma (dermoid cyst)
         Mature cystic teratoma with malignant transformation
   c. Monodermal or highly specialized
      i Struma ovarii
      ii Carcinoid
      iii Others
7. Mixed forms

Table 40.2. Stage distribution FIGO

Stage	No.
Ia	34
Ib	4
Ic	1
IIa	1
IIb	2
III	1
IV	2
Total	45

Table 40.3. Tumor size in relation to recurrences and deaths

Tumor size in cm	No.	Recurrences	Deaths
<5	1	0	0
5–10	4	0	0
10–15	14	4	0
15–20	17	2	2
Total	45	6	2

of the cases, 31 altogether, had a tumor size between 10 and 20 cm in diameter. Of these 31 cases, 6 had recurrences of their disease, and in the group with a tumor size between 15 and 20 cm, a total of 17 patients, 2 died from their disease.

In three cases the tumor ruptured during operation. One of these with a Stage IIb lesion died during radiotherapy after non-radical surgery. The other two with ruptured tumors are alive 15 and 16 years after radiation.

HISTOLOGY

All 45 tumors represented pure dysgerminomas with no admixture of other elements (Fig. 40.1). The number of mitoses, the degree of cellular atypia, the amount of connective tissue, the lymphocyte infiltration and the degree of granulomatous reaction were all studied. Furthermore, poor demarcation of the tumor, infiltration of the tumor capsule and/or in vascular spaces were registered as present or absent.

This attempt at a histopathological subgroup-

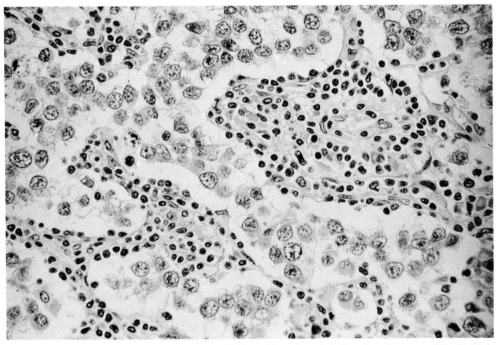

Fig. 40.1. Pure dysgerminoma with large, polygonal cells and lymphocytic infiltration. Courtesy of Dr. V. Abeler.

Table 40.4. Treatment methods and recurrences in 34 Stage Ia dysgerminomas

Treatment	No.	Recurrences	Deaths
Unilateral oophorectomy	4	3	0
Unilateral oophorectomy and inverted half Y (1) field	17	3	0
More radical surgical/radiological treatment	13	0	0

ing was not helpful in identifying high-risk patients. The most important pathologic factor is if the lesion is a pure dysgerminoma, since other germ cell elements give a poorer prognosis (4). Thus, it is always necessary to sample tissue from several parts of the tumor.

TREATMENT

In the earlier years of the study, treatment was radical with bilateral salpingo-oophorectomy with or without hysterectomy and in most cases followed by irradiation. Since the study of Koller and Gjønnæss in 1964 (2) a more conservative approach was used with unilateral oophorectomy followed, as a rule, by ipsilateral pelvic irradiation and irradiation to the lymph nodes alongside the aorta up to Th.12. A summary of the different treatment modalities in Stage Ia in relation to recurrences and deaths from cancer is shown in Table 40.4. As can be seen, three out of four patients where only unilateral oophorectomy was

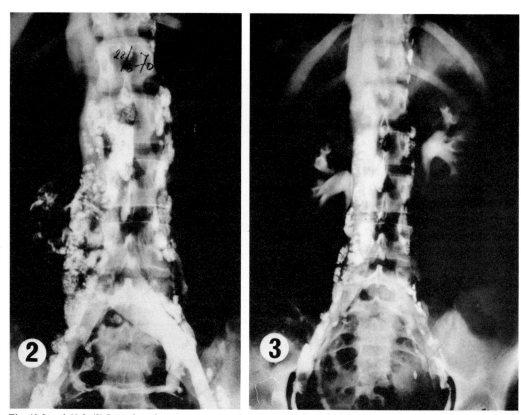

Fig. 40.2 and 40.3. (2) Lymph node metastases to periaortic glands from a right-sided dysgerminoma. 3. Appearance of glands after successful irradiation.

performed, had a recurrence, but could be treated by irradiation. Of the 17 Stage Ia lesions, which received unilateral oophorectomy plus ipsilateral and periaortic irradiation, three recurrences occurred outside the irradiated area. These three cases could also be saved by irradiation to the recurrence site. In the whole series 24 cases all received extended radiotherapy, which means irradiation to the whole pelvis and to the periaortic region. The extreme radiosensitivity of dysgerminoma is clearly shown in our series. Two patients had metastatic disease. One of these had metastases to the periaortic glands, supraclavicular glands, the left axilla and the left breast. She received irradiation with conventional radiotherapy to all these sites and is today alive, 25 years after primary therapy.

Chemotherapy was used in only two cases. One of these was a 16-year-old girl who was originally treated with a unilateral oophorectomy and radiation to an inverted half Y field. Wedge resection of the contralateral ovary was negative. Eight months later, however, a metastasis was found in the contralateral ovary; it was removed, and further radiotherapy was given to complete a pelvic field. One year later metastases were detected in the liver, spleen and bones. The patient was treated with a combination of vincristine 1.5 mg/m^2, adriamycin 50 mg/m^2, cyclophosphamide 500 mg/m^2 and actinomycin D 0.5 mg/m^2 every third week. During this regime the metastases disappeared completely, and the patient is in complete remission eight years later.

Seven patients (15%) had recurrent disease. Of these, six were initially treated conservatively. Two occurred in the first year, two in the second, one in the third and two in the fifth year of follow-up.

Only two patients in this series of 45 cases died of dysgerminoma, one during therapy and the other following unsuccessful treatment for recurrent disease. The actuarial 5-year survival rate for the whole group was 96%, whilst for Stage Ia it was 100%. Thirty-seven patients have been observed for more than five years, and eight patients have had an observation time of between two and four years.

During the later years of the study, we have always performed a wedge resection of the macroscopically normal-looking remaining ovary. Altogether 12 patients have undergone wedge resection, but all specimens were without tumor infiltration. In two of these, dysgerminoma nevertheless developed in the biopsied ovary. Both of these have been successfully treated, one mentioned previously with radiotherapy followed later by chemotherapy, and one by radiotherapy only.

FERTILITY AND OVARIAN FUNCTION

Since therapy, one woman has had three successful pregnancies. One had tubal adhesions and another has been unsuccessful in attempts to become pregnant, but has not been investigated for infertility. The remaining 11 treated conservatively are either too young or have not wanted to become pregnant. With the exception of one 13-year-old girl, all are menstruating regularly.

FUTURE TREATMENT PROTOCOL

We have decided that in the future all young women with an ovarian tumor shall have a blood sample taken for determination of the betasubunit of HCG and alphaphoetoprotein. In pure dysgerminomas these tumor markers will not be elevated. Before operation, X-ray of the lungs, intravenous pyelograms and lymphography shall be performed (Fig. 40.2 and 40.3). It must be realized, however, that in most cases the diagnosis will only be made after the surgery. Since dysgerminomas in almost 90% of the cases are unilateral, we will continue to perform only unilateral salpingo-oophorectomy together with wedge resection of the normal looking contralateral ovary. Postoperatively, irradiation to the ipsilateral pelvic wall and periaortic region will be given. The dose should not exceed 40 Gy. If by lymphography or during operation metastases are found in the periaortic region, then the mediastinal glands shall also receive irradiation. This is in accordance with the treatment of seminomas in the male. With modern high-voltage technique it is easy to shield the normal-looking contralateral ovary, and fertility can be preserved. Surgery alone may be performed if the tumor is less than 5 cm in diameter. Chemotherapy will be restricted to cases with metastases which cannot be adequately treated with radiotherapy.

41
Endodermal sinus tumor

In 1959 and 1965 Teilum (1, 2) published the results of his investigations into the histogenesis and interrelationship of ovarian and testicular tumors of germ cell origin. He claimed that embryonal carcinoma, malignant teratoma, endodermal sinus tumor and mixed mesodermal sarcomas develop from the germ cell (Fig. 41.1). The pure germ cell tumors are the male seminomas and the female dysgerminomas. According to Teilum the so-called endodermal sinus tumor or yolk sac tumor develops from extraembryonic structures.

It has been claimed that endodermal sinus tumor is almost as common as dysgerminoma in girls and young women. This is not our experience. Dysgerminomas are relatively common tumors, while endodermal sinus tumors are extremely rare in Norway. This may, however, be due to the fact that the endodermal sinus tumor is a comparatively new entity and therefore incidence figures are difficult to obtain. During our survey of 63 cases of so-called mesonephroid tumors of the ovary we found that four of these should be classified as yolk sac tumors.

Alphaphoetoprotein (AFP) is characteristically produced by the yolk sac and as such is an excellent tumor marker for this type of tumor. Because the histological picture is now clearly described and AFP may be measured in the blood or by histochemical methods in sections from the tumor, endodermal sinus tumors are recognized more frequently than before.

CLINICAL FEATURES

The cases we have seen had an age range of between 14 and 25 years. As in other larger series (3, 4), we found that the symptoms were uncharacteristic, but usually the patients had an acute abdominal pain or increasing abdominal girth. The duration of symptoms was usually brief, only a few weeks. These tumors can grow extremely rapidly and even with a one-sided tumor (Stage Ia), about 90% of the patients have subclinical spread (3). Bilateral tumors are rare, but spread to pelvic structures or the upper abdomen is common. The tumor growth rate is probably the fastest of any human malignancy, and some patients may have had a normal pelvic examination only a few weeks or months before the removal of a large tumor with intra-abdominal spread. In earlier years, the recommended treatment was bilateral salpingo-oophorectomy with hysterectomy followed by irradiation. However, radiotherapy has no place in this type of tumor, since it is completely radioresistant. It is also as a rule unnecessary to remove the other ovary and the uterus.

Single agent chemotherapy has met with little success. Kurmann and Norris (3) have reported one of the largest series of endodermal sinus tumor comprising a total of 71 cases. Among 65 patients on whom follow-up information was available, the actuarial survival rate was only 13% at three years. Of the neoplasms that recurred, 93% did so within one year, and of those patients who died, 93% did so within two years. This extremely poor prognosis has also been seen in our own few patients. The size and stage of the tumor had prognostic significance, but the patient's age, the mitotic activity and the histologic pattern did not.

HISTOLOGY

The histologic appearance as described in detail by Teilum displays five basic, interrelated growth patterns. The commonest is the reticular pattern composed of a loose meshwork of spaces and channels lined by flattened or cuboidal cells with scanty cytoplasm and indistinct borders (Fig. 41.2). So-called "festoons" are tufted structures,

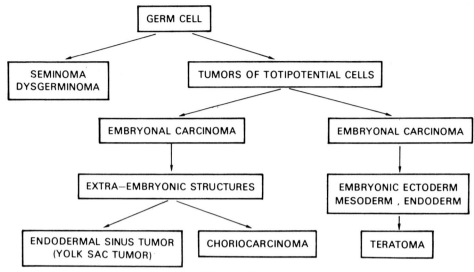

Fig. 41.1. Histogenesis of germ cell tumors after Teilum (1, 2).

which are considered pathognomonic of this neo-plasm. Hyaline bodies are common in the reticular pattern. A so-called polyvesicular vitelline pattern is rarer, being characterized by multiple micro-cysts with flat or columnar epithelial cells having clear cytoplasm lying in dense fibroblastic stroma. Usually, all three patterns coexist in the same tumor. The fourth pattern is of alveolar-glandular type, in which cystic spaces are lined by papillary processes having cuboidal epithelium. The fifth and rarest form is a relatively solid growth of undifferentiated cells resembling embryonal carci-noma. In approximately a third of cases these five growth patterns are mixed. There is no prognostic difference between any of the types (3).

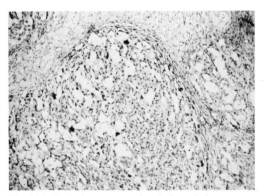

Fig. 41.2. Reticular pattern of endodermal sinus tumor.

The endodermal sinus tumors must be con-sidered to constitute a surgical and therapeutic emergency because of the extremely fast growth rate.

TREATMENT

As mentioned above, radiation and radical sur-gery have not reduced the mortality, and single agent chemotherapy is of little value.

Some hope for cure has appeared in the litera-ture in recent years, however. In a large series of endodermal sinus tumor of the ovary seen in the M. D. Andersen Hospital (4), 21 of 41 patients are alive and well after multiple drug chemo-therapy with a combination of vincristine, acti-nomycin D and cyclophosphamide (VAC). Sixteen of 22 patients treated with this combination have survived for five years. Another combination of drugs which has met with success is vinblastine, bleomycin and cis-platinum. It is of importance to note that if one drug combination fails a re-sponse with another drug combination may give a good response rate. This is in contrast to the epithelial tumors where the first drug combination is that which really matters to get a complete response rate. In epithelial tumors it is seldom that second line chemotherapy is successful.

During chemotherapy with multiple drugs in

endodermal sinus tumor, AFP is an excellent tumor marker and will soon indicate whether the drug combination chosen is successful or not. If there is a slow fall in AFP or, still worse, if the AFP level in blood starts to rise, there should be an immediate change to another combination of chemotherapeutic drugs. There is no doubt that today there is hope for patients with endodermal sinus tumor, a tumor that in earlier days was almost always considered fatal.

42
Malignant (immature) teratoma of the ovary

An ovarian teratoma is a tumor containing tissues derived from all three germ cell layers of the embryo, namely the endoderm, the mesoderm and ectoderm. In the benign teratomas of the ovary all these tissues are mature. Ordinarily they are designed as dermoid cysts. Dermoid cysts are among the most common tumors of the ovary comprising between 10 and 20% of all tumors found in fertile women. These mature cystic teratomas are most commonly found during a routine pelvic examination or as a result of some accident such as torsion. An ordinary X-ray of the pelvis may reveal calcifications, e.g. teeth, and histopathological examination may in addition reveal hair, sebaceous glands, cartilage, skin with its appendices, glandular structures from the endoderm such as the stomach or intestines, and neural components such as nerve elements or glial tissue. As long as all these structures are mature, the tumor must be considered benign.

Only about 1–2% of the teratomas contain immature or embryonic tissue. This immaturity directly reflects the malignant potential for invasion or metastases. A third small group of tumors may be recognized, namely the highly specialized monodermal teratomas, usually consisting of ovarian struma, carcinoid, or a mixture of the two. Presentation in this group is usually an abdominal mass or endocrine disturbances.

The immature solid teratoma occurs almost exclusively in the child or young girl. Any teratoma seen in this age group must be considered malignant until an extensive search by the pathologist has proven otherwise. Robboy and Scully (1) have proposed a simple grading system for these tumors based upon the immaturity of neural tissue.

STAGING

The FIGO staging of ovarian carcinoma may be applied in malignant ovarian teratomas. However, with modern chemotherapy, especially combinations of vincristine, actinomycin D, cyclophosphamide (VAC) or cis-platinum, vinblastine and bleomycin (PVB), it seems that ordinary clinical staging is not so important as the size of the tumor and the level of the two tumor markers HCG and/or AFP (alphaphoetoprotein).

At the Norwegian Radium Hospital we have little experience with these tumors. Since 1974 we have seen eight cases of malignant ovarian teratomas. All of these had Grade 3 lesions. We have treated them with doxorubicin (adriamycin) as a single agent up to the maximum dose of 500 mg/m^2. On this regime all patients are still surviving 4–8 years later.

TERATOMA MATURATION

Maturation of immature or embryonal elements is reported to occur both spontaneously and after several forms of chemotherapy (1). In our own series of eight patients, all of them had palpable disease after operation and also after chemotherapy. Second-look surgery showed, however, that all elements were mature. When possible, these lesions have been excised, but in cases with multiple implantations this has not always been possible. These mature implants have not shown any tendency to grow or to revert to immature elements. Thus, in assessing response to chemotherapy, biopsy of any palpable mass should be performed before concluding that the treatment is unsuccessful, and it may not be necessary to institute a highly complex and toxic regime.

Two cases had immature neural or glial elements. One of these received adriamycin and is still alive 15 years after extensive spread of disease throughout the abdominal cavity. In another patient with glial and neural elements we did not give any therapy, and she is also alive without evidence of active disease five years after it was decided not to give therapy. It is in accordance with the experience of other authors that neural or glial teratomas usually have a very good prognosis.

STRUMA OVARII

In many of the benign dermoid cysts thyroid elements may be found. Significant ectopic thyroid function is rare, and presentation is usually as a non-specific ovarian cystic tumor. The malignancy rate of these tumors is relatively low. Scully (3) states that the malignancy rate is about 5–10%. Surgery is therefore usually sufficient treatment. He points to the fact that pleural and peritoneal effusions, which may be associated with struma ovarii, have been shown to regress after surgery.

We have experience with only one case of malignant struma ovarii, and this developed metastases to the lumbar glands and to the vertebrae L. 4–5.

In this special case, radioactive iodine was used, and the metastases disappeared completely. It seems from this single case that it may be worth trying radioactive iodine in malignant struma ovarii with metastases.

CARCINOID (ARGENTAFFINOMA)

Primary carcinoid of the ovary is very uncommon. We cannot report a single case. In a series, which was collected by Robboy, Scully and Norris in 1975 (4), the presentation of carcinoid of the ovary was a typical "carcinoid syndrome", with flushes, diarrhea or cardiac murmurs associated with either pulmonary stenosis or tricuspid insufficiency. In accordance with Robboy, Scully and Norris these symptoms may occur in the absence of metastases. They have a low grade of malignant potential, and surgery is the treatment of choice. Follow-up is facilitated by series determination of urinary 5-hydroxyindole acetic acid (5-HIAA). Chemotherapy with an alkylating agent or 5-fluorouracil may produce response in metastatic disease. It must be admitted, however, that we still know too little about both the diagnosis and the best treatment of carcinoid tumors because of the rarity of this disease.

43
Embryonal carcinoma of the ovary

The endodermal sinus tumor of the ovary is today recognized as a clinical and histopathological entity different from other germ cell tumors. A pure endodermal sinus tumor produces alphaphoetoprotein, but not human chorionic gonadotrophin.

In 1976 Kurmann and Norris (1) described 15 of what they believed was the female counterpart to embryonal carcinoma of the testis. Embryonal carcinoma of the ovary may be distinguished from the endodermal sinus tumor on the basis of its histologic and immunohistochemical characteristics.

The age of the patients ranged from 4 to 28 years, and seven were prepubertal. Abnormal hormonal manifestations occurred in nine patients and consisted of precocious puberty manifested by bilateral breast development, vaginal bleeding and growth of hair on the vulva in three of the seven prepubertal girls. Amenorrhoea, infertility and mild hirsutism occurred in one postmenarchial woman, and either amenorrhoea or irregular vaginal bleeding occurred in five other women. In four cases the embryonal carcinoma was mixed with either dysgerminoma, endodermal sinus tumor or benign cystic teratoma. In nine of the patients the pregnancy test was positive.

The diameter of the tumor varied between 12 and 25 cm. In all cases so-called syncytio-trophoblastic giant cells were found together with hyaline droplets, and indirect immunoperoxidase method for the localization of human chorionic gonadotrophin (HCG) and alphaphoetoprotein (AFP) was done on formalin fixed paraffin-embedded tissue from 10 neoplasms. HCG was present in all 10 neoplasms, and AFP was found in 7.

The patients were treated with a combination of surgery, radiotherapy and chemotherapy. Different drugs were used. The actuarial survival for the entire group was 39%, and for those with Stage I tumors 50%.

In the Norwegian Radium Hospital we have seen only three cases of embryonal carcinoma during the last 10 years. All patients died within 15 months in spite of treatment with surgery, radiotherapy and chemotherapy. There is no doubt that embryonal carcinoma is a very malignant tumor. Possibly, in the future, modern chemotherapy with either VAC (vincristine, actinomycin D and cyclophosphamide), PVB (cisplatinum, vinblastine and bleomycin) or other drug combinations will give better treatment results.

CHORIOCARCINOMA

This is the rarest of the germ cell tumor group of the ovary. In the literature there are only about 50 cases reported. Choriocarcinoma may occur in the ovary as metastases from gestational choriocarcinoma. We have never seen a primary choriocarcinoma developing from the gonad, but we have seen two examples of gestational choriocarcinoma of the ovary arising from an ectopic pregnancy. Choriocarcinoma of the ovary may, however, represent part of mixed germ cell tumors such as immature teratoma or embryonal carcinoma.

In the literature it is stated that choriocarcinoma of the ovary occurs mainly in the first two decades, and it is suggested it has a slightly better prognosis than the endodernal sinus tumor. However, whereas single agent methotrexate is effective in many cases of gestational trophoblastic disease, this drug does not have the same efficiency in choriocarcinoma originating in germ cells. The trophoblastic elements produce HCG, and in pure cell choriocarcinoma it is a very valuable tumor marker.

It is a disease of young girls, and the symptoms are very similar to those of any other ovarian tumor, with abdominal distension and pain predominating. Endocrine disturbances associated with HCG production may lead to isosexual precocity or menstrual disturbances.

The tumor itself is usually encapsulated and on sectioning there are frequently large hemorrhagic areas.

The management of choriocarcinoma of the ovary is surgery combined with modern combination chemotherapy.

44
Primary invasive cancer of the Fallopian tube

Primary cancer of the Fallopian tube is a rare disease. In the literature, figures between 1.1% and 1.3% for all cases of gynecological cancer have been presented. This means that there are few doctors that can collect a sufficient number of Fallopian tube cancer cases to be used as a guide for both the diagnosis and treatment of this extremely rare disease.

The Fallopian tube epithelium is derived from the same structures in the embryonic life as the surface epithelium of the ovary, the endometrium and the epithelium of the cervix. It is therefore striking that so few tumors develop from the Fallopian tube epithelium compared to the lesions which e.g. develop from the surface epithelium of the ovary. The serous carcinomas of the ovary are common, but the similar carcinomas of the Fallopian tube are extremely rare.

From 1952 through 1975 the Cancer Registry of Norway registered 62 cases of cancer of the Fallopian tube. This is approximately 0.6% of the registered number of cancer of the ovary during the same period. We have surveyed specimens from histological material and compared the histopathological patterns with the notes in the records of these 62 cases.

Forty-two of the 62 cases could be confirmed as definite primary invasive cancer of the Fallopian tube. These patients have been evaluated according to age, parity, earlier gynecological disease, symptoms, stage distribution, histology, treatment and survival. All patients have been followed for more than five years (1).

HISTOLOGICAL MATERIAL AND METHODS

Histological material from all 62 patients was reviewed without knowledge of the clinical course. All cases had to fulfill the following criteria:

1. The tumor should obviously originate in the tubal mucosa.
2. The tumor should be grossly and microscopically mainly located in the tube.

In the cases in which the tubes, ovaries and/or uterus were involved, histological study and size of the tubal carcinoma in relation to the tumor involvement of the other organs were important factors in determining the primary site. Using these criteria, 20 cases were omitted from the series.

The age distribution of the series of 42 patients is shown in Fig. 44.1. The average age for the series was 55 years.

Eighteen of the patients had never been pregnant. Twenty-one patients had from one to seven births, and in three patients there was no information about pregnancy.

Eight patients had a history of early salpingitis, one had been treated by radical vulvectomy for cancer of the vulva, two had been operated for myoma of the uterus, and two had been operated for benign ovarian cysts.

SYMPTOMS

The symptoms of Fallopian tube carcinoma are vague. In our series they were often present for several months, and the most frequent symptom was abnormal bleeding (Table 44.1). Abnormal bleeding was followed by lower abdominal pain, discharge, increased size of the abdomen and other symptoms. The so-called hydrops tubae profluens, which was described in 1915 by Latzko as pathognomonic of cancer of the Fallopian tube, was not found in our series.

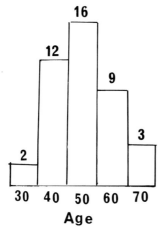

Fig. 44.1. Age distribution of 42 patients with carcinoma of the Fallopian tube.

STAGE DISTRIBUTION

In the absence of an accepted stage distribution for primary cancer of the Fallopian tube, we have used FIGO's stage distribution for ovarian cancer:

Stage I   18.
Stage II   20.
Stage III 4.
Stage IV   0.

HISTOLOGY

The tumors were classified histologically according to the WHO International Classification of tumors. When necessary, new sections were cut and stained with hematoxyline and eosin. Forty of the 42 patients and all 18 cases in Stage I were adenocarcinomas. In Stage I, 10 tumors were localized in the right tube, 6 in the left, and 2 were bilateral. Both of the bilateral tumors were poorly differentiated.

Table 44.1. Symptoms

Bleeding	25
Pain	13
Extended abdomen	5
Discharge	10
Other	4

The specimens were also grouped according to the maximum depth of infiltration in the tubal wall as follows:

1. Tumor limited to the tubal mucosa.
2. Infiltration in the muscularis.
3. Infiltration to the peritoneal serosa.

Furthermore, they were classified according to whether vessel invasion was present or not.

TREATMENT

In no case in this series was the diagnosis made prior to laparotomy. The surgical treatment generally consisted of removal of the tumor, the other adnexa, the uterus and the omentum. Thirty-eight of the 42 patients received additional irradiation to the pelvis or to a pelvic and an abdominal field (not including the liver). Adjuvant chemotherapy with the alkylating agent thio-tepa was given to five patients.

The 5-year survival rate in all stages is shown in Fig. 44.2. Two patients in Stage I died of cancer within six years.

Of the four patients who did not receive any radiotherapy, two of three in Stage I were alive for more than five years, and one Stage III died three months after diagnosis. Five of the 38 irradiated patients received additional chemotherapy with thio-tepa. Of two patients in Stage I, one survived the disease, and one died of cancer after three years. Of two patients in Stage II, one

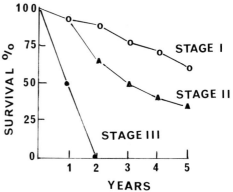

Fig. 44.2. Survival rate related to stage in 42 cases of carcinoma of the Fallopian tube.

is alive and one died of cancer after 18 months. One patient in Stage III died one year after irradiation and chemotherapy.

DISCUSSION

It is difficult with such a rare disease to get enough experience with the treatment. Early diagnosis is, as elsewhere in cancer treatment, of importance. An exact diagnosis before laparatomy is in our opinion almost impossible.

It is remarkable that patients, who presented with poorly differentiated cancer, had a somewhat better prognosis both in Stages I and II than those with moderately to well differentiated cancer. In accordance with cancer of the endometrium most cancers of the Fallopian tube are adenocarcinomas in postmenopausal women, and many of the patients are nulliparae (2, 3, 4). In this group of patients surgical therapy followed by external irradiation gave an overall 5-year survival rate of 43%.

In early Fallopian tube cancer without any signs of macroscopic spread of the tumor, intraperitoneal instillation of radioactive phosporus (P_{32}) may be of value (5). There is no doubt, however, that the overall survival rate for Fallopian tube cancer is low. The tumor is radiosensitive and some form of irradiation should be given to the areas where the tumor has spread. On the other hand, it is also quite clear that modern combined chemotherapy, as in ovarian cancer, with e.g. vincristine, actinomycin D and cyclophosphamide or with cis-platinum, vinblastine and bleomycin may be of value in the future treatment of this extremely rare tumor (6). The rarity of the tumor is surprising. When compared to ovarian carcinoma, the histopathological picture is that of a serous adenocarcinoma and this is the most frequent type of carcinoma in the ovary. It seems as if the Fallopian tube, even if it is frequently affected by inflammatory conditions, does not give rise to invasive carcinoma at a rate that can be compared with endometrial or ovarian carcinoma.

45
Primary malignant tumors of the female urethra

Tumors of the urethra may be referred either to urological departments or to departments of gynecologic oncology. We have reviewed our material of carcinoma of the urethra in three papers, namely in 1968, 1969 and 1983 (1, 2, 3). It is sad to say that no type of treatment used during the years from 1932 to the present day has been successful. The latest retrospective study of 51 cases with histologically verified invasive cancer of the female urethra showed that the disease occurred in most cases after the age of 50.

STAGING

In cases of cancer of the urethra, the so-called TNM system is usually used. T – tumor, N – lymph nodes, M – metastases.

Stage 0 (T1S). – Carcinoma in situ, preinvasive cancer.
Stage I (T1). – Tumor limited to the endothelium or subepithelial growth without invasion to the muscularis. Clinically soft, mobile tumor, e.g. a caruncula with malignant change.
Stage II (T2) or *III* (T3). – Tumor infiltration into the muscularis, either superficial or deep. Clinically indurated, but still mobile without signs of spread.
Stage IV (T4). – Tumor infiltration beyond the urethra with fixation to the pelvis or the vaginal wall.

DIAGNOSIS

Women with urethral cancer are often referred to the gynecologist because of bleeding from the urethra or vagina, or because of tumor has been found in the urethral region. Theoretically it is possible to diagnose a carcinoma of the urethra in situ by urinary cytology, but in practice pre-invasive cancer is often diagnosed histologically following transurethral resection for a bladder neck stenosis. With a urethral caruncula, cytology should always be taken from the lesions itself. Colposcopy is of value in determining the site of biopsy (Fig. 45.1).

Most tumors are squamous carcinomas, occurring in the lower half of the urethra. Adenocarcinomas and transitional cell tumors are relatively rare. This last group usually occurs in the upper half of the urethra.

One must always remember that tumors of the female urethra may occur in conjunction with other urinary tract tumors, or may be spreading from either cervix, vaginal, or corpus cancers. One quite commonly sees suburethral metastases with corpus cancer. It is therefore necessary that all patients with urethral carcinoma have a thorough gynecological investigation to exclude any other genital malignancy. This should include cytological examination of the cervix, colposcopy, biopsy and fractional curettage. From a urological point of view, urinary cytology, urography, urethrocystoscopy with biopsy and urethral pressure profile (4) should be performed in all patients. Most important, however, is palpation under anesthesia (5). The last two examinations may give a clue as to how far up in the urethra the tumor has extended.

During the years 1940–72, 51 cases were treated in the gynecological department of the Norwegian Radium Hospital. This comprised about 80% of the total number registered in the whole country. Only two or three cases each year were admitted.

CLINICAL FEATURES

Two of the patients had been treated for a supposed urethral polyp, one and two years respec-

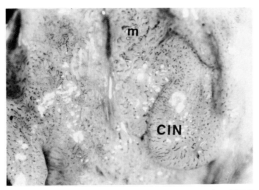

Fig. 45.1. Colposcopic appearance of preinvasive (CIN) and microinvasive (m) carcinoma of the urethra. CIN demonstrates regular punctation pattern. m.: small atypical vessels.

tively before diagnosis of cancer. Three patients had been treated for urethral caruncula, one of them over a period of 15 years. None of these patients had had histological examination of their disease. Most of them had bleeding symptoms or dysuria.

HISTOLOGY

Most of the tumors in the urethra developed in the outer third and were of squamous cell origin. Of the 51 cases, 32 had squamous carcinoma, 10 transitional carcinoma, and 9 adenocarcinoma of the urethra.

STAGING PROBLEMS

The staging of urethral carcinoma in the female has already been described. However, it is difficult to keep to this system for several reasons. There are at least two types of epithelium involved, transitional in the upper part of the urethra and non-keratinizing squamous epithelium in the lower part. When a squamous tumor has started to invade locally, there is no means of distinguishing it from a primary vaginal cancer. Direct and lymphatic spread occur both inside the pelvis, to the obturator and internal iliac lymph nodes, and outside the pelvis to the inguinal nodes.

The site in the urethra is important both as regards direction of spread and also as regards treatment (5). The question of preservation of continence greatly influences the choice of treatment method.

SPREAD

Of the 21 patients in clinical Stage I and II, only 1 had inguinal lymph node metastases. In the 29 patients in Stages III and IV who underwent treatment, 10 had inguinal lymph node metastases, and 2 had lung metastases. Of the 13 patients in Stages I and II who died of cancer, 1 patient had histologically verified inguinal lymph node metastases when the diagnosis was made. Eight of these 13 patients later developed inguinal or pelvic lymph node metastases. Three developed pelvic node metastases, and 1 lung metastases.

TREATMENT

The treatment in this series of 51 cases consisted of surgery, local and external radiotherapy, both separately and in combination. However, the treatment differed so much from patient to patient that a systematic evaluation would not lead to any valid conclusion.

Altogether 72% of the patients died of their disease within two years of observation. It has been reported that radiotherapy alone can give more than 50% 5-year disease free survival in early stages. This does not correspond with our experience. However, it is certain that local and/ or external radiotherapy should always be considered as a main form of treatment. The patients are mostly elderly, and radiotherapy has obvious advantages in avoiding mutilating surgery in older patients. It is our opinion that surgical resection has a definite place only when urethral continence can be preserved. This can be evaluated before operation with urethral pressure profile, cysto-urethroscopy and palpation under anesthesia.

Since half of our patients in the early stages developed inguinal lymph node metastases, inguinal lymphadenectomy or radiotherapy should always be considered.

46
Malignant trophoblastic neoplasia

In the following, the term "malignant tropho-blastic neoplasia" (MTN) is used about cases of invasive mole or true choriocarcinoma with or without metastases.

EPIDEMIOLOGY

The incidence of benign hydatidiform mole, invasive mole and choriocarcinoma varies considerably in different parts of the world, but is much greater in the Orient than elsewhere. In 1965 a study was published about the incidence of trophoblastic disease in Norway in the years 1953–61 (1). In 1952 compulsory registration of all malignant disease in the country was introduced, and consequently it was possible to give the exact number of malignant trophoblastic tumors diagnosed each year within this geographically defined area. To get an estimate about the number of benign hydatidiform moles diagnosed during the study period, information was received from all the pathological institutes in Norway.

The total series consisted of 405 benign hydatidiform moles, 9 invasive moles and 36 choriocarcinomas. The percentage of invasive moles was much less than in a later study from the Norwegian Radium Hospital, which will be reported below. It was concluded that an average of 45 benign moles and 3 malignant trophoblastic tumors were diagnosed each year in Norway during the study period. The frequency of vesicular mole was calculated as approximately 1:1,300 deliveries, and that of malignant trophoblastic tumors as 1:20,000 deliveries. Of the 405 moles, invasive mole developed in three cases (0.74%), and choriocarcinoma in nine cases (2.22%). This means that approximately 3% of benign moles in Norway develop into MTN. This is in accordance with studies from other Western countries. The prognosis for the invasive moles was excellent

with no deaths, while only 27.8% of the patients with choriocarcinoma survived. It must here be mentioned that the treatment during this early study period did not include chemotherapy. Treatment comprised mainly of hysterectomy, in some cases also followed by radiotherapy. It was not found, however, that radiotherapy had any significant influence on the survival. In one patient with multiple lung metastases on the initial examination, spontaneous regression of the metastases occurred after removal of the primary tumor. When the study was performed, the observation time for this patient was 11 years.

The introduction of methotrexate in the treatment of malignant trophoblastic tumors by Li, Hertz and Spencer in 1956 (2), and the use of this chemotherapeutic agent in a few cases in our country in the late 1950s with a definite response, induced an interest in a centralization of treatment of these tumors to the Norwegian Radium Hospital. From 1964 on almost every case of malignant trophoblastic neoplasia has been referred to our unit. During the same years, encouraged by the works by Fernström (3), pelvic arteriography was introduced as a routine procedure in the evaluation of malignant trophoblastic tumors. A preliminary report on the results was published in 1966 (4) and another report of pelvic arteriography in malignant trophoblastic neoplasia was published in 1969 (5). The monitoring of therapy in a series comprising 30 patients was discussed in 1972 (6). All these cases were gestational, and in 16 cases metastases were found.

The histological diagnoses were made on the following criteria:

Choriocarcinoma was diagnosed in hysterectomy specimens and in metastatic deposits on the commonly accepted microscopic findings of trophoblastic malignancy in the absence of villi (Fig.

46.1). In curettings, where invasion may not be evident, the diagnosis was made if the tissue consisted entirely of non-villus malignant trophoblast with or without uterine muscle.

Invasive mole was diagnosed in hysterectomy specimens, metastatic deposits or in curettings showing infiltration by malignant trophoblastic tissue containing chorionic villi (Fig. 46.2). The advent of successful chemotherapy for MTN had resulted in some cases with definite clinical evidence of such a neoplastic process, but without histological confirmation of diagnosis. Such cases were listed as histologically uncertain.

In the earlier years of the study period, monitoring of treatment was performed by determinations of HCG in urine with the hemagglutination inhibition method. From 1968 radioimmunoassay of luteinizing hormone (LH) in serum was used, and in the later years the β-subunit of HCG in serum has been determined.

In cases with an intact uterus, arteriography was performed. The results of our arteriographic findings had already been published in 1969 (5). Pelvic arteriography was found to be simple and safe; it was also concluded that this procedure may be of great help in the early diagnosis and management of MTN located to the myometrium only. Some examples of the arteriographic findings are shown in Figs. 46.3, 4 and 5.

In many cases of molar pregnancy in which the HCG concentration in the urine did not fall to normal levels within the course of 4–8 weeks, pelvic arteriography revealed vascular tumors in the uterus, and in some of these cases curettings were normal without sign of trophoblastic disease. It was concluded that in molar pregnancy in which HCG concentration in the urine did not fall to normal levels within a period of approximately eight weeks, arteriography and curettage should be performed. If arteriography showed a vascular tumor in the uterus, treatment with methotrexate or a combination of methotrexate and actinomycin D was immediately started.

We have now reviewed the total material of malignant trophoblastic neoplasia treated during the years 1964–81.

MATERIAL AND METHODS

During the years 1964–81 a total of 75 cases of MTN were treated in our hospital. This gives an

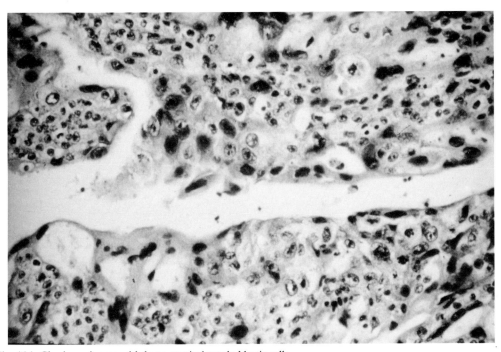

Fig. 46.1. Choriocarcinoma with large atypical trophoblastic cells.

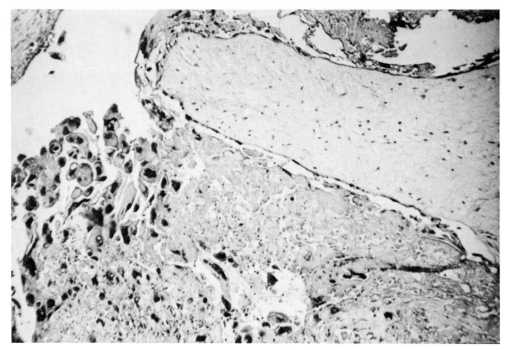

Fig. 46.2. Invasive mole with atypical trophoblastic cells, but with preservation of chorionic villous.

incidence of approximately four cases per year in Norway with a female population of about two million and about 55,000 deliveries each year.

Most of the patients were young, but it is striking that we had seven cases which were postmenopausal. The time interval for these seven cases from menopause to diagnosis of MTN was from two to four years.

The great majority had from one to three pregnancies including the pregnancy which developed into MTN. Many patients had multiple pregnancies, from 5 to 12. This is quite unusual in Norway, the average number of pregnancies during the study period being between two and three. One patient developed MTN in her sixth pregnancy, two in their seventh pregnancy, one in her eighth pregnancy, one in her tenth pregnancy, three in their eleventh pregnancy and two in their twelfth pregnancy. The great majority, 53 cases, had a molar pregnancy before developing MTN. In 15 cases the preceding pregnancy resulted in a spontaneous abortion, and in 7 cases full time delivery.

HISTOLOGY

In seven patients we had only curettings which showed a molar pregnancy, but the course of the disease and especially the study of the HCG and pelvic arteriography confirmed that we were dealing with an invasive mole, in some of the cases with lung metastases. In 38 cases we had in curettings or in hysterectomy specimen a diagnosis of invasive mole and in 30 cases a histologic diagnosis of choriocarcinoma.

SYMPTOMS

The symptoms which made the patient consult a doctor were in 66 cases vaginal bleeding with or without pain. In 3 cases there were lung symptoms with dyspnoea or hemoptysis, and in 3 cases there were neurological symptoms indicating a brain tumor. One patient showed hematuria, and spread to the kidney was found by arteriography.

Altogether 21 patients had lung metastases

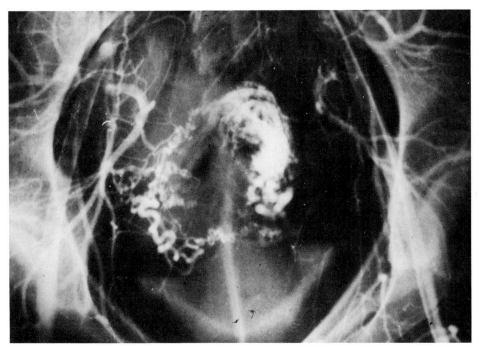

Fig. 46.3. Invasive mole presenting as large, vascular tumor in the left part of the fundus uteri. Note also dilatation and enlargement of uterine vessels.

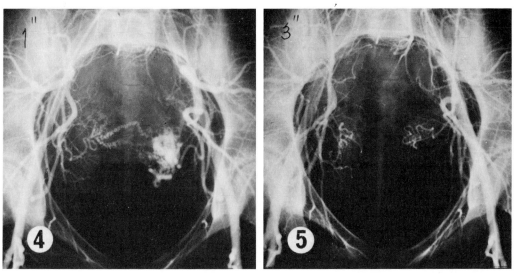

Fig. 46.4 and 46.5. (46.4) Invasive mole. Vascular tumor in left side of uterus. (46.5) Same patient after chemotherapy with methotrexate and actinomycin D. Normal uterine vessels can be seen on both sides.

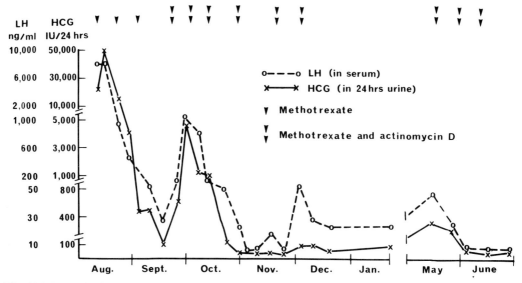

Fig. 46.6. Determination of LH level in serum and HCG values in urine in a case treated first with methotrexate alone, thereafter with methotrexate and actinomycin D. A recurrence was detected earlier by LH determinations than by measurement of HCG in urine.

when examined the first time in our hospital. In addition, nine patients had both lung metastases and metastases to the liver, brain, bone or other places (mediastinum, pericard and kidney). In five cases perforation of the tumor to the abdomen led to shock bleeding. In four of these, hysterectomy was performed immediately. In one case the tumor was resected. This last patient also had lung metastases, but was treated with methotrexate and actinomycin D with success. She has later been delivered of a child by caesarian section.

ARTERIOGRAPHY

In 58 patients pelvic arteriography was performed. In 14 cases this was negative except for an increased vascularity of the uterus, but in 44 cases a typical vascular tumor was found in the uterus.

SURGICAL TREATMENT

In 27 cases hysterectomy was performed. Seven of these were performed before referral to our hospital. In four cases the patient had perforation with bleeding leading to shock. In nine patients persistence of tumor in the uterus or recurrence

of the tumor was found. The hysterectomy was performed because the patient was more than 50 years of age in six cases. One patient demanded hysterectomy herself in spite of the fact that she could have been treated with chemotherapy alone.

CHEMOTHERAPY

At the beginning of the study period many of the patients were treated with methotrexate alone (16 cases). We soon found that it was better to give a combination of methotrexate and actinomycin D, and 58 patients were treated with this combination chemotherapy. In the later part of the study period high or moderate dose methotrexate with leucovorin rescue was given to eight cases. In the last 5–6 years of the study period methotrexate and actinomycin D were, in high-risk cases, combined with vincristine, cyclophosphamide and in one case also with adriamycin.

RESULTS

In our retrospective study we divided the cases into those which by the Charing Cross classification (7) might be considered as high- and medium-risk cases, 29 altogether, and low-risk cases,

46 altogether. None of the low-risk cases have died from their disease although 19 had lung metastases. Of the high- and medium-risk cases, 8 out of 29 died, which gives a mortality rate of 27.6% in this group.

It is remarkable that three of these 8 cases were postmenopausal with an interval between menopause and the detection of MTN of between two and four years. One of the postmenopausal patients was admitted because of hemoptysis. She had lung metastases and was given methotrexate, actinomycin D and vincristine. She tolerated the courses of chemotherapy poorly and there were long intervals between each course because she developed severe mucositis and severe exanthema. Another of the postmenopausal patients had extremely large lung metastases, and she developed lung insufficiency during the first two courses of methotrexate, actinomycin D and vincristine. At autopsy there were also massive metastases to the liver and the gastrointestinal tract. The third postmenopausal patient received only one course of methotrexate and actinomycin D before she died. She was four years postmenopausal and had multiple metastases to the lungs, pericardium and the pelvis. The other 5 high-risk cases all had massive metastases at several sites, and four of them died after only one course of chemotherapy.

When reviewing the material it was of interest to see if we cured more high-risk cases during the later years of the study, than in the earlier study period. Altogether 10 patients were classified as high-risk cases during the last five years from 1977 to 1981. Only one of these died of her disease. It must therefore be concluded that the more aggressive therapy with multiple drugs and high-dose methotrexate has influenced the survival rate remarkably. None of the four patients with liver metastases survived, while two of the four patients with brain metastases were cured. One of these had hemiparesis when she arrived at the hospital, extensive lung metastases, and large metastases to the parametrium. She was treated with high-dose methotrexate, vincristine, cyclophosphamide and adriamycin. She is living and well five years after treatment.

In the low-risk group of patients we have, over the years, used a very simple treatment with a combination of methotrexate 25 mg daily for 3–5 days at intervals of approximately 7–12 days and at the same time, actinomycin D 0.5 mg given in intravenous injection for 4 days. The two drugs have been given simultaneously. We have had few severe complications. The most irritating complication has been mucositis. In low-risk cases we have not used high dose methotrexate with leucovorin rescue. The number of courses has varied from 3 to 11 according to the determination of HCG. In three of the patients, after normal values for HCG in urine were obtained, local recurrence in the uterus occurred within a period of from 4 to 12 months. In all cases arteriography showed a new development of tumor in the uterine wall, in one case in the cervix, and hysterectomy was performed followed by 2–3 courses of methotrexate and actinomycin D. As mentioned previously, none of the 46 low-risk cases have died from their disease.

In accordance with the Charing Cross Group (7) we have found that in the high-risk group with massive metastases where intensive combination chemotherapy is started, one should always be careful in the dosage during the first few courses because of development of lung insufficiency and in the case of those with brain metastases the possibility of edema. In those with brain metastases we usually also give dexametasone.

DISCUSSION

The material here presented is small compared to that of other centers, and we have gained our experience over a long period of time. Through the years the monitoring of therapy has changed from HCG determination in the urine, to LH determination in serum (Fig. 46.6), and in later years to determination of the betasubunit of HCG in serum. Furthermore, at the beginning we believed that we could follow the treatment of intrauterine trophoblastic tumors by arteriography and in this way monitor therapy. In some cases, however, the radiographic findings persisted for a much longer time than the abnormal elevation of HCG. In three cases arteriovenous shunts developed, one of which was closed by operation. In another case, where there was still an arteriographic large vascular tumor in the uterus, hysterectomy was performed, but no viable tumor tissue could be found. We thus stopped the serial arteri-ographic examinations and depended rather upon the determination of betasubunit in serum. We have always given at least two courses of chemo-therapy after the values have become normal. We have not seen recurrences later than one year after completion of therapy. After normalization of the HCG values the patients have been set upon some sort of contraception, as a rule the pill, for at least two years. This form of contraception has not caused any problems with recurrent disease.

We have not used a strict prognostic scoring system, but have experienced that a number of factors seem to affect the risk of a tumor becom-ing drug resistant. These factors are:

1. The age of the patient, the patients above 40 years having a poorer prognosis.
2. The parity also seems to influence the prog-nosis. Multiple pregnancies, i.e. more than four, has a deleterious effect on survival.
3. The antecedent pregnancy also has an influ-ence. Molar pregnancies have a much better prognosis than if MTN develops after abortion or term pregnancy. This may, however, be due to the fact that after abortion and term preg-nancy the interval between the antecedent pregnancy and treatment is usually much longer. There is no doubt that a long interval between antecedent pregnancy and chemo-therapy makes it more difficult to treat the patient.
4. The HCG values at start of treatment are also an important factor. An HCG excretion rate greater than 100,000 i.u./day increases the fatality rate.
5. Finally, of course, the number of metastases, the site of metastases and the largest tumor mass is of great importance.

Taking into account all these factors, we have tried arbitrarily to classify the patients in a high-risk or a low-risk group. This is of cour-se a simplification of the prognostic scoring system recommended by Bagshawe (7). We have not used the drugs hydroxurea, 6-mercap-topurine or VP16 even in high-risk cases. We have used a combination of high/medium dose methotrexate, actinomycin D, vincristine and cyclophosphamide, and as mentioned pre-viously, in one patient with massive lung meta-stases and metastases to the brain, also adri-amycin to achieve a complete remission. It re-mains to be seen if cis-platinum should be added to the combination drug treatment in the very high-risk patients.

CONCLUSION

The regular follow-up of HCG values in serum or urine after evacuation of hydatidiform mole permits early recognition of the need for chemo-therapy. Today it seems as if MTN developing after molar pregnancy should always be cured by a simple chemotherapeutic regime as e.g. metho-trexate combined with actinomycin D. The major problem is presented by the high-risk group. Such cases usually develop after abortion or term preg-nancy. It would be advisable if one could always think about the possibility of malignant tropho-blastic disease after evacuation of an abortion or after full-term pregnancy when bleeding occurs. Determination of the betasubunit of HCG is now easily performed using a radioimmunoassay and is very reliable in determining whether the bleeding after abortion or delivery is caused by trophobla-stic neoplasia.

47
Follow-up and terminal care

FOLLOW-UP

In Chapter 3, "Registration", it was emphasized that a complete image of the cancer situation in a given population could not be achieved without there being some system of compulsory notification of all new cases and all deaths from cancer or other causes. Unfortunately there are few countries or even regions which have such a registration system, so data from many institutions are biased. Referals to hospitals may be dependent upon factors which give a too prestigious picture of the results obtained because advanced cases are refused. The economic situation of the patient is another factor which may influence admittance to hospital. On the other hand, some oncology departments admit every patient living within a geographically defined area, even if it is obvious from the information obtained before admittance that many will die within a relatively short time, regardless of the treatment given. But here it has to be remembered that palliative treatment is of great importance for the patient, her relatives and for the hospital staff.

As mentioned previously, as early as in the 1930s Heyman in Stockholm, Lacassagne in Paris and Voltz in Munich started to collect follow-up data on patients with cervical cancer. The sponsor of this very early and most important task was the League of Nations in Geneva. At the Berlin Congress in September 1985, the nineteenth *Annual Report on the Results of Treatment in Gynecological Cancer* was presented by the editorial staff at Radiumhemmet, Stockholm (1). The Chief Editor is now Dr. Folke Petterson. During the last three decades, the secretaries, Mrs. Hedda Holmberg and Mrs. Sunny Barnekow, have proved that it is possible to get follow-up information from institutions all over the world. The data presented in the nineteenth *Annual Report* show clearly that an international agreement on classification and staging and a close follow-up of all patients can bring us a step closer to the ultimate goal, namely the successful combating of gynecologic cancer.

It must be pointed out, however, that in many countries with a large, migrating population, or in developing countries where patients neglect the advice of doctors to return for regular examination, the data may be misleading. Even in a developed country like the United States, many clinicians are happy if at least 60–70% of their patients show up on scheduled examination days. In Europe, the United States and Australia, about 40–60% of patients in the very early stages of malignant disease, for example cervical intraepithelial neoplasia or microinvasive carcinoma, may drop out from follow-up after 3–6 years.

I still have difficulty when discussing the statistical background of the results of different modalities of treatment of premalignant and malignant disease. Such data cannot be accurately assessed unless we know the exact fate of *all patients – information about recurrences, new malignant disease, deaths from cancer or from other causes.* A statement I often hear from prominent gynecologic oncologists is: "my colleagues within the area our hospital covers will be more than happy to report to us all our mishappenings". This is of course not true. And statistics is not as simple as that.

Another factor of importance is that, unfortunately, pathologists differ in their interpretation of the microscopic picture of the tumor. Furthermore, clinicians may differ widely in their clinical staging. *A systematic up-staging of the disease would give better results stage by stage.* The Cancer Committee of FIGO recommends that: *when it is doubtful to which stage a particular case should be allotted, reference must be made to the earlier stage.*

FOLLOW-UP ROUTINES

The problem of which follow-up routines should be mandatory for the different malignant diseases has never been thoroughly discussed. This is not difficult to understand. Facilities and opinions about the importance of the various types of examination differ very much from country to country and from clinic to clinic within the same region. An ideal situation where all patients attended at regular intervals and underwent the same follow-up examinations can never be reached. This should be kept in mind when comparing the results of treatment; for example those found in the *Annual Report*.

It is probably not necessary to stress that the patient's own story about her complaints should be taken very seriously indeed. Furthermore, a thorough clinical and gynecological examination should always be performed.

In addition, there are certain tumor types which require special examinations—benign and malignant trophoblastic disease for example, where we have a tumor marker which is so sensitive that even microscopic recurrences can be detected. In these patients the β-subunit of HCG in serum should be determined on every scheduled follow-up visit. When malignant trophoblastic disease has been treated, a chest X-ray may also be of value, although HCG determinations are extremely reliable.

In patients treated by surgery for preinvasive or an early stage of invasive cervical carcinoma, a cytologic smear should be taken at the follow-up visits. Gynecologic oncologists with training in colposcopy would also perform this type of examination in such cases. It takes only a few minutes, and should not increase the fee of the doctor as substantially as unfortunately is the case in many countries.

There is great uncertainty as to the value of obligatory cytologic smears in patients treated with radiotherapy in the later stages of cervical cancer. Recurrences after modern expert radiotherapy seldom occur centrally, which is a prerequisite for exenterative procedures. Usually the recurrences are found on the pelvic wall, in the periaortic nodes, or in some cases they are present as distant metastases. Recurrences of advanced cervical cancer within the field of irradiation can seldom be cured, but it may be necessary to perform an exploratory laparotomy to find out whether a pelvic recurrence is central or lateral. In the former case, there is a chance of cure by anterior, posterior or total exenteration.

In the later stages of cervical cancer, even if there are no symptoms or signs of recurrence, it seems reasonable to perform simple X-ray examinations such as urography, X-ray of the lungs and the skeleton during at least the first three years of follow-up. More sophisticated examinations such as ultrasound, CAT-scan or NMR should be performed on indication (cost-benefit!).

Since we have found that CEA is released in a high percentage of metastatic adenocarcinomas of the cervix, we recommend such determinations for all these patients within 2–3 years of treatment. In the majority of squamous cell carcinoma of the cervix, CEA determination on a serial basis is a waste of time and money. However, if the CEA value before treatment is abnormally high, and this value drops to normal or near normal after therapy, it may be of interest to measure CEA at 3–6 months' intervals for about 2–3 years. The problem is, however, that even when we realize a rise in the CEA value indicates a recurrence, it is extremely difficult to know where to search for this often hidden metastatic site. We have for example experienced how a patient with elevated CEA underwent a series of X-ray examinations, scintigraphy, liver scan and liver function tests. She was then re-laparotomized without anything abnormal being detected. A few months later she returned with massive liver metastases. Perhaps in the future nuclear magnetic resonance (NMR) will be of some help in such difficult cases, although I doubt that today any form of chemotherapy would have saved this particular woman's life. NMR is still too expensive, and examination time of a single patient too long for it to be used routinely.

Most cases of corpus carcinoma of the uterus will be treated by surgery or a combination of surgery and radiation. When scheduling a patient with Stages I or II endometrial carcinoma for follow-up, account should be taken of the fact that a certain percentage of these patients, supposedly successfully treated, may show up with lung metastases. The percentage of such cases is small, but nevertheless a chest X-ray should be taken on each visit during the first 2–3 years of follow-up.

In recent years the search for ovarian tumor markers has been intensive. CEA has been found of some value in mucinous carcinomas. Lately determination of serum CA125 has been in focus. The level of CA125 is claimed to reflect both progression and regression of ovarian carcinoma, especially of the serous type. Possibly we are close to a real breakthrough in this field.

PSYCHOSOCIAL PROBLEMS

A patient who has gone through all the phases of physical and psychological problems which always follow in the wake of cancer, needs a lot of understanding and help not just from her doctor, nurses, and social workers, but above all from her family and friends. For many people the word "cancer" still means inevitable death.

Fortunately, more and more experts and lay people have become aware of the difficulties that face the patient even when the chances of permanent cure are high. Radical surgery, radiotherapy and chemotherapy influence the physical strength of the body, but perhaps still more the psychosocial situation. For women treated for gynecologic cancer, an unnecessary problem is often caused because neither she nor her partner are given any information about future sexual life. Many people still believe that cancer is a contagious disease. The doctor and other hospital personnel, especially the nurses, must from the very beginning inform the patient of the nature of her disease, which examinations have to be performed, the type of treatment necessary, possible complications that may arise, and also the difficulties she may have to face after coming home from hospital.

During the follow-up period, the patient should be helped to build up both her physical an psychical strength. Questions about adequate nutrition may arise, especially after radiotherapy and chemotherapy. Recommendations concerning diet and physical exercise should be given.

TERMINAL CARE

When I started my career in gynecologic oncology, it was common for a recurrence—especially one which could not be cured by further therapy—to be refused admittance. Fortunately this situation has changed radically in the last two decades. Palliative treatment of the dying patient is now very much in the focus of modern medicine.

Compared with malignant tumors at many other sites, the results of treatment in gynecologic cancer must be characterized as good. Nevertheless, about 30% of patients with either cervix or endometrial carcinoma, all stages taken into account, still return with an incurable recurrence. For ovarian cancer, this figure is even higher, approximately 60%.

There are many philosophies about how the terminally-ill patient should be cared for. It is fashionable today to talk about the so-called "hospice system" or the "team approach", in which the gynecologic oncologist, specially trained nurses, social workers, the family physician and the patient's family all cooperate to make her as comfortable as possible during the last days of her life. The hospice system also allows for the patient to be admitted to special clinics designed for terminally-ill cases. Unfortunately, the hospice system is impractical in most places, particularly in developing countries. Nevertheless, the philosophy of the system is important, and it should be pointed out that the gynecologic oncologist is always a central person in the care of the terminally-ill woman.

Terminal care aims to ease the physical discomfort of the patient, and to help her with any psychological problems. And she should preferably be treated in her home or in a nearby clinic so that it is possible for her family and friends to see her often.

It is our philosophy that at the time of primary treatment, almost all patients should be given some hope of cure. But when a recurrence occurs, and it becomes evident that the disease has entered a phase that is threatening to life, then the patient has the right to know the truth. It is remarkable how tremendously strong women can be when they are facing death. I cannot help admiring them, although it should not be forgotten that the majority of terminally-ill patients need our help to go through the different phases of the understanding that all of us eventually have to face death.

Articles and books by Kübler-Ross (2, 3) and a chapter in McGowan's book on gynecologic oncology (4) do much in this respect.

Unfortunately, women with incurable genital cancer frequently suffer tremendous pain. *Relief of pain* is therefore a most important aspect of the treatment. Neither additional radiotherapy, chemotherapy with single or multiple drugs, nor neurosurgery can act as a substitute for *morphine*. The fear of making a dying cancer patient dependent on morphine should never be considered. It should also be stressed that to keep a patient free from pain, it is necessary to administer the pain-relieving drugs some time *before* the pain returns, and not after it. Morphine can be given orally, either alone or in mixtures with other drugs; It can be used in subcutaneous intermittent injections, and in epidural injections. There are so many practical considerations when deciding upon the type of pain relief that it is impossible to give exact advice. There is no doubt that spinal blockade with for example phenol, or neurosurgical methods can give a relatively long-lasting pain-free period.

The patient will often be given some medication, usually cytostatics, that hopefully may reduce the size of the tumor. In most situations, however, chemotherapy cannot prolong life by more than a few months. When it is obvious that the drugs are no longer effective, it is my sincere belief that one of most important duties of the gynecologic oncologist is to stop treatment. Reports on cooperative trials with new drugs are numerous. As mentioned previously, the effect of a new regime is usually measured by the response rate—complete response (CP) and partial response (PR). More and more clinicians, however, have become aware of the fact that even though some multiple drug regimes may prolong life for a few months, the concept of quality of life must be taken into consideration. Clinical trials are necessary, but many of the trials set up today for terminally-ill patients are doomed to failure. Let us die with dignity, not as "clinical trial subjects".

Bibliography

References to ch. 1

1. Asvall JE, Eker R. Cancer control in Norway. Oslo: Oslo University Press, 1974.

References to ch. 2

1. Series of League of Nations Publications. III. Health. 1929. III. 5. Publications Department. Geneva: League of Nations, 1929.
2. Heyman J, ed. Annual report on the results of radiotherapy in cancer of the uterine cervix. Geneva: League of Nations Health Organization, 1937:1.
3. Heyman J. Atlas. Stockholm: PA Norstedt and Sons, 1980.
4. UICC. TNM classification of malignant tumors. 3rd ed. Geneva, Switzerland.
5. Manual for staging of cancer. Chicago, Illinois: American Joint Committee, 1977.
6. Kottmeier H-L, Kolstad P, McGarrity K, Pettersson F, Ulfelder H, eds. Annual report on the results of treatment in gynecological cancer. Stockholm: Radiumhemmet, 1982:18.

References to ch. 3

1. Pedersen E, Magnus K. Cancer registration in Norway. The incidence of cancer in Norway 1953–58. Oslo: The Norwegian Cancer Society, 1959.
2. Incidence of cancer in Norway 1972–76, 1977, 1978, 1979, 1980. Oslo: The Norwegian Cancer Society, 1981.
3. Trends in cancer incidence in Norway 1955–1967. Oslo: Universitetsforlaget, 1972.
4. The Cancer Registry of Norway. Survival of cancer patients. Cases diagnosed in Norway 1968–75. The Norwegian Cancer Society, 1980.

References to ch. 4

1. International society for the study of vulvar disease. New nomenclature for vulvar disease. Obstet Gynecol 1976;47:122.
2. Jeffcoate TNA, Woodcock AS. Premalignant conditions of the vulva with particular reference to chronic epithelial dystrophies. Br Med J 1961;2:127.
3. Friedrich EG, Jr. Vulvar disease. Philadelphia, London, Toronto: WB Saunders Company, 1976.
4. Stening M. Cancer and related lesions of the vulva. Sydney: ADIS Press, 1980.
5. Way S. Malignant disease of the vulva. Edinburgh: Churchill Livingstone, 1982.

References to ch. 5

1. Friedrich EG, Jr. Intraepithelial neoplasia of the vulva. In: Coppleson ME, ed. Gynecologic oncology. London: Churchill Livingstone, 1981.
2. Hay DM, Cole FM. Postgranulomatous epidermoid carcinoma of the vulva. Am J Obstet Gynecol 1970;129:525.
3. Stening M. Cancer and related lesions of the vulva. Sydney: ADIS Press, 1980.

References to ch. 6

1. Paget J. On disease of the mammary areola preceding cancer of the mammary gland. St. Bartholomew's Hospital Reports 1874;10:87.
2. Dubreuilh W. Paget's disease of the vulva. Br J Dermatol 1901;13:403.
3. Helwig EB, Graham JH. Ano-genital (extramammary) Paget's disease. A clinico-pathological study. Cancer 1963;16:387.
4. Taylor PT, Stenwig JT, Klausen H. Paget's disease of the vulva. A report of 18 cases. Gynecol Oncol 1975;3:46.
5. Friedrich EG, Jr. Intraepithelial neoplasia of the vulva. In: Coppleson ME, ed. Gynecologic oncology. London: Churchill Livingstone, 1981.
6. Julian CG, Callison J, Woodruff JD. Plastic management of extensive vulvar defects. Obstet Gynecol 1971;38:193.

References to ch. 7

1. Richart RM. Natural history of cervical intraepithelial neoplasia. Clin Obstet Gynecol 1967;10:748.
2. Woodruff JD, Julian C, Puray T, Mermut S, Katayama P. The contemporary challenge of carcinoma in situ of the vulva. Am J Obstet Gynecol 1973;115:677.
3. Bernstein SG, Kovacs BB, Townsend DE, Morrow P. Vulvar carcinoma in situ. Obstet Gynecol 1983;61:304.
4. Iversen T, Abeler V, Kolstad P. Squamous cell carcinoma in situ of the vulva. A clinical and histopathological study. Gynecol Oncol 1981;11:224.
5. Hensen D, Tarone R. An epidemiologic study of cancer of the cervix, vagina and vulva based on third national cancer survey in the United States. Am J Obstet Gynecol 1977;129:525.
6. Friedrich EG, Jr. Intraepithelial neoplasia of vulva. In: Coppleson ME, ed. Gynecologic oncology. London: Churchill Livingstone, 1981.

References to ch. 8

1. Annual report on the results of treatment in gynecological cancer. Stockholm: Radiumhemmet, 1982:18.
2. Stening M. Cancer and related lesions of the vulva. Sydney: ADIS Press, 1980.
3. Way S. Malignant disease of the vulva. London: Churchill Livingstone, 1982.
4. Iversen T, Aalders JG, Christensen A, Kolstad P. Squamous cell carcinoma of the vulva: A review of 424 patients, 1956–74. Gynecol Oncol 1980;9:271.
5. Way S. Carcinoma of vulva. Am J Obstet Gynecol 1960;79:692.
6. Iversen T, Aas M. The lymph drainage from vulva. Gynecol Oncol 1983;16:179.
7. Iversen T. Squamous cell carcinoma of the vulva with special reference to the lymph drainage. Trondheim: Tapir, 1982.
8. Krupp PJ, Lee FYL, Bohm JW, Batson HWK, Diem JE, Lamire JE. Prognostic parameters and clinical staging criteria in epidermoid carcinoma of the vulva. Obstet Gynecol 1975;46:84.
9. Friedrich EG, Jr, di Paola GR. Postoperative staging of vulvar carcinoma: A retrospective study. Int J Gynecol Obstet 1977;15:270.
10. Iversen T. The value of groin palpation in epidermoid carcinoma of the vulva. Gynecol Oncol 1981;12:291.
11. Iversen T. Irradiation and bleomycin in the treatment of inoperable vulval carcinoma. Acta Obstet Gynecol Scand 1982;61:195.
12. Fuchs WA. Diagnosis of cancer metastases in lymph nodes. In: Fuchs WA, Davidson JW, Fischer HW, eds. Lymphography in cancer. Berlin: Springer Verlag, 1969.
13. Hagen S, Björn-Hansen R. Lymphography in the treatment of carcinoma of the vulva. Acta Radiol Stockholm: 1971;11:609.
14. Kinmonth JB, Taylor GW, Harper PK. Lymphangiography. A technique for its clinical use in the lower limb. Br Med J 1955;1:940.
15. Way S. The anatomy of the lymphatic drainage of the vulva and its influence on the radical operation for carcinoma. Ann R Coll Surg Engl 1948;3:187.
16. Wharton JT, Gallager S, Rutledge FN. Microinvasive carcinoma of the vulva. Am J Obstet Gynecol 1974;118:159.
17. Iversen T, Abeler V, Aalders JG. Individualized treatment of Stage I carcinoma of the vulva. Obstet Gynecol 1981;57:85.
18. Basset A. L'epithelioma primitif du clitoris. Paris: G. Steinheil, 1912:180.
19. Taussig FJ. Cancer of vulva: analysis of 155 cases 1911–40. Am J Obstet Gynecol 1940;40:764.
20. Morley GW. Infiltrative carcinoma of the vulva: Results of surgical treatment. Am J Obstet Gynecol 1976;124:874.
21. Morris J, McLean. A formula for selective lymphadenectomy. Obstet Gynecol 1977;50:152.
22. Frischbier HJ, Thomsen K. Treatment of cancer of the vulva with high energy electrons. Am J Obstet Gynecol 1971;111:431.
23. Frankendal B, Larsson L-G, Westling P. Carcinoma of the vulva. Results of an individualized treatment schedule. Acta Radiol Ther 1973;12:165.
24. Dahle T. Carcinoma of the vulva and subsequent successful pregnancy. Acta Obstet Gynecol Scand 1959;38:448.

References to ch. 9

1. Abeler V, Iversen T. Malignant melanoma of the vulva, in press.
2. Clark WH, Jr. A classification of malignant melanoma in man correlated with histogenesis and biologic behaviour. In: Montagua W, Hu F, eds. Advances in biology of the skin, the pigmentary system. London: Pergamon Press Ltd, 1967.
3. Breslow A. Thickness, cross-sectional areas and depth of invasion in the prognosis of cutaneous melanoma. Ann Surg 1970;172:902.
4. Morrow CP, DiSaia PJ. Malignant melanoma of the female genitalia: A clinical analysis. Obstet Gynecol Surv 1976;31:233.
5. Veronesi V, Adamus J, Bandiera DC, et al. Inefficiency of immediate node dissection in stage I melanoma of the limbs. N Engl J Med 1977;297:627.

References to ch. 10

1. Brown GR, Fletcher GH, Rutledge FN. Irradiation of in situ and invasive squamous cell carcinomas of the vagina. Cancer 1971;28:1278.
2. Hummer WK, Mussey E, Decker D, Dockerty MB. Carcinoma in situ of the vagina. Am J Obstet Gynecol 1970;10:1109.
3. Furmel JD, Merril JA. Recurrence after treatment of carcinoma in situ of the cervix. Surg Gynecol Obstet 1963;117:15.
4. Townsend DE. Intraepithelial neoplasia of vagina. In: Coppleson M, ed. Gynecologic oncology. London: Churchill Livingstone, 1981.
5. Herbst AL, Ulfelder H, Poskanzer DC. Adenocarcinoma of the vagina. Association of maternal stilbestrol therapy with appearance in young women. N Engl J Med 1971;284:878.
6. Herbst AL, Robboy SJ, Scully RE, Poskanzer DE. Clear cell adenocarcinoma in the vagina and cervix in girls: Analysis of 170 registry cases. Am J Obstet Gynecol 1974;119:713.

References to ch. 11

1. Cruveilhier: Cited by Brack CB, Merritt RI, Dickson RJ. Primary carcinoma of the vagina. Obstet Gynecol 1958;12:104.
2. Messelt OT. Primary carcinoma of the vagina. Surg Gynecol Obstet 1952;95:1.
3. Houghton CRS, Iversen T. Squamous cell carcinoma of the vagina: A clinical study of the location of the tumor. Gynecol Oncol 1982;13:365.
4. Plentl AA, Friedman EA. Lymphatic system of the female genitalia. Philadelphia: WB Saunders, 1971.
5. Herbst AL, Green TH, Ulfelder H. Primary carcinoma of the vagina. An analysis of 68 cases. Am J Obstet Gynecol 1970;106:210.
6. Prenpree T, Viravanthana T, Hanson GS, Wirenberg MJ, Cuccia CA. Radiation management of primary carcinoma of the vagina. Cancer 1977;40:109.

References to ch. 12

1. Rigoni-Stern D. Fatti Statistici Relativi alle Maltie Cancerose. Giorn Servire Progr Pathol Terap 1842;2:507.
2. Gagnon F. Contribution to the study of the etiology and prevention of cancer of the cervix of the uterus. Am J Obstet Gynecol 1950;60:516.
3. Towne JE. Carcinoma of the cervix in nulliparous and celibate women. Am J Obstet Gynecol 1955;69:606.
4. Rotkin ID. A comparison review of key epidemiological studies in cervical cancer related to current searches for transmissible agents. Cancer Res 1973;33:1353.
5. Coppleson M, Reid BL. Aetiology of squamous carcinoma of the cervix. Obstet Gynecol 1968;32:432.
6. Coppleson M, Pixley E, Reid B. Colposcopy. A scientific and practical approach to the cervix in health and disease. Springfield, Illinois: Charles C Thomas, 1971.
7. Johannisson E, Kolstad P, Söderberg G. Cytologic, vascular, and histologic patterns of dysplasia, carcinoma in situ and early invasive carcinoma of the cervix. Acta Radiol (Suppl 258) 1966.
8. Rapp F, Jenkins FJ. Genital cancer and viruses. Gynecol Oncol 1981;12:525.
9. Rawls WE, Inamoto K, Adam E, Melnick JL, Green GH. Herpesvirus type 2 antibodies and carcinoma of the cervix. Lancet 1970;2:1142.
10. Syrjänen KJ. Female genital infections by human papilloma virus and their association with intraepithelial neoplasia and squamous cell carcinoma. The Cervix and the Lower Genital Tract 1984;2:103.
11. Magnus K, ed. Trends in cancer incidence. Washington, New York, London: Hemisphere Publishing Corporation, 1982.
12. The Cancer Registry of Norway. Geographical variations in cancer incidence in Norway 1966–75. The Norwegian Cancer Society, 1978.
13. Dahle T. Transtubal spread of tumor cells in carcinoma of the body of the uterus. Surg Gynecol Obstet 1956;103:332.
14. Messelt OT. Radiation changes in carcinoma of the cervix as revealed by cytology and their role in determining prognosis. Acta Un Int Cancer 1958;14:367.
15. Franzén S, Giertz G, Zajicek J. Cytological diagnosis of prostatic tumors by transrectal aspiration biopsy: a preliminary report. Br J Urol 1960;32:192.
16. Kjellgren O, Ångström T, Bergman F, Wiklund D-E. Fine-needle aspiration biopsy in diagnosis and classification of ovarian carcinoma. Cancer 1971;28:967.
17. Sanner T, Bergsjø P, Koller O, Kolstad P, Pihl A. Technical modification of the 6-phosphoglucomate dehydrogenase test of the vaginal fluid. Am J Obstet Gynecol 1967;98:800.
18. Sanner T, Bentzen H, Kolstad P, Nordbye K, Pihl A. The alleged usefulness of 6-phosphogluconate dehydrogenase determinations in screening for uterine cancer. Acta Obstet Gynecol Scand 1970;49:371.
19. Koller O. The vascular patterns of the uterine cervix. Oslo: Universitetsforlaget, 1963.
20. Kolstad P. Vascularization, oxygen tension and radiocurability in cancer of the cervix. Oslo: Universitetsforlaget, 1964.
21. Bergsjø P. Radiation-induced early changes in size and vascularity of cervical carcinoma. Acta Radiol (Suppl 274) 1968.
22. Kolstad P, Stafl A. Atlas of colposcopy. 3rd ed. Oslo: Universitetsforlaget, Baltimore: University Park Press, London: Churchill Livingstone, 1982.

References to ch. 13

1. Williams J. Cancer of the uterus. In: Harveian Lectures for 1886. London: Lewis, 1888.
2. Rubin IC. The pathological diagnosis of incipient carcinoma of the uterus. Am J Obstet Dis Women Child 1910;62:668.
3. Reagan JW, Hamonic MJ. The cellular pathology in carcinoma in situ: A cytohistopathological correlation. Cancer 1956;9:385.
4. Wied G, ed. Proceedings of the first international congress of exfoliative cytology, Vienna 1961. Philadelphia: Lippincott, 1962.
5. Richart RM. Natural history of cervical intraepithelial neoplasia. Clin Obstet Gynecol 1967;10:748.
6. Kolstad P. Carcinoma of the cervix stage O. Am J Obstet Gynecol 1966;96:1098.
7. Kolstad P. Diagnosis and management of precancerous lesions of the cervix uteri. Int J Gynecol Obstet 1970;8:551.
8. Kolstad P. Vascular changes in cervical intraepithelial neoplasia and invasive cervical carcinoma. Clin Obstet Gynecol 1983;26:938.
9. Hollyock VE, Chanen W. Electrocoagulation diathermy for the treatment of cervical dysplasia and carcinoma in situ. Obstet Gynecol 1976;47:196.
10. Chanen W. Radical electrocoagulation diathermy. In: Coppleson M, ed. Gynecologic oncology. London: Churchill Livingstone, 1981.
11. Crisp WE, Asadourian L, Romberger W. Application of cryosurgery to gynecologic malignancy. Obstet Gynecol 1967;30:668.
12. Richart RM, Townsend DE, Crisp W, et al. An analysis of "long-term" follow-up results in patients with cervical intraepithelial neoplasia treated by cryotherapy. Am J Obstet Gynecol 1980;137:823.
13. Duncan J. The Semm cold cogulator in the management of cervical intraepithelial neoplasia. Clin Obstet Gynecol 1983;26:996.
14. Dorsey JH, Diggs ES. Microsurgical conization of the cervix by carbon dioxide laser. Obstet Gynecol 1979;54:565.
15. Larsson G. Follow-up after laser conization. Am Chir Gynecol 1983.
16. Kolstad P, Klem V. Long-term follow-up of 1121 cases of carcinoma in situ. Obstet Gynecol 1976;48:125.
17. Bergsjø P, Evans J. Radiation sensitivity of intraepithelial carcinoma of the cervix. Am J Obstet Gynecol 1971;109:879.

References to ch. 14

1. Mestwerdt G. Die Früdiagnose des Kollum-Karzinoms. Zentralbl Gynäk 1947;69:198.
2. Mestwerdt G. Elektive Therapie des Mikrokarzinoms am Collum Uteri? Zentralbl Gynäk 1951;73:558.

3. Jordan J, Sharp F, Singer A, eds. Pre-clinical neoplasia of the cervix. London: Royal College of Obstetricians and Gynaecologists, 1982.
4. Kolstad P. Carcinoma of the cervix stage Ia. Am J Obstet Gynecol 1969;104:1015.
5. Iversen T, Abeler V, Kjørstad KE. Factors influencing the treatment of patients with Stage Ia carcinoma of the cervix. Br J Obstet Gynaecol 1979;86:593.
6. Kolstad P, Abeler V, Iversen T, Kjørstad KE. Microinvasive carcinoma of the cervix. Definition and treatment problems. Clin Oncol 1982;1:335.
7. Kolstad P, Iversen T. Microinvasive (Stage Ia) carcinoma of the cervix. Follow-up study of 561 cases. In press.
8. Coppleson M. Preclinical invasive carcinoma of cervix: clinical features and management. In: Coppleson M, ed. Gynecologic oncology. Edinburgh: Churchill Livingstone, 1981.
9. Burghardt E, Holzer E. Diagnosis and treatment of microinvasive carcinoma of the cervix uteri. Obstet Gynecol 1977;49:641.
10. Lohe KJ, Burghardt E, Hillemanns HG, Kaufmann C, Ober KG, Zander J. Early squamous cell carcinoma of the uterine cervix. Gynecol Oncol 1978;6:31.

References to ch. 15

1. Gray LH. Radiobiologic basis of oxygen as modifying factor in radiation therapy. Am J Roentgen 1961;85:803.
2. Koller O. The vascular patterns of the uterine cervix. Oslo: Universitetsforlaget, 1963.
3. Kolstad P. Vascularization, oxygen tension, and radiocurability in cancer of the cervix. Oslo: Universitetsforlaget, 1964.
4. Evans JC, Bergsjø P. The influence of anemia on the results of radiotherapy in carcinoma of the cervix. Radiology 1965;84:709.
5. Bergsjø P, Christensen OJ, Kolstad P. Oxygen tension in cancer of the cervix following administration of vasodilator drugs during oxygen inhalation. Cancer 1967;20:1625.
6. Bergsjø P, Evans JC. Tissue oxygen tension of cervix cancer. Comparison of effects of breathing a carbon dioxide mixture and pure oxygen. Acta Radiol Ther 1968;7:1.
7. Bergsjø P. Radiation-induced early changes in size and vascularity of cervical carcinoma. Acta Radiol (Suppl 274) Stockholm 1968.
8. Kolstad P. Intercapillary distance, oxygen tension and local recurrence in cervix cancer. Scand J Clin Lab Invest (Suppl 106) 1968;22:145.
9. Bergsjø P, Evans JC. Oxygen tension of cervical carcinoma during the early phase of external irradiation. Measurements with a Clark micro electrode. Scand J Clin Lab Invest (Suppl 106) 1968;22:159.
10. Bergsjø P, Kolstad P. Clinical trial with atmospheric oxygen breathing during radiotherapy of cancer of the cervix. Scand J Clin Lab Invest (Suppl 106) 1968;22:167.
11. Hyperbaric oxygen and radiotherapy: A medical research council trial in carcinoma of the cervix. Br J Radiol 1978;51:879.
12. Cater DB, Silver IA. Quantitative measurements of oxygen tension in normal tissues and in the tumors of patients before and after radiotherapy. Acta Radiol 1960;53:233.

References to ch. 16

1. Bergsjø P, Kolstad P. Pain as a prognostic symptom in cancer of the cervix. Acta Obstet Gynecol Scand (Suppl 6) 1964;42:32.
2. Kolstad P. The relation between stage, pain, roentgenological and operative findings in cancer of the cervix. Acta Obstet Gynecol Scand (Suppl 6) 1964;42:35.
3. Kjørstad KE, Børmer O, Martimbeau P. Isotope nephrography in carcinoma of the uterine cervix Stage Ib. Acta Radiol (Ther) 1977;16:219.
4. Rüttimann A. Progress in lymphology. Stuttgart: Georg Thieme Verlag, 1967.
5. Kolbenstvedt A, Knudsen OS. A method for lymphographic and histologic correlation. Experience from 300 patients treated by pelvic lymphadenectomy. Gynecol Oncol 1974;2:9.
6. Kolbenstvedt A. A critical evaluation of foot lymphography in the demonstration of the regional lymph nodes of the uterine cervix. Gynecol Oncol 1974;2:24.
7. Kolbenstvedt A, Kolstad P. Pelvic lymph node dissection under peroperative lymphographic control. Gynecol Oncol 1974;2:39.
8. Kolbenstvedt A. Normal lymphographic variations of lumbar iliac and inguinal lymph vessels. Acta Radiol 1974;15:662.
9. Kolbenstvedt A. Projection difference index in diagnosis of lymph node metastases. Acta Radiol 1975;16:200.
10. Kolbenstvedt A. Lymphography in the diagnosis of metastases from carcinoma of the uterine cervix stages I and II. Acta Radiol 1975;16:81.
11. Wiljasalo M. Lymphographic differential diagnosis of neoplastic diseases. Acta Radiol (Suppl 247) 1965.
12. zum Winkel K, Müller H. Technik, Auswertung und röntgenologische Kontrolle der abdominalen Isotopenlymphographie. Der Radiologe 1965;5:381.
13. Gitsch E, Philipp K. Fortschritte in der Radioisotopenchirugie des Zervixkarzinoms. Zentralbl Gynaekol 1981;103:807.
14. Iversen T, Aas M. Pelvic lymphoscintigraphy with 99 m Tc-colloid in lymph node metastases. Eur J Nucl Med 1982;7:455.

References to ch. 17

1. Abbé R. The use of radium in malignant disease. Lancet 1913:524.
2. Bergsjø P, Kristiansen P. Treatment method and dose distribution in radiotherapy of carcinoma of the cervix. Acta Radiol (Ther) 1968;7:181.
3. Pettersson F, Kolstad P, Ludwig H, Ulfelder H, eds.

Annual report on the results of treatment in gynecological cancer. Stockholm: Radiumhemmet, 1985:19.
4. Annual report on the results of radiotherapy in cancer of the uterine cervix. Stockholm: PA Norstedt, 1941:4.
5. Bergsjø P, Evans JC. Late radiation reactions in cancer of the cervix. Acta Obstet Gynecol Scand (Suppl 7) 1965;43:90.
6. Kottmeier H-L, Gray MJ. Rectal and bladder injuries following radiation treatment of carcinoma of the cervix. Am J Obstet Gynecol 1961;82:74.

References to ch. 18

1. Meigs JV. Surgical treatment for cancer of the cervix. New York: Grune and Stratton, 1954.
2. Annual report on the results of radiotherapy in cancer of the uterine cervix. Stockholm: PA Norstedt, 1941:4.
3. Annual report on the results of treatment in gynecological cancer. Stockholm: Radiumhemmet, 1982:18.
4. Schjøtt-Rivers E. Can the results of irradiation in cancer of the uterine cervix be improved by prophylactic hysterectomy? Acta Obstet Gynecol Scand 31 (Suppl 7).
5. Schlink H. Cancer of the female pelvis. J Obstet Gynaecol Br Emp 1960;67:402.
6. Stallworthy J. Radical surgery following radiation treatment for cervical carcinoma. Ann R Coll Surg Engl 1964;34:161.
7. Dahle T. Combined radiological-surgical treatment of carcinoma of the cervix. Surg Gynecol Obstet 1959;109:1.
8. Koller O. Clinical trials on the treatment of cervical carcinoma Stage I. National Cancer Institute Monographs, 1964;15:95.
9. Kolstad P. Lymph node metastases in cancer of the cervix Stage Ib. Austr NZ J Obstet Gynaecol 1968;8:107.
10. Rampone JF, Klem V, Kolstad P. Combined treatment of Stage Ib carcinoma of the cervix. Obstet Gynecol 1973;41:163.
11. Kjørstad K, Martimbeau PW, Iversen T. Stage Ib carcinoma of the cervix. The Norwegian Radium Hospital; Results and complications. Urinary and gastrointestinal complications. Gynecol Oncol 1983;15:42.
12. Martimbeau PW, Kjørstad K, Kolstad P. Stage Ib carcinoma of the cervix. The Norwegian Radium Hospital 1968–70: Results of treatment and major complications. I. Lymphedema. Am J Obstet Gynecol 1978;131:389.
13. Clark JG. A more radical method of performing hysterectomy for cancer of the uterus. Bull Johns Hopkins Hosp 1895;6:120.
14. Wertheim E. Zur Frage der Radikaloperation beim Uteruskrebs. Arch Gynaek 1900;65:1.
15. Okabayashi H. Radical abdominal hysterectomy for cancer of the cervix uteri. Surg Gynec Obst 1921;33:335.
16. Gusberg SB. Operative treatment of carcinoma of the cervix. In: Gusberg SB, Frick HC eds Corscadens gynecologic cancer. Baltimore: Williams & Wilkins Co, 1970;246–261.

References to ch. 19

1. Martzloff KH. Relative malignancy of cancer of the cervix uteri as indicated by the predominant cancer cell type. Bull Johns Hopkins Hosp 1923;34:141,184.
2. Broders AC. Carcinoma grading and practical applications. Arch Pathol 1926;2:376.
3. Wentz WB, Reagan JW. Survival in cervical carcinoma with respect to cell type. Cancer 1959;12:384.
4. Beecham JB, Halvorsen T, Kolbenstvedt A. Histologic classification, lymph node metastases, and patient survival in Stage Ib cervical carcinoma. An analysis of 245 uniformly treated cases. Gynecol Oncol 1978;6:95.
5. Riotton G, Christopherson WM, eds. International histological classification of tumors. Geneva: WHO, 1973.
6. Baltzer J, Lohe KJ, Köpcke W, Zander J. Histological criteria for the prognosis in patients with operated squamous cell carcinoma of the cervix. Gynecol Oncol 1982;13:184.
7. Stendahl W. A histopathological malignancy grading system for indication of prognosis in invasive squamous cell carcinoma of the uterine cervix. Acta Universitatis Uppsaliensis. Doctoral thesis. Uppsala University, 1981.

References to ch. 20

1. Andras EJ, Fletcher GH, Rutledge F. Radiotherapy of carcinoma of the cervix following simple hysterectomy. Am J Obstet Gynecol 1973;115:647.
2. Davy M, Bentzen H, Jahren R. Simple hysterectomy in the presence of invasive cervical cancer. Acta Obstet Gynecol Scand 1977;56:105.

References to ch. 21

1. Kjørstad K. Early stage cervical cancer. Diagnosis and treatment of high risk patients with particular reference to the use of carcinoembryonic antigen. Thesis. The Norwegian Radium Hospital, 1984:211.
2. Kottmeier H-L, Kolstad P, McGarrity K, Pettersson F, Ulfelder H, eds. Annual report on the results of treatment in gynecological cancer. Stockholm: Radiumhemmet, 1982:18.

References to ch. 22

1. Kolstad P. Value and complications of periaortic irradiation in advanced cervical cancer. In: Morrow CP ed. Recent clinical developments in gynecologic oncology. New York: Raven Press, 1983:33.
2. Kottmeier H-L, Kolstad P, McGarrity K, Pettersson F, Ulfelder H, eds. Annual report on the results of treatment in gynecological cancer. Stockholm: Radiumhemmet, 1982:18.
3. Kolbenstvedt A, Kolstad P. Pelvic lymph node dissection under peroperative lymphographic control Gynecol Oncol 1974;2:39.

References to ch. 23

1. Kottmeier H-L. Surgical and radiation treatment of carcinoma of the uterine cercix. Acta Obstet Gynecol Scand (Suppl 2) 1964:43.
2. Lindell A. Carcinoma of the uterine cervix. Incidence and influence of age. Acta Radiol (Suppl 92) 1962.
3. Rampone JF, Klem V, Kolstad P. Combined treatment of Stage Ib carcinoma of the cervix.
4. Kjørstad K. Carcinoma of the cervix in the young patient. Obstet Gynecol 1977;50:28.
5. Gynning I, Johnsson J-E, Alm P, Tropé C. Age and prognosis in Stage Ib squamous cell carcinoma of the uterine cervix. Gynecol Oncol 1983;15:18.

References to ch. 25

1. Iversen T, Talle K, Langmark F. Effect of irradiation on the foeto-placental tissues. Acta Radiol Oncol 1979;18:129.

References to ch. 26

1. Bergsjø P. Adenocarcinoma cervicis uteri. Acta Obstet Gynecol Scand 1963;42:85.
2. Kjørstad K. Adenocarcinoma of the uterine cervix. Gynecol Oncol 1977;5:219.

References to ch. 27

1. Gold P, Freedman SD. Specific carcinoembryonic antigens of the human digestive system. J Exp Med 1965;122:467.
2. LoGofero P, Crupey J, Hansen HJ. Demonstration of an antigen common to several varieties of neoplasia. N Engl J Med 1971;285:138.
3. Reynoso G, Chu TH, Holyoke D, et al. Carcinoembryonic antigen in patients with different cancers. JAMA 1972;220:361.
4. Hansen HJ, Snyder JJ, Miller E, et al. Carcinoembryonic antigen (CEA) assay. A laboratory adjunct in the diagnosis and management of cancer. Human Pathol 1974;5:139.
5. Khoo SK, Mackay EV. Carcinoembryonic antigen in cancer of the female reproductive system: Sequential levels and effect of treatment. Aust NZ Obstet Gynecol 1973;3:1.
6. Khoo SK, MacKay EV. Carcinoembryonic antigen by radioimmunoassay in the detection of recurrence during long-term follow-up of female genital cancer. Cancer 1974;34:542.
7. Van Nagell JR, Pavlik EJ, Gay EC. Tumor markers in gynecologic cancer. In: van Nagell, Barber, eds. Modern concepts of gynecologic oncology. Boston, Bristol, London: John Wright PSG Inc, 1982.
8. Kjørstad KE. Early stage cervical cancer. Diagnosis and treatment of high risk patients with particular reference to the use of carcinoembryonic antigen. Thesis. The Norwegian Radium Hospital, Oslo: 1984.
9. Kjørstad KE, Ørjasæter H. Studies on carcinoembryonic antigen levels in patients with adenocarcinoma of the uterus. Cancer 1977;40:301.
10. Kjørstad KE, Ørjasæter H. Carcinoembryonic antigen levels in patients with squamous cell carcinoma of the cervix. Obstet Gynecol 1978;51:536.
11. Kjørstad KE, Ørjasæter H. The prognostic value of CEA determinations in the plasma of patients with squamous cell cancer of the cervix. Cancer 1982;50:283.
12. Kjørstad KE, Ørjasæter H. The prognostic value of CEA determinations in patients with adenocarcinoma of the uterine cervix. Gynecol Oncol 1984.
13. Kjørstad KE, Ørjasæter H. Clinical significance of low pretreatment values of CEA in patients with squamous cell carcinoma of the cervix. In press.
14. Kolstad P. Microinvasive carcinoma of the cervix. A follow-up study of 567 patients. In Morrow CP, Smart GE (eds.) Gynecological Oncology. Berlin, Heidelberg, London, Tokyo: Springer Verlag, 1985.

References to ch. 29

1. Fox H. Atypical hyperplasia and adenocarcinoma of the endometrium. In: Morrow CP, Bonnar J, O'Brian TJ, Gibbons W, eds. Recent developments in gynecological oncology. New York: Raven Press 1984.
2. Bergsjø P. Progesterone and progestational compounds in treatment of advanced endometrial carcinoma. Acta Endocrinol. 1965;49:412.
3. Novak ER, Woodruff JO. Gynecologic and obstetric pathology. Philadelphia: Saunders, 1974.
4. Kjørstad KE, Welander C, Halvorsen T, Grude T, Onsrud M. Progestagens as primary treatment in premalignant changes of the endometrium. In: Brush, King, Taylor, eds. Endometrial cancer. London: Balliére Tindall, 1978.

References to ch. 30

1. Kottmeier L-H, Kolstad P, McGarrity K, Petterson F, Ulfelder H, eds. Annual report on the results of treatment in gynecological cancer. Stockholm: Radiumhemmet, 1982:18.
2. Bergsjø P, Nilsen PA. Carcinoma of the endometrium. A study of 256 cases from the Norwegian Radium Hospital. Am J Obstet Gynecol 1966;95:496.
3. Nilsen PA, Koller O. Carcinoma of the endometrium in Norway 1957–60 with special reference to treatment results. Am J Obstet Gynecol 1969;105:1099.
4. Onsrud M, Kolstad P, Norman T. Postoperative external pelvic irradiation in carcinoma of the corpus Stage I: A controlled clinical trial. Gynecol Oncol 1976;4:222.
5. Aalders J, Abeler V, Kolstad P, Onsrud M. Postoperative external irradiation and prognostic parameters in Stage I endometrial carcinoma. Obstet Gynecol 1980;56:419.
6. Creasman WT, Boronow RC, Morrow CP, DiSaia PJ, Blessing J. Adenocarcinoma of the endometrium; its metastatic lymph node potential. A preliminary report. Gynecol Oncol 1976;4:239.

7. Rutledge F. The role of radical hysterectomy in adenocarcinoma of the endometrium. Gynecol Oncol 1974;2:331.
8. Iversen T, Holter J. Radical surgery in Stage I carcinoma of the corpus. Br J Obstet Gynecol 1981;88:1135.
9. Engeset A. Irradiation of lymph nodes and vessels. Oslo: Universitetsforlaget, 1964.

References to ch. 31

1. Dahle T. Transtubal spread of tumor cells in carcinoma of the body of the uterus. Surg Gynecol Obstet 1956;103:332.
2. Creasman WT, DiSaia PJ, Blessing J, Wilkinson RH, Johnson W, Weed JC. Prognostic significance of peritoneal cytology in patients with endometrial cancer and preliminary data concerning therapy with intraperitoneal radiopharmaceuticals. Gynecol Oncol 1981:60.
3. Yazigi R, Piver S, Blumenson L. Malignant peritoneal cytology as prognostic indicator in Stage I endometrial cancer. Obstet Gynecol 1983;62:359.

References to ch. 32

1. Onsrud M, Aalders JG, Abeler V, Taylor P. Endometrial carcinoma with cervical involvement (Stage II): Prognostic factors and value of combined radiological-surgical treatment. Gynecol Oncol 1982;13:76.
2. Kottmeier H-L, Kolstad P, McGarrity K, Pettersson F, Ulfelder H, eds. Annual report on the results of treatment in gynecological cancer. Stockholm: Radiumhemmet, 1982:18.
3. Boronow RC, Morrow CP, Creasman WT, DiSaia PJ, Blessing JA. Surgical-pathologic staging of FIGO Stage I endometrial carcinoma.

References to ch. 33

1. Kottmeier H-L, Kolstad P, McGarrity K, Pettersson F, Ulfelder H, eds. Annual report of the results of treatment in gynecological cancer. Stockholm: Radiumhemmet, 1982:18.
2. Aalders JG, Abeler V, Kolstad P. Clinical Stage III as compared to subclinical intrapelvic uterine spread in endometrial carcinoma. Gynecol Oncol 1983;17:64.

References to ch. 34

1. Aalders JG, Abeler V, Kolstad P. Stage IV endometrial carcinoma: A clinical and histopathological study of 83 patients. Gynecol Oncol 1984;17:75.
2. Bruckner HW, Deppe G. Combination chemotherapy of advanced endometrial cancer with adriamycin, cyclophosphamide, 5-fluorouracil and medroxyprogesterone acetate. Obstet Gynecol (Suppl 50) 1977:105.
3. Quinn MA, Campbell JJ, Murray R, Pepperell RJ. Treatment of advanced endometrial cancer with tamoxifen and aminogluthethimole In: Morrow CP, Bonnar J, O'Brian TJ, Gibbons WF, eds. Recent clinical developments in gynecologic oncology. New York: Raven Press, 1983.

References to ch. 35

1. Aalders JG, Abeler V, Kolstad P. Recurrent adenocarcinoma of the endometrium: A clinical histopathological study of 379 cases. Gynecol Oncol 1984;17:85.

References to ch. 36

1. Ober WB. Uterine sarcomas: Histogenesis and taxonomy. Ann NY Acad Sci 1959;75:568.
2. Kempson RL, Bari W. Uterine sarcomas: Classification, diagnosis and prognosis. Hum Pathol 1970;1:331.
3. Kolstad P. Adjuvant chemotherapy in sarcoma of the uterus: A preliminary report. In: Progress in cancer research and therapy. New York: Raven Press, 1983:24.
4. Omura GA, Blessing JA. Chemotherapy of Stage III, IV and recurrent uterine sarcomas; a randomized trial of adriamycin versus adriamycin + DTIC. AACR Abstract No. 103. Proc AACR/ASCO 1978.

References to ch. 37

1. Serov SF, Scully RE, Sobin LM. Histological typing of ovarian tumors. In: International histological classification of tumors, No. 9. Geneva: WHO.
2. Doll R, Muir C, Waterhouse J, eds. Cancer incidence in five continents. International Union Against Cancer. Berlin: Springer Verlag, 1972.
3. Kolstad P, Beecham J. Epidemiology of ovarian neoplasia. Proceedings of the American-European Conference on the Ovary, Montreux, Switzerland 1974. Amsterdam: Excerpta Medica.
4. Franceschi S, LaVecchia C, Mangioni C. Familial ovarian cancer: Eight more families. Gynecol Oncol 1982;13:31.
5. Fathalla MF. Factors in the causation and incidence of ovarian cancer. Obstet Gynecol Surg 1972;27:751.
6. The Cancer Registry of Norway. Survival of cancer patients. Cases diagnosed in Norway 1968–75. The Norwegian Cancer Society, 1980.

References to ch. 38

1. Kolstad P, Davy M, Scheinert H. Individualized treatment of ovarian neoplasia. Proceedings of the American-European Conference on the Ovary, Montreux, Switzerland, 1974. Amsterdam: Excerpta Medica.
2. Kottmeier H-L, Kolstad P, McGarrity K, Pettersson F, Ulfelder H, eds. Annual report on the results of treatment of gynecological cancer. Stockholm: Radiumhemmet, 1982:18.
3. Kjellgren O, et al. Fine needle aspiration biopsy in diagnosis and classification of ovarian carcinoma. Cancer 1971;28:967.

4. Iversen T, Klem V, Stenwig J. Fine needle aspiration cytology in ovarian cancer (in Norwegian). Tidsskr Nor Lægeforen 1979;99:1446.
5. Asmussen M, Miller A. Gynecological urology. London: Blackwell Scientific Publications, 1983.
6. Aure JChr, Høeg K, Kolstad P. Radioactive colloidal gold in the treatment of ovarian carcinoma. Acta Radiol Ther 1971;10:399.
7. Kolstad P, Davy M, Høeg K. Individualized treatment of ovarian cancer. Am J Obstet Gynecol 1977;18:617.
8. Aure JChr, Høeg K, Kolstad P. Clinical and histologic studies of ovarian carcinoma. Long-term follow-up of 990 cases. Obstet Gynecol 1971;37:1.
9. Teilum G. Endodermal sinus tumor of the ovary and testis. Comparative morphogenesis of the so-called mesonephroma ovarii (Schiller) and extraembryonic (yolk sac-allantoic) structures of the rat's placenta. Cancer 1958;12:1092.
10. Sampson JA. Endometrial carcinoma of the ovary. Arch Surg. 1925;10:1.
11. Schiller W. Mesonephroma ovarii. Am J Cancer 1939;35:1.
12. Morrow CP. Malignant and borderline epithelial tumors of ovary: clinical features, staging, diagnosis, intraoperative assessment and review of management. In: Coppleson M, ed. Gynecologic oncology. Fundamental principles and clinical practice. London: Churchill Livingstone, 1981.
13. Munnell EW. The changing prognosis and treatment in cancer of the ovary. Am J Obstet Gynecol 1968;100:790.
14. Griffiths CT. Surgical resection of tumor bulk in the primary treatment of ovarian carcinoma. Natl Cancer Inst Monogr 1975;42:101.
15. Davy M. The role of isotopes in the treatment of ovarian cancer. In: Grundman E, ed. Carcinoma of the ovary. Stuttgart: Gustav Fischer Verlag, 1983.
16. Dembo AJ, Busch RS. Radiation therapy of ovarian carcinoma. In: Griffiths CT, Fuller AF, eds. Gynecologic oncology. Boston, The Hague: Martinus Nijhoff Publishers, 1983.
17. Boye et al. Whole-body distribution of radioactivity after administration of ^{32}P colloids. Br J Radiol 1984;57:395.
18. Kjørstad KE, Welander C, Kolstad P. Preoperative irradiation in stage III carcinoma of the ovary. Acta Obstet Gynecol 1977;56:449.
19. Welander C, Kjørstad KE, Kolstad P. Postoperative irradiation and chemotherapy in patients with advanced ovarian cancer. Acta Obstet Gynecol Scand 1978;57:161.
20. Lewis GCJr, Blessing J, Kellner JR. Clinical trials in gynecologic oncology: Cooperative group research. In: Griffiths CT, Fuller AJ, eds. Gynecologic oncology. Boston, The Hague: Martinus Nijhoff Publishers, 1983.
21. Davy M, et al. Early stage ovarian cancer: The effect of adjuvant treatment with a single alkylating agent. In press.

References to ch. 39

1. Kolstad P, Beecham JC. Epidemiology of ovarian neoplasia. Proceedings of the American-European Conference on the Ovary, Montreux, 1974. Amsterdam: Excerpta Medica.
2. Stenwig JT, Hazekamp JT, Beecham JB. Granulosa cell tumors of the ovary. A clinicopathological study of 118 cases with long-term follow-up. Gynecol Oncol 1979;7:136.
3. Andersson WR, Levine AJ, MacMillan D. Granulosa-theca cell tumors: Clinical and pathologic study. Am J Obstet Gynecol 1971;110:32.
4. Sjöstedt S, Wahlén T. Prognosis of granulosa cell tumors. Acta Obstet Gynecol Scand (Suppl 6) 1961;40:3.
5. Norris HJ, Taylor HB. Prognosis of granulosa-theca tumors of the ovary. Cancer 1968;21:255.
6. Fox H, Agrawal K, Langley FA. A clinicopathologic study of 92 cases of granulosa cell tumor of the ovary with special reference to the factors influencing prognosis. Cancer 1975;35:231.
7. Gusberg SB, Kardon P. Proliferative endometrial response to theca-granulosa cell tumors. Am J Obstet Gynecol 1971;111:633.

Reference to ch. 40

1. Ahnfelt P. Dysgerminoma ovarii. Nord Med 1951;45:1006.
2. Koller O, Gjønnæss H. Dysgerminoma ovarii. Acta Obstet Gynecol Scand 1964;43:268.
3. Aalders JG, Davy M, Stenwig JT. Dysgerminoma of the ovary. In press.
4. Norris HJ, Adam, E. Malignant germ cell tumors of the ovary. In: Coppleson M, ed. Gynecologic oncology. London: Churchill Livingstone, 1981.

References to ch. 41

1. Teilum G. Endodermal sinus tumors of the ovary and testis; comparative morphogenesis of the so-called mesonephroma ovarii (Schiller) and extraembryonic (yolk-sac-allantois) structures of the rat's placenta. Cancer 1959;12:1092.
2. Teilum G. Classification of endodermal sinus tumors (mesoblastoma vitellium and so-called "embryonal carcinomas" of the ovary). Acta Pathol Microbiol Scand 1965;64:407.
3. Kurmann RJ, Norris HJ. Endodermal sinus tumor of the ovary. A clinical and pathologic analysis of 71 cases. Cancer 1976;38:2404.
4. Gershenson DM, Del Juneo G, Herson J, Rutledge F. Endodermal sinus tumor of the ovary. The MD Anderson experience. Obstet Gynecol 1983;61:194.

References to ch. 42

1. Robboy SJ, Scully RE. Ovarian teratoma with glial implants on the peritoneum. Hum Pathol 1970;1:643.
2. DiSaia P, Saltz A, Kagan AR, Morrow CP. Chemotherapeutic retroconversion of immature teratoma of the ovary. Obstet Gynecol 1977;49:346.
3. Scully RE. Recent progress in ovarian cancer. Hum Pathol 1970;1:73.

4. Robboy SJ, Scully RE, Norris HJ. Primary trabecular carcinoid of the ovary. Obstet Gynecol 1977;49:202.

Reference to ch. 43

1. Kurmann RJ, Norris HJ. Embryonal carcinoma of the ovary. Cancer 1976;38:2420.

References to ch. 44

1. Asmussen M, Wright PB, Abeler V. Primary invasive cancer of the Fallopian tube. In press.
2. Schiller HM, Silverberg SG. Staging and prognosis in primary carcinoma of the Fallopian tube. Cancer 1971;28:389.
3. Benet JL, White GW, Fairey RN, Boyes DA. Adenocarcinoma of the Fallopian tube. Obstet Gynecol 1977;50:654.
4. Roberts JA, Lifshitz S. Primary adenocarcinoma of the Fallopian tube. Gynecol Oncol 1982;13:301.
5. Phelps HM, Chapman K. Role of radiation therapy in treatment of primary carcinoma of the uterine tube. Obstet Gynecol 1974;43:669.
6. Boronow RC. Chemotherapy for disseminated tubal cancer. Obstet Gynecol 1973;42:62.

References to ch. 45

1. Brennhovd IO. Carcinoma urethrae et penis. Tidsskr Nor Lægeforen 1968;6:557.
2. Skjæraasen E. Cancer of the female urethra. Acta Obstet Gynecol Scand 1969;48:589.
3. Asmussen M, Haveland H. Primary malignant tumors of the female urethra. A retrospective study of 51 cases. In press.
4. Asmussen M, Ulmsten U. The role of urethral pressure profile measurement in female patients with urethral carcinoma. Ann Chir Gynaecol In press.

5. Asmussen M, Miller A. Clinical gynaecological urology. Oxford: Blackwell Scientific Publications, 1983.

References to ch. 46

1. Kolstad P, Hognestad J. Trophoblastic tumorsin Norway. Acta Obstet Gynecol Scand 1965;44:80.
2. Li MC, Hertz R, Spencer DB. Effect of methotrexate therapy upon choriocarcinoma and chorioadenoma. Proc Soc Exp Biol Med 1956;93:361.
3. Fernström I. Arteriography of the uterine artery. Acta Radiol (Stockh) (Suppl 122) 1955.
4. Kolstad P, Liverud K. Arteriography and chemotherapy in malignant trophoblastic disease. Acta Obstet Gynecol Scand (Suppl 9) 1966;45:135.
5. Kolstad P, Liverud K. Pelvic arteriography in malignant trophoblastic neoplasia. Am J Obstet Gynecol 1969;105:175.
6. Kolstad P, Høeg K, Norman N. Malignant trophoblastic neoplasia. Monitoring of therapy. Acta Obstet Gynecol Scand 1972;51:275.
7. Bagshawe KD, Begent RHJ. Trophoblastic tumors: clinical features and management. In: Coppleson M, ed. Gynecologic oncology. London: Churchill Livingstone, 1981.

References to ch. 47

1. Pettersson F, Kolstad P, Ludwig H, Ulfelder H, eds. Annual report on the results of treatment in gynecological cancer. Stockholm, Sweden: Radiumhemmet, 1985;19.
2. Kübler-Ross E. On death and dying. New York: Macmillan, 1969.
3. Kübler-Ross E. On death and dying. Bull Am Coll Surg 1975;60:12.
4. McGowan L, ed. Gynecologic oncology. New York: Appleton-Century-Crofts, 1978.